# Neurological Pathophysiology

# Neurological Pathophysiology

SVEN G. ELIASSON, M.D., Ph.D.
ARTHUR L. PRENSKY, M.D.
WILLIAM B. HARDIN, Jr., M.D.

New York
OXFORD UNIVERSITY PRESS
London        1974        Toronto

The cover illustration is a diagrammatic view of the three basic types of central nervous system circuitry. The column on the left represents the cerebral and cerebellar cortex (designed for repetitive feedback, oscillation, association, and power functions). The center column represents such nerve net and nuclear structures as the diencephalon, brain stem, and spinal cord gray matter (designed for the spread of information, the concentration and dissemination of nervous impulses). The column on the right represents white matter with its glia (designed to carry information accurately across relatively long distances without cross-talk). These are the structural substrates that carry out all central neurophysiological activities.

Copyright © 1974 by Oxford University Press, Inc.
Library of Congress Catalogue Card Number: 74-79621
Printed in the United States of America

# Preface

When the incisive mind of the academically inclined teacher confronts his students' blunt demands for clinical relevance, the apparent impasse generally gives way to a pathway that leads through superfluous details toward relevant facts. Five years of experience teaching the course, Pathophysiology of the Nervous System, at Washington University and listening to the criticisms of our students has convinced us that this book, which is the result of such interaction, is an acceptable compromise. As such, it should not interfere with the viewpoints of the basic scientists or the experienced clinicians. It is hoped that it describes the pathological mechanisms behind clinical neurological disorders and will serve thereby as a point of origin for teachers of similar courses in pathophysiology. Practicing neurologists, neurosurgeons, and neuropsychiatrists may wish to use this book to refresh their memories and rejuvenate their approaches to clinical subjects. Teachers and students in advanced courses in neurophysiology including the fields of physical and occupational therapy, as well as students for advanced degrees in the biological sciences, may wish to review select chapters. The book, however, is primarily for the medical student who is in the transitional, and therefore difficult, period between the basic and the clinical sciences.

Washington University                                        S.G.E.
St. Louis, Missouri                                          A.L.P.
May 1974                                                     W.B.H.

# Contents

vii

# 2

## Disorders of Nerve and Muscle, 49

# 3

## Disturbances of Autonomic and Visceral Function, 94

# 6

# 13

# Neurological Pathophysiology

# 1

# Developmental Disorders of the Central Nervous System

## NORMAL BRAIN DEVELOPMENT

ARTHUR L. PRENSKY

### Introduction

Insults to the developing nervous system are discussed in a separate section of this text because their effects on neurological function are not only determined by the size and location of the lesion and its underlying etiology (the essential determinants of the pathophysiological effects of disease of the mature nervous system), but by other factors unique to the immature nervous system. The effects of disease of the developing nervous system also depend upon (1) the stage of neurological development at which the insult initially takes place, (2) the rate of progression of disease in relation to the rate of acquisition of neurological function, and (3) the ability of the immature nervous system to compensate for the effects of a restricted lesion. During its period of rapid growth, whether *in utero* or soon after birth, the brain is particularly susceptible to injury by a variety of toxic, metabolic, and infectious agents, which might not permanently or severely damage the mature brain. Generally, the major effect of an agent is on the developmental events that are most active at the time of the insult. If the lesion is extensive, involving large areas of the neuraxis, and lasts a long period of time, all further neurological development may cease or be distorted. If the

3

lesion is restricted both in time and space, the clinical abnormality may be limited. For example, isolated hemiparesis may be seen with porencephalic cysts or spastic diplegia resulting from hypoxemia *in utero* or at birth unassociated with other significant neurological disease. An even more striking example is the failure of neural tube closure that results in a meningomyelocele or, less frequently, an encephalocele without any other evidence of damage to brain development thereafter.

Many other examples of the relationship between disease and the state of the development of the nervous system will be presented in succeeding sections of this chapter. In order to fully comprehend this dynamic interrelationship, it is necessary to have some idea of the normal anatomical and biochemical maturation of the nervous system and the physiological and clinical tools by which we can measure the progress of normal maturation.

## Anatomical development

By the end of the first month of gestation, the basic configuration of the brain is already determined. The crown to rump length of the human embryo is only 3 mm at this time, but the neural tube has already developed its cervical and mesencephalic flexures that will mark the limits of the hind brain separating it from spinal cord and prosencephalon, respectively. The lateral outpouchings of the prosencephalic vesicle are present, although the prosencephalon is still a holosphere. By the end of the second month, the beginnings of the paired hemispheres are apparent, but there is still a midline rhinic lobe and a single ventricle. During the third month of fetal life, the hemispheres are recognizable, the thalamus is strikingly enlarged, and the cerebellum begins to appear. By the end of the third month, the lateral ventricles are separate except for their connections with the third ventricle via the foramen of Monro; the external surface of the hemispheres is still smooth. Fissuration commences in the fourth fetal month with the lateral fissure of the cerebrum, which eventually becomes the Sylvian fissure (separating the temporal lobe from the rest of the cerebrum) and the posterolateral fissure of the cerebellum (separating the nodulus and flocculus from the vermis). By the end of the fourth month, the major divisions of the cerebral and cerebellar hemispheres are recognizable, but secondary and tertiary fissures are still lacking. These sulci increase during the last trimester of fetal life, and fissuration is essentially completed in the first 2 years of postnatal life.

If the immature brain is sectioned sagittally from the external to the ventricular surface, it will be found to consist of three layers: namely, the outer marginal layer, the mantle layer, and the matrix layer. It is in the matrix layer next to the ventricle that all the cells of the nervous system originate and begin the process of multiplication and differentiation into neurons and glia. Cells destined to be neurons migrate through the mantle layer into the marginal zone and eventually form the cerebral cortex. The neuronal complement of most of the cerebral cortex appears to be complete before birth, although some studies in animals indicate a continuing migration and multiplication of neurons in the hippocampus and the olfactory bulb after birth. Multiplication and migration of glial cells continues in infancy and childhood, however. In the cerebellum, the situation is quite different. Although the full complement of Purkinje cells exists before birth, there is considerable multiplication of cerebellar granule cells during infancy. At birth, the cerebellar granule cells are situated on the external surface of the cerebellar cortex and form the external granule cell layer. They divide during postnatal life and migrate internally to lie beneath the Purkinje cells. Thus, the cerebellum is especially vulnerable to postnatal insults that interfere with cell multiplication.

Although extensive proliferation of neurons in postnatal life is limited to the cerebellum, the human brain is undergoing remarkable growth during infancy and early childhood. The most obvious manifestation of these changes is in brain weight. The average weight of the brain in the neonate is 350-400 gm. By the end of one year, the weight has increased two and one-half-fold and weighs approximately two-thirds the weight of the average male adult brain (1500 gm). The remaining growth occurs during the next 10 to 12 years of life when there is an enormous increase in the brain's functional capacities. Investigations in animals and humans suggest that the major postnatal events that account for considerable brain enlargement are an increase in the number of glial cells in both white and gray matter; an increase in the thickness of the cerebral mantle correlated with the development of neuropil formed by the outgrowth of neuronal dendrites and elongation and increased branching of axons; and an increase in the length and diameter of axons in the white matter and the associated development of the myelin sheath. Myelin sheaths, with the exception of dorsal and ventral roots and certain segments of the spinal cord, are thin and sparse at birth but rapidly become the predominant membrane of the white matter. The development of myelin within the nervous system is uneven. Primary projection areas such as visual, auditory, and thalamocortical sensory pathways, as well as the corticospinal tract, are myelinated relatively early in life, whereas axonal pathways between association areas of the cerebral cortex are myelinated later. Myelination is a process that continues within the cortex, particularly in association areas, into the fifth and sixth decades of life. With growth of the neuropil, there is an increase in the number of synapses, both axonal-somatic (which predominate at birth) and axonal-dendritic (which predominate in adult life).

## Biochemical maturation

Some of the major biochemical changes that occur as the brain matures can be roughly correlated with morphological development. The increase in deoxyribonucleic acid (DNA) in developing brain correlates with the increase in numbers of cells. In sampling small areas of the brain during development, however, this biochemical measure is not always a reliable index of cell replication, since increasing amounts of DNA may reflect migration of new cells into particular regions. Another obstacle in relating DNA levels to morphological changes in nervous system is that the DNA contents of neurons and glial and ependymal cells is roughly the same; consequently, this biochemical index does not distinguish between cell populations whose composition and functions may be radically different.

The studies by Winick and his associates suggest that, in the brain (as in other organs), a period of cellular hyperplasia marked by a rapid increase in DNA is followed by a period of cellular hypertrophy during which the relative increase in ribonucleic acid (RNA) and protein exceeds that of DNA. The RNA and protein content of the brain appear to correlate roughly with cell growth, although it is unclear if either biochemical index represents a particular parameter of such growth as cell surface or cytoplasmic area. The relationship of the period of hyperplasia to hypertrophy relative to birth varies from species to species, occurring prenatally in the guinea pig and almost entirely postnatally in the rat. In the human cerebrum, hyperplasia of glial cells continues postnatally and hypertrophy is the predominant postnatal event in the neuronal population.

Several of the major changes in the chemical composition of the maturing brain can be attributed to myelination. As myelination proceeds, the water content of the white matter per unit fresh weight of tissue drops rapidly from 88-90% to 65-70%. The lipid content of the white matter increases. Before the onset of myelination, lipids account for just under one-third of the total solids in white matter; after myelination is complete, lipids account for about two-thirds of the solids. Although all classes of lipid accumulate during myelination, certain lipids are more likely to be associated with the myelin membrane; these are the galactose-containing glycolipids, cerebroside and sulfatide, and a protein-lipid complex, containing a high proportion of neutral amino acids soluble in organic solvents, known as proteolipid. Cerebroside, sulfatide, and proteolipid are found in high concentration in white matter and in myelin but are certainly not limited to this membrane. Nevertheless, they are reasonable indices of myelination, and their increase in white matter during development roughly parallels the increase in myelin.

Because myelin is a membrane that can be isolated relatively easily, changes in its chemical composition with age have been thoroughly studied in a number of species. During development, there are changes in the intrinsic chemical composition of the membrane that theoretically would tend to make it more physically stable with age. As the membrane matures, choline phosphoglyceride (lecithin) decreases, while cerebroside and sphingomyelin increase as a percentage of the total lipid. There is also a change in the protein content of the membrane: a decrease in proteolipids and an increase in the basic protein fraction from 16 to 27% of the total protein in the myelin membrane. The fatty acid composition of lipid classes in myelin also changes with maturation. Studies of various species suggest that, with age, the average chain length of the fatty acids increases, the proportion of hydroxy to non-hydroxy fatty acids also increases, and there is a decrease in the relative amount of unsaturated fatty acids. This suggests that long chain, saturated hydroxy fatty acids tend to promote the stability of myelin, since it is the most stable membrane in the nervous system.

The concept that the mature nervous system is unable to replace lost neurons, although true, leads to an invalid conclusion as to its degree of stability. The continuous replacement of cells noted in such organs as skin and intestine is minimal in the nervous system and, for the most part, limited to glial elements. But there is a rapid turnover of lipids and protein in the membranes that comprise both the developing and mature nervous system. Myelin, in spite of its relative physical stability, exhibits a relatively rapid biochemical turnover of phospholipids, particularly lecithin whose half-life may be as short as 16 days. Thus, membranes of even the mature nervous system are susceptible to injury by metabolic insults.

Virtually every constituent of the nervous system changes in quantity and concentration during development. The changes in levels of enzyme activity, of amino acids, of amine content, and of electrolyte concentration are not as clearly related to the morphological development of the nervous system as some of the biochemical indices previously discussed. We assume that such alterations during development have functional importance with regard to neural activity, but, as yet, it has not been possible to relate any specific change in an enzyme or biochemical substrate to a particular functional event in the maturing nervous system. Several general statements, however, may be made about biochemical maturation. (1) Enzyme activities and substrate levels may vary markedly from one area of the brain to another. Their rates of development may also vary considerably, depending upon the area of brain investigated. (2) Changes in the amount of a substrate or the level of enzyme activities in an area of brain or whole brain may occur very rapidly. This is true not only for an increase in content of a molecular species relative to wet weight, e.g., glutamic acid in rat brain, which doubles between the 14th and the 21st day of postnatal life, but also for a decrease in some compounds, e.g., proline, which drops two and one-half-fold relative to wet weight during the same period. (3) The "safety factor" of any single brain constituent is unknown. That is, it is unclear to what degree changes in levels of enzyme reactivity or substrate concentration result in observable changes in cerebral function. (4) Increasing evidence indicates that the development and maintenance of normal brain function depends more upon the relationship of the concentration of groups of interrelated compounds in a given area of brain than upon the absolute levels of any single chemical constituent. Such relationships are controlled by a multiplicity of metabolic pathways that influence the synthesis and breakdown of these compounds.

To sort out the factors responsible for the concentration of a single amino acid in a given area of brain at any point during development, we must examine the transport systems that regulate the rate of entry of that amino acid into the brain from plasma and the systems that regulate its rate of exit. Knowledge of the rate at which the amino acid is used locally for protein synthesis, or formed locally by catabolism of proteins, and of its intermediary metabolism, is also essential. For example, the rate at which tyrosine is transformed into dopamine and norepinephrine, 5-hydroxytryptophan into serotonin, and glutamic acid into $\gamma$-aminobutyric acid (GABA) certainly influences the level of these amino acids in brain tissue.

The rapid rise in glutamate levels in rat brain during the second and third weeks of development is an excellent example of the complex problem of assigning responsibility for such changes to a specific biochemical event during maturation. While the concentration of glutamate is rapidly rising in the brain, there is no evidence that free glutamate can be transported from plasma against a gradient. But there is a rapid exchange between plasma and brain glutamate. During this time, glutamate incorporation into protein increases as does the conversion of glutamate to both glutamine and GABA. Glutamate is capable of re-entering the tricarboxylic acid (TCA) cycle and can be used as a substrate for energy metabolism, but there is no indication that during maturation there is a significant change in the amount of glutamate so metabolized. It would seem, therefore, that the rate of synthesis of glutamate must rapidly increase. In the rat, for example, the period of rapid increase in the concentration of free glutamate in brain does coincide with a rapid increase in the ability of the brain to incorporate carbon derived from glucose into dicarboxylic amino acids, but there is a concomitant decrease in the incorporation of carbon from short chain keto acids. This period also coincides roughly with the time of maximal dendritic growth and synaptic proliferation in the rat. The concentration of free glutamate in nerve endings is particularly high, and the presence of such "storage depots" may account for increasing levels of the amino acid with maturation.

Because such oxidative enzymes of the TCA cycle as succinic dehydrogenase are not well developed in immature brain, the complete oxidation of glucose is restricted in immature animals, and much of the adenosine triphophate (ATP) formed from the utilization of glucose is the product of anaerobic glycolysis that converts glucose into lactic acid. Since the immature brain is extremely active, metabolically, it would seem that other substrates must be available both for synthesis and for energy metabolism. We mentioned previously that glutamate and other dicarboxylic amino acids can be used as a source of energy, if glucose is restricted. Other work indicates that both acetate and short chain keto acids are more effectively used by the immature brain than by the adult brain for the synthesis of structural lipids and proteins. With increasing age, the brain depends more upon glucose for these syntheses.

## Electrical maturation

The two most commonly used electrical measurements of physiological maturation of the human nervous system are evoked cortical potentials in response to specific sensory stimuli and the electroencephalogram. Hunt and Goldring (1951) were the first to trace the maturational pattern of the evoked cortical response by studying the visual response of rabbits from 1 to 21 days after birth. The initial response to a visual stimulus is surface negative, but, as the animal matures, a surface positive response of short latency and increasing amplitude develops. The fatigability of the response also decreases with age. Initial surface positivity, decreased latency, and decreased fatigability are characteristics of the maturational development of evoked response in all species and all primary sensory areas (i.e., visual, auditory, or somesthetic). The decrease in latency seems clearly related to the myelination of primary sensory pathways. Other developmental parameters in the evoked response are less clearly related to anatomical events, although the change from a predominantly surface negative to a surface positive wave may be related to the increasing number of axonal-dendritic synapses in more superficial cortical layers as the telencephalon matures. In addition to the positive-negative wave complex of short latency, which is eventually seen in primary cortical sensory areas, the more mature animals have "secondary discharges" of longer latency and wider cortical distribution, which reflect the development of associational pathways within the hemisphere.

The electroencephalogram represents the organization of large numbers of neurons to produce repetitive rhythmic patterns of electrical discharge. The major features that characterize the development of electrical potentials with age are (1) the rapid decrease in the duration of periods of relative electrical silence; (2) an increase in the frequency and amplitude of resting activity, which, in the neonate and young infant, is generally of low voltage (10-40 $\mu$V) and in the 4-7/second frequency range. With age, this basic frequency rises to 8-9/second and finally to 10-12/second in the majority of the normal population. Also, with maturation, this basic resting frequency is increasingly localized in the occipital area, and its rhythmicity is better defined, approaching a regularly repeating sinusoidal wave form; (3) synchrony over identical areas of both hemispheres becomes more obvious; and (4) it becomes easier to differentiate a resting tracing from a sleep tracing and the tracings of various stages of sleep. Whereas the maturation of electrical potentials can be described in some detail, correlation of electroencephalographic changes with age to either anatomical or biochemical ontogenetic events has never been successfully accomplished. In addition, it is very hazardous to predict intellectual development and behavioral maturation from electroencephalographic changes. A certain proportion of normal adults never develop a regular posterior sinusoidal rhythm in the 8-13/second (alpha) range. This has very little relation to their intellectual competence.

## Developmental landmarks

As might be expected, clinical measures of maturation are even less related to underlying anatomical and biochemical events. The newborn may be said to function without a telencephalon. Many infants who have no cerebral cortex (anencephalics) have been mistaken for normal infants. Such anencephalics may even smile and exhibit seizure activity, normal postures, and movement at birth. Only when one attempts to demonstrate responses to visual stimuli do their responses begin to differ. This is difficult to demonstrate in the neonate without special equipment and conditioning of the young infant to respond. By 1 month of age, however, visual pathways are sufficiently developed so that the normal infant will follow a moving object for very brief periods of time, whereas the anencephalic will not. The normal development of the infant is characterized by the loss of flexor tone, the disappearance of reflexes such as the Moro and tonic neck response, which reflect organization at a diencephalic or midbrain level, and the acquisition of skills that increasingly require cortical and cerebellar control. This includes reaching for objects, first with the whole hand and then with the finely opposed finger and thumb, transfer of objects, sitting, and standing. Finally, walking and the rudiments of speech develop in the second year of life. Control of motor functions, development of language, and learning of new skills continue throughout childhood and adolescence, and, for many, learning continues into old age despite the fact that by gross measurements the anatomical, chemical, and physiological parameters that characterize the adult brain are fully developed by 15 to 16 years of age. The microchemistry and physiology of learning, therefore, remain little known areas of neurological development. Numerous maturational tables outlining motor, sensory, and social milestones during the early years of life have been constructed and can be found in pediatric texts.

It is essential to know the stage of development of the brain in evaluating the clinical manifestations of a lesion. Certain neurological symptoms, such as seizures, tend to undergo a high rate of remission as the nervous system matures. Others, such as the manifestations of antenatal or perinatal forebrain injury, may not be apparent in the young infant whose functional capabilities are at the level of hindbrain activities. Only when the child matures and more complex behavior patterns emerge do many significant clinical neurological signs resulting from brain injury much earlier in development become apparent; therefore, it is necessary to be aware of the behavioral correlates of increasing physiological capabilities as well as the processes that determine cerebral maturation. Such relationships will be illustrated later.

## General references

Altman, J. and G. P. Das. 1966. Autoradiographic and histological studies of postnatal neurogenesis I. A longitudinal investigation of the kinetics, migration and transformation of cells incorporating tritiated thymidine in neonate rats, with special reference to postnatal neurogenesis in some brain regions. J. Comp. Neurol. 126:337-360.

Davison, A. N., M. L. Cuzner, N. L. Banik, and J. Oxberry. 1966. Myelogenesis in the rat brain. Nature 212:1373-1374.

Davison, A. N., J. Dobbing, R. S. Morgan, and G. Payling Wright. 1959. Metabolism of myelin: The persistence of (4-$^{14}$C) cholesterol in the mammalian central nervous system. Lancet I:658-660.

Dodge, P. R. 1964. Neurologic history and examination. Pages 1-64 in T. W. Farmer, ed. Pediatric neurology. Harper & Row (Hoeber), New York.

Eeg-Olofsson, O. 1970. The development of the electroencephalogram in normal children and adolescents from the age of 1 through 21 years. Acta Paediat. Scand. Suppl. 208:4-46.

Ellingson, R. J. 1964. Studies of the electrical activity of the developing brain. Pages 26-53 in W. A. Himwich and H. E. Himwich, eds. The developing brain. Prog. Brain Res. Vol. 9, Elsevier, Amsterdam.

Fois, A. 1961. The electroencephalogram of the normal child. Charles C. Thomas, Springfield, Ill. 124 pp.

Folch, J. 1955. Composition of the brain in relation to maturation. Pages 121-136 in H. Waelsch, ed. Biochemistry of the developing nervous system. Academic Press, New York.

Himwich, W. A., ed. 1970. Developmental neurobiology. Charles C. Thomas, Springfield, Ill. 770 pp.

Illingworth, R. S. 1966. The development of the infant and young child: Normal and abnormal. 3rd ed., Williams & Wilkins, Baltimore. 378 pp.

Minkowski, A., ed. 1967. Regional development of the brain in early life. F. A. Davis, Philadelphia. 539 pp.

Paoletti, R. and A. N. Davison, eds. 1971. Chemistry and brain development. Plenum Press, New York/London. 457 pp.

Sidman, R., I. L. Miale, and N. Feder. 1959. Cell proliferation and migration in the primitive ependymal zone; an autoradiographic study of histogenesis in the nervous system. Exp. Neurol. 1:322-333.

Winick, M. 1968. Changes in the nucleic acid and protein content of the human brain during growth. Pediat. Res. 2:352-355.

# UNDERNUTRITION

MARVIN A. FISHMAN AND ARTHUR L. PRENSKY

Investigation of the effects of undernutrition on the developing nervous system has clearly illustrated the problems that arise when one tries to define in detail the pathophysiological basis of a relatively diffuse, nonspecific development insult. Nutritional deprivation can be produced in experimental animals by a variety of techniques, and the morphological and biochemical consequences of the insult can be carefully evaluated. A favorite experimental animal has been the rat, because the brain of this animal is relatively immature at birth and since there is considerable multiplication of both neurons and glial cells in the first 3 weeks of postnatal life. Extensive myelination of the cerebrum does not begin until the second postnatal week. Therefore, the infant rat is extremely susceptible to nutritional deprivation. Morphological and biochemical studies of rats that have been nutritionally deprived from the day of birth indicate that the major effects of the insult are similar to those found in the human infant: (1) a reduction in brain weight, which is considerably less severe than the reduction in body weight; (2) a reduction in cell number, which is most apparent in the cerebellum; (3) a reduction in the lipid contents of the brain, which is most pronounced in those lipid classes closely associated with the myelin sheath; and (4) a decrease in cortical width, associated with a reduction in the complexity of the neuropil.

Although extraneous variables can be restricted in experimental animals, it is still not possible to demonstrate whether the deficiency in myelin noted in nutritionally deprived rats is the result of failure of mature oligodendroglial cells to synthesize the membrane at a normal rate, whether the deficiency is in the maturation of oligodendroglial cells, or whether the deficiency is in the total number of oligodendroglial cells. All three events probably contribute to the final reduction in the amount of myelin present. Reduction in the amount of myelin may also be related to a failure in axonal growth, since the thickness of the myelin sheath and, thus, the amount of myelin depends directly upon the diameter of the axon.

Even greater difficulties arise if one tries to single out a specific biochemical abnormality as the cause of failure of development of these morphological parameters of brain growth. Undernutrition is associated with alterations in normal levels of numerous substrates in brain, including amino acids and putative neuro-transmitters. Incorporation of labeled carbon from glucose into proteins and lipids is reduced. Transcriptional and translational control of protein synthesis may be impaired. It is not clear, however, that any one of these biochemical abnormalities is, by itself, responsible for the morphological changes noted.

The striking resistance of the mature brain to severe undernutrition and the relative resistance of the developing brain to this insult, as compared to other body organs, is extremely interesting. It is possible that the effects of undernutrition are least severe in those organs whose rate of cell replication during the time of the insult is least rapid. Recovery from undernutrition does appear to be related to the timing of the insult in relationship to cell replication. If the period of undernutrition ends before the postnatal period of relatively rapid cell replication ends, i.e., about 10 to 12 days in the rat and about 3 to 4 months in the human, considerable or even total recovery from the insult appears to be possible. Similarly, if undernutrition begins after the period of rapid cell replication has ceased, cell growth may be transiently affected, but again almost total recovery can be achieved after the period of food deprivation ends. Such experiments emphasize two general principles of neurological growth: (1) rapid cell replication appears to be a programmed event with a definite time course, which cannot be modified significantly. Thus, if large numbers of cells fail to divide at their expected time during development because of a transient insult, it cannot be assumed that they will divide at an accelerated rate once the insult has ceased. The underlying mechanisms that control the rate of multiplication of both neurons and oligodendroglial cells in brain are unknown, but they definitely appear to be time dependent and to cease as the animal matures. (2) In contrast to rapid cell replication, cell hypertrophy appears to be less time restricted. Undernutrition allows growth to resume upon refeeding. The growth rate is such that normal weights are eventually reached. Both biochemical and anatomical measurements of morphological development are too coarse to allow us to say whether such accelerated growth involves all cells or whether all cells finally assume a normal morphological configuration.

## General references

Agrawal, H. C., M. A. Fishman, and A. L. Prensky. 1971. A possible block in the intermediary metabolism of glucose into proteins and lipids in the brains of undernourished rats. Lipids 6:431-433.

Barnes, R. H., A. U. Moore, I. M. Reid et al. 1967. Learning behavior following nutritional deprivation in early life. J. Amer. Diet. Assoc. 51: 34-39.

Bass, N. H., M. G. Netsky, and E. Young. 1970. Effect of neonatal malnutrition on the developing cerebrum. Arch. Neurol. 23:289-313.

Benton, J. W., H. W. Moser, P. R. Dodge et al. 1966. Modification of the schedule of myelination in the rat by early nutritional deprivation. Pediatrics 38:801-807.

Cragg, B. G. 1972. The development of cortical synapses during starvation in the rat. Brain 95:143-150.

Culley, W. J. and R. O. Lineberger. 1968. The effect of undernutrition on the size and composition of the rat brain. J. Nutrition 96:375-381.

Fishman, M. A., A. L. Prensky, and P. R. Dodge. 1969. Low content of cerebral lipids in infants suffering from malnutrition. Nature 221:552-553.

Klein, R. E., H. E. Freeman, J. Kagon et al. 1972. Is big smart? The relation of growth to cognition. J. Health and Soc. Behav. 13:219-225.

Winick, M. 1969. Malnutrition and brain development. Pediatrics 74:667-679.

## CONGENITAL MALFORMATIONS OF THE CENTRAL NERVOUS SYSTEM

PHILIP R. DODGE

Congenital malformations are structural defects present at birth. Warkany has stated that they may be gross or microscopic, located on the surface of the body or within it, familial or sporadic, hereditary or non-hereditary, and single or multiple.

Certain malformations of the nervous system are apparent on casual inspection at birth (e.g., anencephaly) or may be suspected to exist even before birth (e.g., hydrocephalus). Other malformations of the cerebral cortex will be manifested later in infancy or childhood by such functional disorders as mental retardation or epilepsy. Others may be discovered by special examination. For example, certain retinal malformations will escape notice unless there is an ophthalmoscopic examination, and air encephalography is necessary to demonstrate such gross ventricular distortions as occur with agenesis of the corpus callosum. Although inborn errors of metabolism represent molecular malformations, they are usually not discussed in this context.

### Etiology

The etiology of most congenital malformations is unknown. A malformation can be inherited according to Mendelian principles (more often as a dominant than a recessive trait), or it can be acquired during gestation. Nutritional deficiencies, such noxious agents as drugs, and infectious organisms have all been implicated in the etiology of congenital malformation of the nervous system of animals and man. The same malformation can originate from different mechanisms; for example, hydrocephalus secondary to narrowing of the Sylvian aqueduct can result from inflammation of the ventricular wall or from the expression of a sex-linked gene.

The interaction of several factors seems probable in the etiology of many malformations. Caution must be exercised, lest the physician accept readily an attractive theory of causation that explains certain but not all features of a given malformation. The associated malformations that comprise the relatively common myelomeningocele–Arnold-Chiari–hydrocephalus syndrome complex are a case in point. The basic fault is unknown, and most of the theories contrived to explain the defect at best describe certain mechanical forces, which may determine the ultimate form of the malformation. Even in these theories, there has been a notable tendency for investigators to be simplistic. For example, the theory that traction exerted by the tethered cord in the myelomeningocele could account for the caudal displacement of the rhombencephalon (portions of the cerebellum and medulla) failed to take into account the observation that both malformations may exist early in fetal life (10 weeks gestational age) before the disproportionate linear growth of the vertebral column over the spinal cord occurs. Furthermore, the elongation of the brain stem seen in the Arnold-Chiari malformation can exist, in the absence of myelomeningocele and a change in the course of the spinal roots. The actual data seem most consistent with a basic embryological fault, admitting some modification of the final form of the defect as the result of patterns of growth and hydrodynamic forces. The increased occurrence of these defects in particular families suggests the possibility of a genetic determinant, but no simple pattern of inheritance has emerged.

## Embryogenic considerations

Studies of normal embryogenesis in a wide variety of animal species have indicated that there is remarkably little individual variation in ontogenetic development within a given species. The development of the nervous system occurs systematically and is linked to the time following conception. Brief insults during embryogenesis can restrict future development of the organ. In experimental animals, it is possible to apply noxious influences over a short time period at various stages of embryogenesis and produce different developmental defects. A standardized dose of radiation at 9 to 10 days of gestation in the rat produces anencephaly. Microcephaly occurs with radiation at 18 days, and, 3 days later, malformation of the cerebellum results. Most noxious agents or deficiency states known to produce malformations experimentally do not affect humans in such a discrete manner, so it is rarely, if ever, possible to determine precisely whether a teratogen was present. Certain malformations, however, cannot result from factors operating after a particular point in embryogenesis. This is the principle of termination periods enunciated by Schwalbe early in this century. The point is well illustrated by the various human dysraphic states (myeloschisis, myelomeningocele, and anencephalus) that result from incomplete closure of the neural tube. Because the process of closure is normally completed before the end of the 4th week of embryonic life in the human, these malformations must originate before this time. The responsible factors may not cease their action after this time, but they must begin before the 4th week.

A number of other developmental phenomena illustrate the termination principle. By the end of 11 to 12 weeks of gestation, the shape of the developing human brain resembles, in broad outline, that of the fully developed organ. Coronal sections during this early developmental period demonstrate the dramatic interior changes occurring over these first weeks of life (Fig. 1-1). Before about 7 weeks of gestational age, the cavity of the forebrain is essentially a rounded tube. Bilateral evaginations appear at this time and result ultimately in the fully formed lateral ventricles connected to the central or third ventricle by the foramina of Monro. The human malformation, holoprosencephaly, reflects a failure of development beyond a single tube or ventricle. Clearly, this means that the factors responsible for the malformation were operative before that time, when outpouchings from the primitive ventricle should have occurred.

Cellular proliferation by mitosis and migration of cells outward from the periventricular zone is basic to the growth and develop-

**BRAIN DEVELOPMENT — HUMAN**

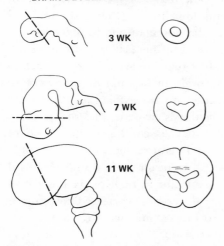

**Fig. 1-1** Embryonic brain development in the human.

ment of the brain. Studies in mice suggest that DNA synthesis occurs in the neuroepithelial cells around the ventricle and that these
cells migrate inward to the subependymal area where they continue
to divide and then move toward the cortical mantle in waves, each
wave passing through the layers of cells deposited by earlier migrations. The result is a multilayered cortical arrangement in which
the cells nearest the surface are those that arrived most recently.
Excessive amounts of vitamin A fed to the pregnant mouse during
ontogeny may interfere with this pattern, and other agents are
known to cause similar alterations. Cortical cellular migrations in
man are thought to occur primarily during the earliest weeks of
post-conceptual life, so that disorganization of the pattern of cortical
lamination must derive from events transpiring before this process
is normally completed. Examples of such disorganization in man
are numerous. Islands of gray matter (heterotopias) may be found
in the white matter. Such abnormalities are seen most often in mentally retarded individuals, in whom the etiology is obscure; heterotopias occur also in such well-defined conditions as neurofibromatosis. Cellular migration occurs very late in the regions near the
lateral ventricle and in the cerebellum, where movement of some
cells from the external granular layer to the granular regions is

delayed until the first year of postnatal life. The late development of
the cerebellum probably accounts for the fact that radiation and
other teratogens may influence its development late in ontogeny.

The convoluted surface of the cerebral hemispheres is characteristic of adult man. The gyri and sulci that impart this appearance to
the external surface of the human brain make their first appearance
at about 4 months of gestational life with the Sylvian fissure. By the
end of month 5, the Rolandic fissure is evident and the primary
temporal and frontal fissures have developed. Later the Island of
Reil (insula) becomes visible on the lateral surface, but, during the
rest of life, it is buried beneath the posterior frontal and temporal
lobes. This entire process of convolution formation is the consequence of accelerated growth of the cerebral cortex. The result is
a brain possessing much more cortical tissue than it would if its
surface were smooth (as is characteristic of many animal species).

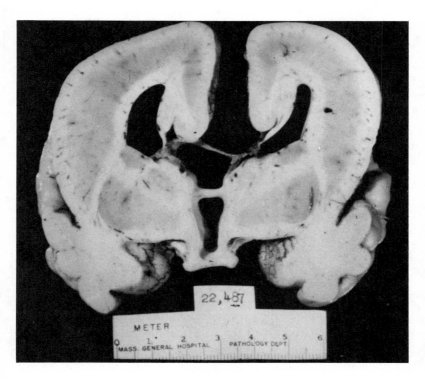

**Fig. 1-2**

Rarely, the process of fissurization is impaired, and varying degrees of agyria (lissencephaly) result (Fig. 1-2). More commonly, disturbances in gyral pattern are less dramatic and take the form of absence of certain gyral fissures and increase (macrogyria) or decrease (microgyria) in size. Given the normal time period for the unfolding of the cortical ribbon, agyria must have its origins before month 5 of fetal life. Shrinkage of gyri (eulegyria) can result from disease at any period of life, once the gyri are formed. Such shrinkage can be distinguished from microgyria by the fact that the cortical tissue is usually very firm due to the gliosis that accompanies the shrinking.

Agenesis of the corpus callosum was cited above as a defect possibly producing no clinical symptoms; it may be an incidental finding at autopsy. If discovered early in life, it is usually because such dramatic nonspecific symptoms as developmental retardation and seizures led to air encephalography, although abnormalities of cortical development probably underlie these symptoms (Fig. 1-2). Normally, the development of the corpus callosum proceeds caudally from its point of origin in the lamina terminalis at about month 4 of fetal life. Its formation takes place over a considerable period of time, thus allowing for the variety of partial defects known to result from its defective development. Usually, these localized defects are posterior in location.

## Brain tissue destruction in utero

Once the brain has more or less assumed its fully formed shape, disease processes would not be expected to significantly influence the migration of neurons, the formation of ventricular cavities, or the elaboration of cerebral convolutions. Rather, one would anticipate pathological reactions similar to those encountered in postnatal life.

This is, in fact, true, but certain characteristics of the developing brain make it especially vulnerable to tissue destruction with resulting cavity formation. The fetal brain is gelatinous and friable. Underlying these physical characteristics are:

1. High water content: About 90% of the brain weight is water in late fetal life as compared to 70% in the adult brain.

2. Low lipid content: In general, there is an inverse relationship between the amount of water and lipid, primarily myelin, in the brain during development. As the myelin membrane develops, the

water content drops. There is little myelin lipid in the fetal brain, and the concentrations of water in the cortex and white matter of the cerebrum are about the same. The fully myelinated, postnatal brain is firmer than the fetal brain.

3. Limited cell numbers and processes: The number of cells increases through gestation into postnatal life. The majority of neurons are formed early by mitotic division and migrate within the nervous system. The increase in neurons after birth is probably minimal in man, except in the cerebellum. Supporting glial cells, however, continue to increase in number during the first 6 postnatal months and probably account for the increasing total cell numbers demonstrated by the DNA method of study. Glial cells and their fibers give support to the cerebral tissue. In response to injury, the immature astroglia react less efficiently than do mature glial cells, and this limits their capacity for scar tissue formation and, thus, enhances cavity formation.

Early in their development, neurons exhibit a paucity of processes, but, as they mature, increasing numbers of dendritic branchings appear, and complex synaptic relationships among neurons are established. This permits a greater diversity of neural function together with solidification of cortical tissue.

4. Relatively few blood vessels: The vascularity of the brain increases throughout development, giving more and more support to the brain.

Cavities formed in the developing brain may vary considerably in size. Porencephaly is the term most often used to refer to anomalous cavities that generally extend from the ventricular system to cortical surfaces (Fig. 1-3). The edges of these cavities are often overgrown with tissue. Usually unilateral, they may occasionally be bilateral and symmetrical. Bilateral defects or clefts, called schizencephaly, may represent altered development dating back to an earlier period in embryogenesis. Porencephalic and schizencephalic lessions usually occur in the area of the middle cerebral arteries. It may be that their occlusion leads to infarction and subsequent dissolution of immature brain tissue with cavity formation. Occlusion of fetal common arteries in the monkey can lead to cerebral cavity formation mimicking porencephaly or to anencephaly, a condition in which most of the brain above the diencephalon is reduced to a transparent membrane but without the marked cranial enlargement seen in

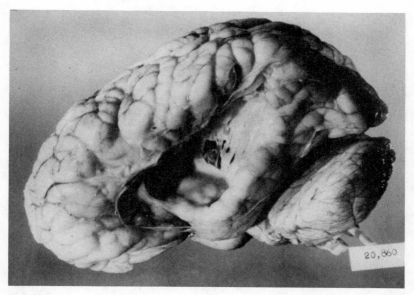

**Fig. 1-3**

hydrocephalus. Confirmation of the vascular etiology of these lesions has not been firmly established in the human, since preservation of the main intracranial vessels is occasionally reported in hydranencephaly. Other etiological possibilities include necrotizing infections and trauma. Hydrostatic influences are almost certainly of importance in determining the final form and extent of these cystic malformations. Because the force exerted on the walls of the diverticulum is equal to the pressure times the surface area ($F = P \times CM^2$), it is possible that a cavity may increase in size even at low pressures. At times, a porencephalic cyst may displace the brain to the opposite side with subsequent thinning of the overlying bone (Fig. 1-4). A pulsative vascular factor has been incriminated because choroid plexectomy on one side prevents enlargement of the ventricle on that side. The process of dissolution of tissue and cavity formation seems to be accelerated in obstructive hydrocephalus, which shares much in common with hydranencephaly except that destruction of the brain occurs in the latter condition in the absence of marked cranial enlargement and impaired cerebrospinal fluid circulation.

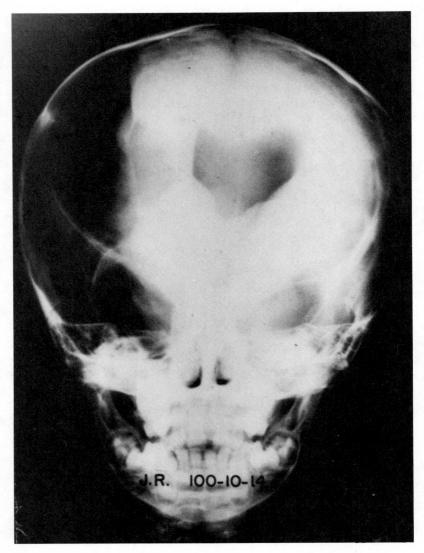

**Fig. 1-4**

## General references

Laurence, K. N. and Weeks, R. 1971. Abnormalities of the central nervous system. Pages 25-86 *in* A. P. Norman, ed. Congenital abnormalities in infancy. 2nd ed. Blackwell Scientific Publications, Oxford.

Warkany, Josef. 1971. Congenital malformations, notes and comments. Year Book Medical. Chicago.

## NEUROLOGICAL DISORDERS OF THE NEONATAL PERIOD

### JOSEPH VOLPE

This section will deal with certain important neurological disturbances of the newborn period (seizures, apneic spells, and jitteriness) and with the major insults affecting the neonate (hypoxic-ischemic injury, intracranial hemorrhage, and neonatal hypoglycemia—as the prototype of metabolic insults).

### Seizures

Seizures are a frequent and often dramatic occurrence in the neonatal period. Unlike seizures in older infants, neonatal seizures do not usually represent a medical emergency, since the convulsive activity in the neonate only rarely interferes with respiratory activity. Nevertheless, it is critical to determine the etiology of the spells rapidly and to treat them, since they often reflect significant illness.

The types of seizures in newborns differ considerably from those observed in older infants, and the types in premature babies differ from those in full term babies. Among both full term and premature newborn infants, most seizures are fragmentary, manifested only by tonic horizontal deviation and/or jerking of the eyes; tonic posturing of a limb; repetitive blinking or fluttering of the eyelids; drooling, sucking, or other oral-buccal movements; apnea; or clonic movements of a limb, which migrate to another part of the body in a random fashion. These spells resemble isolated aspects of generalized seizures in older infants. They become repetitive focal clonic or hemiclonic seizures occasionally and generalized tonic seizures with intermittent clonic movements rarely. The type of seizure rarely helps determine the etiology. For example, focal seizures in the neonate can accompany metabolic disturbances or generalized structural disease of the nervous system. Types of etiology in order of decreasing frequency are (1) perinatal hypoxic-ischemic injury, (2) subarachnoid hemorrhage, (3) hypoglycemia, (4) central nervous system infection, and (5) congenital cerebral anomaly.

Although the pathophysiological mechanisms underlying the distinctive pattern of neonatal seizures are not clearly understood, certain neuroanatomical and neurophysiological data do bear upon this problem. The most critical neuroanatomical processes occurring during the period from month 6 of gestation to the early postnatal months are the so-called organizational events. These events are characterized by the attainment of proper orientation, alignment, and layering of cortical neurons; the elaboration of axonal and dendritic ramifications; and the establishment of synaptic connections. The completion of these processes is probably required for the propagation of a generalized seizure in the adult central nervous system, and their immaturity probably accounts for the fragmentary nature of neonatal seizures. The relatively advanced development of limbic cortex and the connections of this region to diencephalon and brain stem may underlie the predominance of oral-buccal phenomena, oculomotor abnormalities, and apnea as manifestations of neonatal seizure. Purpura and co-workers have emphasized the role of neurophysiological development in the genesis of seizures in the newborn kitten. Their work has demonstrated that inhibitory synaptic activities are predominant early and that the excitatory activities that develop later may account for the relative rarity of generalized seizure activity in the neonate.

## Apneic spells

In the neonatal period, apneic spells have long been considered possible forerunners of brain injury, but a quantitative nature of the relationship has never been established. It is a frequent clinical problem and one that demands the immediate attention of the physician. Apneic spells in small infants are related to the irregular respiratory pattern known as periodic breathing. A discussion of the latter will help in understanding the former.

### PERIODIC BREATHING

In its typical form, periodic breathing occurs in 30 to 50% of premature infants, and similar irregularities of respiration occur at one time or another in nearly all small infants. Classically, the pattern consists of a period of apnea of 5 to 10 seconds followed by ventilation of 10 to 15 seconds at a rate of 50-60 respirations/minute. The over-all respiratory rate is 30-40/minute. During the period of apnea, no changes in heart rate, color, or body temperature occur, in con-

trast to apneic spells. The pattern is more common when the infant
is awake, and the frequency of periodic breathing is greater the
smaller the infant and decreases markedly after week 36. Only minor blood gas changes have been noted in association with periodic
breathing, and these not consistently. In cases not complicated by
apneic spells, the prognosis is uniformly good.

Apneic spells are periods of apnea of more than 20 seconds, which
may or may not be accompanied by bradycardia and cyanosis. With
prolonged monitoring, it has been found that at least 25% of babies
in a premature intensive care unit have such spells. The spells seem
to occur only in conjunction with periodic breathing. Bradycardia
and cyanosis are followed by hypotonia and unresponsiveness—the
former occurring in most premature infants after 20 seconds and
the latter after 45 seconds. For smaller infants, the time periods
may be much shorter. The important clinical settings that are associated with the development of apneic spells are, in decreasing order of frequency:

1. Extreme immaturity, especially with changes in skin temperature, after feeding, or with rectal or nasopharyngeal stimulation.
2. Pulmonary insufficiency with hypoxia, usually from respiratory
   distress syndrome but also due to pulmonary infection or hemorrhage.
3. Metabolic aberrations, especially hypoglycemia, hypocalcemia,
   acidosis, or hyperbilirubinemia.
4. Sepsis.
5. Central nervous system disease, including seizures but almost
   always accompanied by other subtle manifestations of seizure
   activity (see above).

It is now clear that apneic spells and periodic breathing are uniformly related to a disturbance of regulation characteristic of the
premature infant. Periodic breathing appears at a time when the
regulatory system(s) within the central nervous system is maturing.
We may speculate that the locus of this system is the cerebrum, since
periodic breathing is remarkably similar to the Cheynes-Stokes
breathing of older patients (caused by lesions situated bilaterally
in the hemispheres) and since brain-stem structure and function are
relatively well developed in the premature infant. Periodic breathing results in apneic spells when this vulnerable developing regula-

tory system suffers any of the insults listed above, just as other developing systems, e.g., that of glucuronyl transferase, may similarly decompensate when so damaged.

## Jitteriness

The remarkable state of jitteriness is characteristically a disorder of the neonatal period and it rarely, if ever, occurs in similar form at a later age. It may be defined as a movement disorder with qualities primarily of tremulousness but occasionally also of clonus. It is usually easy to distinguish jitteriness from seizure phenomena if the following points are kept in mind. (1) Jitteriness is not accompanied by abnormalities of gaze or extraocular movement, seizures usually are; (2) jitteriness is exquisitely stimulus-sensitive, seizures are not; and (3) the dominant movement in jitteriness is tremor, i.e., the alternating movements are rhythmic, of equal rate and amplitude, but the dominant movement in seizure is clonic jerking, i.e., the movements have a fast and slow component.

The pathogenesis of jitteriness is entirely unknown, and often its clinical significance is comparably obscure. It does seem clear that the disorder represents a generalized disturbance of neurons within the central nervous system and not a peripheral neuromuscular phenomenon. This notion is supported by the fact that clinical settings that produce seizures also result in jitteriness. The classical etiologies of jitteriness are hypoxia, hypoglycemia, hypocalcemia, and drug withdrawal states. The outcome is determined by the neuropathological state producing the jitteriness.

## Hypoxic-ischemic injury

This is a serious clinical problem because hypoxic and/or ischemic injuries cause by far the greatest number of severe nonprogressive neurological deficits in the perinatal period. These neurological deficits usually occur in combination and include mental retardation, seizure disorders, spasticity, choreoathetosis, and ataxia. Patients afflicted with these deficits constitute the majority of children with "cerebral palsy."

Hypoxic-ischemic insults are concomitants of a wide variety of neonatal diseases. Hypoxia (or, more accurately, hypoxemia) occurs most commonly in association with birth asphyxia, recurrent apneic spells, and severe respiratory disease. Ischemia, that is, diminished perfusion of the brain (usually associated with systemic hypotension), occurs most commonly following cardiac arrest or severe bradycardia associated with birth asphyxia or recurrent apneic spells, severe cardiac failure, as in congenital heart disease, and vascular collapse associated with sepsis.

Considerable insight into the pathophysiological events underlying hypoxic-ischemic perinatal brain injury has been obtained from recent studies of birth-related phenomena in the human and subhuman primate. Studies have been made of the relationship between uterine contractions and the fall in heart rate that is synchronous with the peak of the contraction (type I dips). Although this bradycardia is associated with changes in the fetal electroencephalogram, which can be produced in experimental animals by hypoxia, the role of type I dips in the pathogenesis of hypoxic-ischemic injury to human brain occurring at the time of birth is unknown. Fetal bradycardia that has its onset during uterine contraction but reaches a maximum 30 to 60 seconds after the completion of the contraction (type II dips), however, is of definite clinical importance. The fetus that exhibits delayed bradycardia is usually severely asphyxiated at birth. Work in subhuman primates has documented that type II dips are associated with fetal hypoxia, hypotension, and acidosis. The central feature of this constellation is hypoxia; correction of fetal hypoxia ends the bradycardia.

The evolution of brain injury associated with hypoxic-ischemic events during birth of the subhuman primate has been studied. By a variety of means that result in reduction of placental blood flow, investigators have produced delayed bradycardia, hypotension, hypoxia, hypercapnia, and acidosis in the fetus. These insults resulted in neuropathological lesions very similar to those described below for the full term human newborn.

At least four basic lesions can be recognized. Two are associated primarily with hypoxemia: cortical necrosis and status marmoratus of basal ganglia and thalamus. Two are associated primarily with ischemia: "watershed" infarcts and periventricular leukomalacia. The lesions often occur in combination, but one of the four is usually dominant.

CORTICAL NECROSIS

This is the hallmark of a hypoxemic injury. There is necrosis of the neurons of the cerebral and cerebellar cortices. In the cerebral cortex, the deeper cortical layers, especially in depths of sulci, are affected. In the cerebellar cortex, the Purkinje cells are destroyed. In mild cases, only the hippocampal cerebral cortex (neurons of Sommer's sector and Purkinje cells) are affected; in more severe cases, the injury involves the cerebral cortex more diffusely. The clinical sequelae are readily predicted from the location of the lesions—mental retardation, seizures, and spasticity from the cerebral lesions and ataxia from cerebellar lesions. Rarely ataxia dominates the clinical picture.

STATUS MARMORATUS (ÉTAT MARBRE, MARBLED STATE)

This lesion is probably related to hypoxemic injury, but other pathogenic factors may be operative, e.g., traumatic delivery with consequent stasis in the Galenic system of veins. Status marmoratus refers to a distinctive change in the basal ganglia (striatum and pallidum) and thalamus, which develop the gross appearance of marbling. The microscopic features are neuronal loss, glial fibrosis, and hypermyelination. The latter causes the marbled appearance and, remarkably, seems due to myelination around glial fibrils. It is this lesion that underlies most of the cases of congenital athetosis (not associated with kernicterus). Mental retardation may develop secondary to either thalamic disease or concomitant cortical injury.

"WATERSHED" INFARCTS

These infarcts are a result of ischemia occurring in the full term or older infant. The lesions are in the border zones of the three major cerebral arteries (anterior, middle, and posterior), regions most vulnerable to a drop in perfusion pressure, i.e., watershed regions. Necrosis of cortex and subcortical white matter thus extends in a band over the superomedial aspect of the cerebral convexity (between the anterior and middle cerebral arteries) to the posterior parieto-occipital region (between the anterior, posterior, and middle cerebral arteries). The concept that these affected regions, in fact, represent a watershed is supported by recent studies. Profound systemic hypotension was produced in the monkey by pharmacological means, while normal arterial oxygen saturation was maintained by mechanical ventilation. Typical watershed lesions in the cerebrum in the distribution just described were ascribed to the sharply reduced cerebral blood flow. The clinical sequelae in human infants include motor deficits, especially in the hip-shoulder distribution, and deficits in higher cortical function.

### PERIVENTRICULAR LEUKOMALACIA

This is the ischemic lesion of prematurity. It is the most common neuropathological lesion of premature infants seen at autopsy, and in 75% or more of all cases it occurs in premature infants. It affects primarily the periventricular region in the corona radiata. The premature infant does not have a watershed over the cortex because some of the interarterial loops that connect the major cerebral arteries during early fetal development are still present in the last trimester of gestation. The periventricular watershed is located deep in the hemisphere between the distribution of the middle cerebral artery and the choroidal vessels and also between certain subependymal branches of the middle cerebral artery. Since the infarcts are located near or within the descending corticospinal tract fibers from the leg areas of the motor cortex, spastic diplegia, the most common motor deficit occurring after prematurity, may be a sequela.

## Intracranial hemorrhage

Intracranial hemorrhage is a very frequent clinical occurrence in the newborn period. Three types are of clinical importance: subdural hemorrhage, primary subarachnoid hemorrhage, and periventricular hemorrhage.

### SUBDURAL HEMORRHAGE

This is almost exclusively a traumatic lesion of large, full term infants. Trauma etiology depends on the relationship of the size of the fetal head to the size of the birth canal, the rigidity of the birth canal, and the duration and type of labor and delivery. Thus, subdural hemorrhage occurs most often when the baby is relatively large and/or the birth canal is relatively small; when pelvic structures are relatively rigid, as in a primaparous or an elderly multiparous mother; when the duration of labor is unusually brief and does not allow enough time for dilation of the pelvic structures, or unusually long, subjecting the head to prolonged compression and molding; when the head must pass through a birth canal not gradually adapted to it, as in foot or breech presentations; or when delivery requires difficult forceps extraction. These circumstances result in excessive molding of the head, particularly with frontal-occipital elongation. The result is stretching of the falx and tentorium, possible tearing of the tentorium or falx, and stretching and tearing of the lateral or straight sinuses or the vein of Galen and/or its tributaries. Extreme vertical molding underlies most tears of superficial cerebral veins and subdural hemorrhage over the convexities.

### PERIVENTRICULAR HEMORRHAGE

This lesion of premature infants occurs most frequently in association with severe, prolonged hypoxia, accompanying severe birth asphyxia or respiratory distress syndrome. The hemorrhage often occurs 2 to 3 days after the most severe hypoxia. The hemorrhage emanates from terminal veins of the Galenic system, draining the cerebral white matter, the striatum, and the thalamus; it is primarily intracerebral and only secondarily intraventricular.

The pathogenesis of periventricular hemorrhage relates to the venous drainage of the affected areas and the effects of hypoxia on these veins. The terminal veins of the Galenic system are located in the gelatinous subependymal germinal matrix, an area with very little supportive tissue. The germinal matrix is nearly exhausted by term. Stasis and subsequent rupture of these vessels are especially likely to occur at the level of the foramen of Monro, where the periventricular tributaries from the striatum and centrum semiovale to the paired internal cerebral veins change their direction of flow at a sharp angle. Hypoxia further predisposes to hemorrhage because it is associated with venous congestion and endothelial injury. Moreover, the walls of vessels in the premature infant are unusually thin and fragile, and this contributes to the propensity for rupture, together with the hemodynamic and anatomical factors just described.

The most common clinical syndrome noted in babies who suffer periventricular hemorrhage is a sudden catastrophic neurological deterioration characterized by coma, fixed and dilated pupils, flaccid quadriparesis, and respiratory arrest, all evolving in minutes to an hour or so. If death does not ensue, severe neurological sequelae remain. No therapeutic maneuver is helpful, although attempts to prevent increased cerebral venous pressure (i.e., avoidance of high positive pressure respirators) are probably indicated.

SUBARACHNOID HEMORRHAGE

This is more commonly a lesion of the premature than the full term infant. Unlike the arterial subarachnoid hemorrhage of older patients, this is a venous hemorrhage that can result from birth trauma or hypoxia, and often both. The relationship of the hypoxemic insult to the development of the hemorrhage is similar to that described for intraventricular hemorrhage. When hypoxia is the major pathogenetic factor, the hemorrhage occurs 48 to 72 hours after the most severe hypoxia. Three major clinical syndromes can result. First, minimal or no symptoms may be apparent, as in the large number of "normal" neonates with blood in the cerebrospinal fluid. Second, seizures may occur in an otherwise "normal" infant. Prognosis in the first two categories is excellent. Third, a massive subarachnoid hemorrhage may be accompanied by coma and respiratory failure, evolving in hours. This is a rare event, often with permanent sequelae.

## Neonatal hypoglycemia

Hypoglycemia in the neonatal period is an important cause of injury to the developing nervous system. Because of the myriad of hormonal and metabolic factors that influence carbohydrate metabolism, a great many disorders can lead to hypoglycemia. A practical classification of etiologies based on pathophysiology includes four groups: (1) infants of diabetic mothers or erythroblastotic infants in whom hyperinsulinism occurs secondary to hyperplasia of pancreatic islets (the disorder is manifested by abundant tissue deposition of glycogen and fat and by high absolute levels of insulin); (2) infants demonstrating intrauterine malnutrition or undernutrition (e.g., small for gestational age) in whom relative hyperinsulinism is thought to occur (they have diminished tissue levels of glycogen); (3) infants who have high metabolic needs (as in severe respiratory disease) and diminished substrate stores (as in prematurity); and

(4) infants with the variety of genetic, hormonal, or metabolic defects that can lead to hypoglycemia. The last group is very small compared to the first three, and we will confine our discussion to the more common problems.

Neonatal hypoglycemia (i.e., glucose below 20 mg% in the premature or 30 mg% in the full term infant) is a common clinical problem. The incidence in infants of overtly diabetic mothers is 50%, in infants of mothers with gestational diabetes 20%, and in low birth weight infants, at least 6%. The incidence of symptoms associated with the hypoglycemia is quite different, however; in infants of diabetic mothers it is only 10 to 20%, and in the low birth weight infants it is 60 to 90%. This difference is probably related to the duration of the hypoglycemia, which is relatively brief (first hours of life) in the infants of diabetic mothers and often prolonged (first days of life) in the low birth weight infants. A study of 151 neonates demonstrated a direct relation between the incidence of symptoms, the duration of hypoglycemia, and the delay before onset of therapy.

The clinical manifestations of neonatal hypoglycemia are diverse, and the index of suspicion for this entity must, therefore, be very high when a physician is dealing with any neonate who is not doing well. The most common presenting sign is jitteriness, which occurs in about 80% of the cases; if the hypoglycemia persists, seizures will occur in 10 to 30% of the cases. Other common neurological signs are hypotonia, stupor, and apnea.

The neuropathological changes in hypoglycemia are impressive. Severe degenerative changes occur in neurons at virtually every level of the nervous system. The disease does not show the predilection for depths of sulci or arterial border zones in the cerebral cortex that hypoxia and ischemia do. Particularly significant is the involvement of anterior horn cells, which may be the locus of neuronal loss underlying the marked hypotonia that can occur as a sequela. The mental retardation, spasticity, and seizures seen in varying combinations as sequelae of hypoglycemia are presumably related to the cerebral involvement. Approximately 50% of hypoglycemic neonates with seizures will have such neurological sequelae on followup. Affected babies whose symptoms do not include seizures have about a 15% incidence of sequelae. Asymptomatic neonates have little or no increased risk of neurological sequelae.

## General references

Berman, P. H. and B. Q. Banker. 1966. Neonatal meningitis: A clinical and pathological study of 29 cases. Pediatrics 38:6.

Brown, J. K., F. Cockburn, and J. O. Forfar. 1972. Clinical and chemical correlates in convulsions of the newborn. Lancet I:135.

DeReuck, J., A. S. Chattha, and E. P. Richardson, Jr. 1972. Pathogenesis and evolution of periventricular leukomalacia in infancy. Arch. Neurol. 27:229.

Koivisto, M., M. Blanco-Sequeiros, and V. Krause. 1972. Neonatal symptomatic and asymptomatic hypoglycaemia. A follow-up study of 151 children. Devel. Med. Child. Neurol. 14:603.

# INHERITED METABOLIC AND DEGENERATIVE DISORDERS OF THE DEVELOPING BRAIN

ARTHUR L. PRENSKY

## Introduction

The etiology of most degenerative diseases of the developing brain is not yet known. In the past 30 years, however, it has become increasingly apparent that many of these relentlessly progressive disorders represent disturbances in intermediary metabolism, often the result of a mutation in a single enzyme. Although it is possible that other mechanisms may underlie these diseases (e.g., slow viruses or chronic ingestion of toxic substances), the close relationship between degenerative disorders of developing brain and inborn errors of metabolism warrant that they be considered together.

## Degenerative diseases: General characteristics

Degenerative diseases of the developing nervous system fall into three broad groups: (1) diffuse disease that primarily involves gray matter; (2) diffuse disease that primarily involves white matter; and (3) system disease. By system disease we mean the degeneration of a particular chain of nuclei and tracts, which are functionally interrelated.

Diseases that predominantly involve gray matter are frequently ushered in by the early onset of seizures. Loss of cognitive and social abilities generally precedes and exceeds the loss of motor control, although the latter inevitably follows. In contrast, the diseases that primarily involve white matter are usually characterized by infrequent seizures, if any at all, and involvement of cerebellar and corticospinal function is initially predominant over general intellectual deterioration.

It should be easier to recognize a system disease than a diffuse disease, since, by definition, only one facet of neurological function is heavily involved. This is not so true early in infancy, however, since the evaluation of "intellectual" function in the first months of life is made almost entirely on the basis of motor control. Therefore, a disease that only affects the lower motor neurons, e.g., Werdnig-Hoffman's disease, may lead the casual observer to believe that the infant is also intellectually retarded. And, in older infants and children, some diffuse diseases of gray and white matter may initially impair motor control to a degree that suggests a system disease.

## Neuronal storage disease

The best understood of the degenerative diseases of the nervous system are those caused by an enzymatic defect that interrupts the normal catabolism of one of the structural components of nervous tissue. Investigation of the pathology of such disorders often shows that destruction of the normal architecture of the nervous system is accompanied by evidence of excessive accumulation of the affected metabolite. Most of these diseases preferentially involve gray matter, and the pathological evidence of metabolite accumulation is characterized by swollen, distended neurons with eccentrically placed nuclei. Occasionally, swelling of glial cell cytoplasm, collections of abnormal material in pockets of degenerating myelin or in perivascular spaces, and collections of material in thickened meninges can be seen. Because of these pathological features, such disorders were known as "storage diseases" long before the biochemical pathways responsible for such accumulations were known. Neuronal loss, axonal degeneration, and disruption of myelin also occur, but frequently (as in Tay-Sachs disease) the histological abnormalities do not appear to be severe enough to account for the marked functional deterioration of the patient.

The currently recognized storage diseases of the nervous system involve the accumulation of lipids or carbohydrates. In the majority

CERAMIDE:   $CH_3-(CH_2)_{12}-C=C-CH-CH-CH_2$

with structure showing $H$, OH, NH (OH), and $R-C=O$

A: __PHOSPHOSPHINGOLIPIDS__

1. CERAMIDE $-O-P-C-C-NH_3^{(+)}$

CERAMIDE AMINOETHYLPHOSPHONATE

2. CERAMIDE $-O-P-O-CH_2-CH_2-N(CH_3)_3$

SPHINGOMYELIN
(NIEMANN-PICK'S DISEASE)

B: __GALACTOSPHINGOLIPIDS__

1. CERAMIDE – GALACTOSE
   CEREBROSIDE
   (GLOBOID CELL LEUKODYSTROPHY)

2. CERAMIDE – GALACTOSE – $SO_4$
   SULFATIDE
   (METACHROMATIC LEUKODYSTROPHY)

C: __GLUCOSPHINGOLIPIDS__

1. CERAMIDE – GLUCOSE
   GLUCOCEREBROSIDE
   (GAUCHER'S DISEASE)

2. CERAMIDE – GLUCOSE – GALACTOSE
   CERAMIDE LACTOSIDE OR CYTOSIDE

3. CERAMIDE – GLUCOSE – GALACTOSE – GALACTOSE
   CERAMIDE TRIHEXOSIDE
   (FABRY'S DISEASE)

4. CERAMIDE – GLUCOSE – GALACTOSE – GALACTOSE – GALACTOSAMINE
   GLOBOSIDE

5. CERAMIDE – SUGARS – NANA
   THE GANGLIOSIDES

TABLE 1-1    *The Sphingolipids*

of these diseases, there are defects in the catabolism of sphingolipids (Table 1-1), which are normal cellular constituents. When excessive amounts of a sphingolipid are stored within a neuron, it combines with other lipids and, possibly, proteins within the cell to form extraneous membranous inclusions to distend the cytoplasm; these first interrupt the function of the cell and eventually destroy it. Membranous cytoplasmic inclusions in neurons also occur in disturbances of mucopolysaccharide metabolism, whereas in the glycogen storage diseases large vesicles containing glycogen are found. The exact mechanisms by which such storage interferes with cell functions have not yet been defined, although initially they may interfere with lysosome activity.

## WHITE MATTER STORAGE DISEASE

Whereas storage disorders predominantly affect the nerve cell, excessive accumulation of metabolites in white matter is common in several of these diseases (particularly metachromatic leukodystrophy, type II glycogenosis, and Tay-Sachs disease). Such accumulations in white matter are associated with a greater destruction of myelin than could be accounted for by destruction of axons with accompanying Wallerian degeneration and probably reflect a primary involvement of glial cells and myelin as well as neurons and axons. In metachromatic leukodystrophy, there is a great increase in the sulfatide content of white matter. In this disease, the myelin membrane (which normally contains sulfatide) is primarily involved, and isolated myelin contains a great excess of sulfatide. Once again, it is not clear how an excess of such a compound as sulfatide normally found in the membrane interferes with myelination of the nervous system. A distinction has been proposed between dysmyelinating diseases and demyelinating diseases. In the dysmyelinating diseases, it is assumed that the myelin formed is abnormal; thus, the rate of synthesis of the membrane is reduced, or, because of its abnormal physical configuration, it is more likely to be destroyed. Metachromatic leukodystrophy would be a typical example of this group of diseases. The demyelinating disorders presumably involve the excessive destruction of a normal myelin membrane. At present there is little evidence to suggest that this distinction between dysmyelinating and demyelinating disease is necessarily valid.

EXTRACEREBRAL STORAGE

There is every reason to believe that the storage disorders that involve the nervous system are generalized diseases and involve other organs of the body as well. In many instances, however, the accumulated metabolite occurs in such small amounts outside the nervous system that it fails to interfere with function and, thus, fails to produce symptoms or signs of systemic disease. Nevertheless, some storage disorders affect other organs of the body to such a degree as to indirectly interfere with neurological function. In rare instances, the function of the liver is sufficiently impaired by excessive storage (i.e., in Niemann-Pick's disease or in GM-1 gangliosidosis) to interfere with cerebral activity. Usually though, liver function remains relatively intact despite the fact that the organ is enormously enlarged. In other disorders, notably Farber's disease, inanition is severe, and central nervous system growth may possibly be delayed by poor nutrition. Although there is excessive accumulation of sulfatide in the kidney in metachromatic leukodystrophy, and early in the history of this disease the diagnosis can be established by examining the urine of suspected patients for metachromatic granules, renal function usually is not seriously impaired. In another of the sphingolipidoses, Fabry's disease, renal impairment can be so severe as to result in a uremic encephalopathy. Glycogen storage diseases, particularly type I, which do not directly involve the central nervous system, may nevertheless result in severe impairment of cerebral function; this is often progressive, as a result of repeated episodes of hypoglycemia. Acute deterioration may occasionally be seen in children suffering from Hurler's (type I) form of mucopolysaccharidosis because of storage of mucopolysaccharide in the meninges, where it can impede the flow of cerebrospinal fluid; this can result in acute hydrocephalus.

Storage disorders were originally delineated on the basis of their clinical features; their classification was further clarified by histological and histochemical studies of the nervous system and, finally, by biochemical studies of involved tissue. Such biochemical studies initially were based on the isolation of stored metabolites from the tissues obtained either at autopsy or by brain biopsy. In recent years, however, the ability to define the enzymatic basis of many of these diseases during life has expanded the physician's potential to diagnose, classify, and possibly prevent many of the storage disorders that affect the nervous system. Since these are systemic diseases, the enzymatic deficiency responsible for the central nervous system dysfunction can often be found in more easily accessible tissues or in body fluids. Thus, for example, there is a severe reduction in hexosaminidase A in the serum of patients with classical Tay-Sachs disease and of aryl sulfatase A in the urine and white blood cells of patients with metachromatic leukodystrophy.

The ability to diagnose a storage disorder by testing for the enzymatic defect permits diagnosis at an early age, often without the use of biopsy material. Potential patients can be identified *in utero*. In many instances, carriers of the defective gene can be detected easily, since their enzyme levels fall mid-way between the normal population and those afflicted with the disorder. In addition to these practical advantages, the enzymatic identification of storage disorders has resulted in a clearer appreciation of the range and heterogeneity of these diseases. Phenotypically identical disorders may be the result of different genotypes. Once again, Tay-Sachs disease is a classic example. There are now three identifiable forms of Tay-Sachs disease, which appear to be phenotypically similar if not identical. The most common form is the result of a hexosaminidase A deficiency in which levels of total hexosaminidase remain normal. In the second form, total hexosaminidase is reduced, and there is a deficiency of both A and B isoenzymes. In the third form, despite the massive accumulation of Tay-Sachs ganglioside in brain tissue, no hexosaminidase deficiency can be established, and it can only be assumed that, for reasons yet to be determined, the function of this enzyme is impaired in the nervous system. It has also been possible, through the use of enzymatic techniques, to identify a fourth form of Tay-Sachs disease that begins later in life—in early childhood rather than early infancy—and has a considerably slower course. This disease, which is phenotypically quite different from classical Tay-Sachs disease both in its age of onset and rate of progression, appears to be a similar disorder genetically in that there is a hexosaminidase A deficiency. This deficiency is not as severe as that in classical Tay-Sachs disease, which probably accounts for the difference in onset and progression.

### Degenerative disorders of white matter

Diseases that predominantly or exclusively involve the white matter of the brain in a diffuse manner during development have been termed leukodystrophies regardless of the basis of the disorder. Metachromatic leukodystrophy, to use a familiar example, is a storage disorder in which there is an increased amount of sulfatide in white matter and myelin resulting from an absence of aryl sulfatase A. Another leukodystrophy, Krabbe's disease, is also the result of a catabolic enzyme defect. Here the principal abnormality is not the inability to remove sulfate from galactose but to hydrolyze the galactose from ceramide (sphingosine + fatty acid). In this disorder, however, there is only a relative increase in galactoceramide (cerebroside) in the white matter. Absolute levels are much lower than those found in normal brain, probably because myelin, which contains most of the cerebroside in white matter, is destroyed very rapidly or not synthesized at a normal rate.

Metachromatic and Krabbe's leukodystrophies are the only two diffuse disorders of white matter characterized by a definite enzymatic disturbance. Other diffuse disorders of white matter are still characterized by their pathological features. Most appear to involve myelin in excess of other white matter elements, but, in some disorders, e.g., Seitelberger's neuraxonal leukodystrophy, the axon appears to be the principal site of pathology; in yet another disorder, Alexander's leukodystrophy, the abnormalities of white matter suggest there may be an error in metabolic processes within astrocytes. Recently it has become clear that many of these disorders affecting central white matter also affect the peripheral nerve, resulting in abnormally slow nerve conduction times; in nerve biopsies, the material may, in some instances, have pathological features sufficiently distinctive to identify the disease.

## System diseases

With rare exceptions, the causes of system diseases are unknown. Why a group of functionally related cells in the nervous system preferentially deteriorates, while the remainder of the central nervous system functions normally, has never been successfully explained. These diseases were originally called "abiotrophies," a term that suggests that at some early time in embryogenesis the early destruction of these cells was somehow programmed into their function. There is no experimental confirmation of this concept. It has not been possible to show that in any of the system diseases the chromosomal pattern of affected cells differs from that of the normal cell population or that defects in regulator genes (or other as yet undefined factors) reduce one or more gene products in the affected cells. A second possibility exists: cells that have related functions in the nervous system share one or more unique and essential metabolic pathways, which may be of trivial importance to cells elsewhere in the body. An inherited metabolic disorder involving such a pathway would result in a limited form of degeneration in the central nervous system. Technical difficulties have hampered the investigation of these hypotheses, but recent advances in the growth of neural explants in culture may make investigations of these disorders more feasible.

The possibility of a toxic etiology has frequently been raised for those system diseases with a sporadic inheritance. The ability of manganese or carbon disulfide (and, more recently, poisoning by the phenothiazines) to produce progressive tremor and rigidity, of mercury to mimic progressive spinal muscular atrophy or cerebellar degeneration, and of cyanide to mimic Leber's optic atrophy, makes such speculations reasonable.

It is more likely that the system diseases also represent metabolic disorders, with expression limited to those cell populations, which, for unknown reasons, are greatly at risk. This would certainly appear to be the case in Wilson's disease, a hereditary disorder that initially involves basal ganglia and cerebellar functions. This disease is the most intensively investigated of all the hereditary system diseases, yet the exact mechanisms responsible for neurological deterioration are unknown. It is associated with an increased deposition of copper, particularly in the basal ganglia. Apart from the nervous system, there is extensive damage to the liver and, to a lesser degree, the kidney, producing early cirrhosis and renal tubular disease. In most patients, there is a reduction of a plasma copper-binding protein, ceruloplasmin, which is believed to leave copper ions free to be deposited in liver and brain, and particularly in the basal ganglia. It is not clear, however, that the deposition of copper in brain is primarily responsible for the neurological symptoms and signs of Wilson's disease, since chronic cirrhosis with high blood ammonia levels may produce similar symptoms and signs. Thus, it is not clear to what degree the cerebral dysfunction noted in Wilson's disease is secondary to hepatic deterioration. It is not certain that excess copper causes cell death in the central nervous system, or, if it does, by what mechanisms. Nevertheless, the treatment of this disorder with such chelating agents as penicillamine, to remove excess free copper from the body, slows or arrests progress of the disease. Wilson's disease, therefore, represents a treatable system disease in which there is a hereditary biochemical defect in a carrier protein for copper, suggesting that in other conditions restricted degeneration of the nervous system may be linked to a hereditary metabolic disturbance.

In Refsum's syndrome, restricted degeneration of the nervous system is again associated with an inherited metabolic abnormality. This disease was once classified with the broad group of familial ataxias because of pronounced signs of cerebellar degeneration, although an associated peripheral neuropathy, sensori-neural deafness, and retinitis pigmentosa were also recognized as part of the syndrome. Over a decade ago, Klenk and his co-workers found that Refsum's syndrome was actually a metabolic disease associated with an enormous accumulation of a tetramethylhexadecanoic acid (phytanic acid). Patients lack the appropriate decarboxylase for converting odd chained fatty acids to even. The syndrome, however, differs from other lipid storage diseases in that the body is not capable of synthesizing the stored compound. The sole source of phytanic acid in the human is the dietary ingestion of phytol. This raises the possibility that dietary restrictions may impede the progress of this disease.

## Hereditary metabolic diseases

There are a number of hereditary metabolic diseases in which neurological function is either acutely or chronically affected, but the central nervous system does not show evidence of storage, and the clinical and pathological picture is not that of a degenerative disease. Most of these disorders involve disturbances in amino acid or carbohydrate metabolism. Their acute neurological symptoms usually include ataxia, stupor, coma, and convulsions, whereas mental retardation, often unassociated with other pronounced neurological symptoms or signs, is the most devastating chronic manifestation.

Acute disturbances of neurological function occurring in the course of these diseases are usually the result of intermittent ketosis or acidosis, as in maple syrup urine disease, methylamalonic aciduria, proprionic acidemia, and isovaleric aciduria; hypoglycemia, as in methylmalonic aciduria, galactosemia, and in certain of the glycogen storage diseases or hereditary fructose intolerance; and hyperammonemia, as in disturbances in the metabolism of amino acids of the urea cycle and in hereditary protein intolerance. Abnormalities in other classes of metabolites may exert an acute toxic effect on neurological function but as yet have not definitely been identified during the course of disease.

The cause of mental retardation in these disorders remains speculative. The most thoroughly studied of the disturbances in amino acid metabolism is phenylketonuria. Despite years of intensive investigation in humans and animals, it has not been possible to define the cause(s) of the severe retardation phenylketonuric patients

suffer when untreated. The fact that dietary restriction of phenylalanine, if instituted early in life, results in considerable improvement
in mental function in the great majority of these patients is an indication that the accumulation of the amino acid itself, or of some
by-product, plays an important role in the neurological disability.
The following mechanisms by which high serum levels of a single
amino acid such as phenylalanine might impair brain growth and
function have been suggested:

1. High serum levels of a single amino acid distort the serum pattern of other amino acids by mechanisms as yet undetermined. High
levels of an amino acid, e.g., phenylalanine, can also interfere with
the transport of other amino acids into the brain, particularly those
neutral amino acids that share a common transport system with phenylalanine. In animals with experimental hyperphenylalaninemia,
levels of several amino acids, notably the branched chain amino
acids leucine, isoleucine, and valine, are extremely low (less than
one-third the levels found in controls). Other neutral amino acids
are affected to a lesser degree. A decrease in the concentration of
amino acids available for protein synthesis may slow the rate of protein synthesis, since the rate may be substrate dependent. Protein
synthesis is also reduced *in vitro* in ribosomal preparations, presumably because of impaired amino acid transport and/or a decrease in
the activity of enzymes needed to activate amino acids to be incorporated into the peptide chain. The effect may be even more fundamental in that high concentrations of one amino acid or reduced
concentrations of other amino acids, notably tryptophan, may actually interfere with the structure and function of brain polyribo-
somes necessary for protein synthesis. Although these are reasonable
suppositions, they are yet to be proved conclusively.

2. Phenylalanine in high concentrations in animal models appears to interfere with the incorporation of labeled glucose into nucleic acids, amino acids, and lipids. Several investigators have found
deficits in lipid biosynthesis without concomitant deficits in the incorporation of such labeled precursors as ${}^3$H-cytidine into RNA or
concomitant decreases in brain DNA or protein. This supports the
concept that the major effect of hyperphenylalaninemia may be on
the process of myelination, and specifically on the formation of the
lipids composing the myelin sheath. Results of other studies are
consistent with the hypothesis that high levels of phenylalanine also

interfere with the intermediary metabolism of glucose, possibly by inhibiting the function of the enzyme pyruvate kinase.

3. High levels of phenylalanine result in low levels of tyrosine, the amino acid precursor of such catecholamine neuro-transmitters as dopamine and norepinephrine. It also results in low levels of brain tryptophan and serotonin by several mechanisms: the hydroxylation of tryptophan in liver is inhibited, the transport of 5-hydroxytrypto-phan across the blood-brain barrier is inhibited, and the decarboxy-lation of 5-hydroxytryptophan to 5-hydroxytryptamine (serotonin) is also inhibited by high phenylalanine levels in serum and brain. Whether defects in transmitter function play a serious part in the mental retardation seen in this disorder remains speculative.

4. The accumulation of phenylalanine may result in the activation of alternate pathways to produce such neurotoxic substances as phenylethylamine. This possibility is theoretically sound, but has yet to be demonstrated as important either in humans or in animal models. Furthermore, the effects of high levels of phenylethylamine are usually acute rather than chronic.

This brief summary of some of the possible mechanisms by which brain development may be slowed in phenylketonuric patients or hyperphenylalaninemic animals illustrates the general problem of understanding how disorders on intermediary metabolism lead to neurological defects. Any explanation of the mechanisms by which high serum levels of phenylalanine, for example, exert their effect on brain must take into consideration several clinical observations. (1) Children of phenylketonuric or severely hyperphenylalaninemic mothers are almost always retarded, although they do not have the metabolic defect. Therefore, high levels of phenylalanine *in utero* result in permanent brain damage despite normal levels after parturition. (2) Dietary therapy that lowers serum levels of phenylalanine improves the neurological function of phenylketonuric patients. (3) These lowered serum levels need not be continued after the sixth to eighth year of life. Thereafter, high levels of phenylalanine in the serum do not appear to damage cerebral function.

## Vitamin-dependent diseases

Diseases that can be partially or fully corrected by ingestion of enormous amounts of a vitamin are known as vitamin-dependent diseases. An apoenzyme (protein) may not react properly with its co-factor (vitamin) to form an enzyme for several possible reasons: (1) the improper absorption of the cofactor; (2) its failure to be trans-ported properly to the cell and across the cell membrane; (3) a change in the structure of the enzyme protein to make binding with the cofactor less efficient than with competing substrates; or (4) an in-ability of the vitamin to be converted into its functional form as a cofactor. Disorders in which large doses of pyridoxine appear to ameliorate the biochemical disorder (e.g., xanthurenic aciduria, homocysteinuria, and cystathianinuria) seem to result from a struc-tural defect in the apoenzyme rather than any general defect in the transport of pyridoxine or the conversion of pyridoxine into its active form, since patients with these disorders usually have only a single metabolic defect and not defects in all the processes for which pyridoxine is a known cofactor. On the other hand, the form of methylmalonic aciduria responsive to $B_{12}$ appears to result from the failure to convert the ingested form of $B_{12}$, cyanocobalamin, into its active form, 5-deoxyädenosyl cobalamin. Similarly, in Leigh's encephalopathy (a progressive disorder characterized by abnormali-ties in cranial nerve function and respiration, vomiting and muscle weakness), a substance excreted in the urine may block the conversion of thiamine pyrophosphate to thiamine triphosphate. This can be partially corrected in some patients, for limited periods of time, by the administration of very large doses of thiamine.

Pharmacological doses of vitamins, often 100 times the minimal daily requirement, exert beneficial effects by the law of mass action in several ways: they may shift a reaction in favor of the formation of an active cofactor; they may favor a combination of cofactor and apoenzyme in the presence of competitors; or they may accelerate an alternate pathway for the catabolism of the stored metabolite. In the latter instance, there would be no direct effect on the defec-tive enzymatic reaction resulting in the original accumulation of the metabolite.

Treatment of hereditary metabolic diseases involving the central nervous system consists either of restricting the accumulated metab-olite in the diet, if it is a compound that cannot be synthesized in the body, or accelerating removal of the metabolite by enhancing the activity of degradative pathways through the use of pharmaco-logical doses of potential cofactors or, in the case of metallic ions, by binding them to chemicals not found in the body that are rapidly excreted. The direct replacement of defective enzymes is not yet possible. Recent experimental work in this area is encouraging, however. In tissue cultures, it is possible to grow defective cell lines with other cells that have the missing enzyme and, in many instances, correct the biochemical defect in the defective cells. This presumably occurs by diffusion of the enzyme through the media into the abnormal cell. The repeated infusion of enzymatic material *in vivo* is, of course, complicated by the hazards of developing an immune reaction. Furthermore, it may be particularly difficult for infused enzymatic material to enter the brain, although it may enter other tissues. A much more satisfactory method of introducing the required enzyme into the body involves the transplantation of organs from genetically intact humans. These organs then continue to function normally in the host, producing the needed enzymatic material. This has already been successfully employed on several occasions in the treatment of Fabry's disease in which the enzyme defect, although generalized, most seriously interferes with renal function. Kidney transplantation in patients with this disorder can be life-saving. It is still not clear that organ transplantation, when feasible, will result in increased concentrations of a defective enzyme in brain and thus allow for the correction of those metabolic diseases that primarily affect the nervous system.

## General references

Bernsohn, J. and H. J. Grossman, eds. 1971. Lipid storage diseases: Enzymatic defects and clinical implications. Academic Press, New York/London, 316 pp.

Bickel, H., F. P. Hudson, and L. I. Woolf, eds. 1971. Phenylketonuria and some other inborn errors of amino acid metabolism. Georg-Thieme Ver Bag, Stuttgart, 336 pp.

Brady, R. O. 1968. Enzymatic defects in the sphingolipidoses. Adv. Clin. Chem. 11:1-19.

Brady, R. O., J. F. Tallman, W. G. Johnson, et al. 1973. Replacement therapy for inherited enzyme deficiency: Use of a purified ceramidetrihexosidase in Fabry's disease. New Eng. J. Med. 289:9-14.

Brady, R. O. 1973. Abnormal biochemistry of untreated disorders of lipid metabolism. Fed. Proc. 32:1660-1667.

Glazer, R. I. and G. Weber. 1971. The effects of L-phenylalanine and phenylpyruvate on glycolysis in rat cerebral cortex. Brain Res. 33:439-450.

Haymond, M. W., I. E. Karl, R. D. Feigin, et al. 1973. Hypoglycemia and maple syrup urine disease: Defective gluconeogenesis. Pediat. Res. 7:500-508.

Hsia, D. Y-Y. 1966. Inborn errors of metabolism: Part I: Clinical aspects. 2nd ed., Year Book Medical, Chicago, 396 pp.

Morrow, G. III and L. A. Barness. 1972. Combined vitamin responsiveness in homocystinuria. J. Pediat. 81:946-954.

Nadler, H. L. 1972. Allotransplantation for the treatment of inborn errors of metabolism. Ann. Intern. Med. 77:314-316.

Nyhan, W. L., ed. 1967. Amino acid metabolism and genetic variation. McGraw-Hill, New York, 495 pp.

Prensky, A. L., S. Carr, and H. W. Moser. 1968. Development of myelin in inherited disorders of amino acid metabolism. Arch. Neurol. 19:552-558.

Rosenberg, L. E., A-C. Lilljequist, and Y. E. Hsia. 1968. Methylmalonic aciduria: Metabolic block localization and vitamin $B_{12}$ dependency. Science 162:805-807.

Rosenberg, L. E. 1969. Inherited aminoacidopathies demonstrating vitamin dependency. New Eng. J. Med. 281:145-152.

Sloan, H. R. 1970. Tissue culture studies in the lipid storage disorders. Chem. Phys. Lipids 5:250-260.

Snyder, R. A. and R. O. Brady. 1969. The use of white cells as a source of diagnostic material for lipid storage diseases. Clin. Chim. Acta 25:331-338.

Stanbury, J. B., J. B. Wyngaarden, and D. S. Frederickson, eds. 1972. The metabolic basis of inherited disease. 3rd ed. McGraw-Hill, New York, 1778 pp.

# 2
# Disorders of Nerve and Muscle

## DISTURBANCES OF PERIPHERAL NERVE FUNCTION

W. M. LANDAU AND S. G. ELIASSON

### Physiological aspects

In principle, the most direct correlations in neurology should be those between clinical phenomena of peripheral nerve disease and anatomical and physiological basic knowledge, for the peripheral nerve trunk includes all input pathways for somatic sensation and somatic reflex behavior and all output pathways for control of striated muscle and other peripheral effector structures. To some extent, the effects of peripheral nerve disease on impulses normally conducted into or out of the nervous system are analogous to the effect of cutting a major telephone trunk cable on a communication system. The model fails to be a satisfactory generalization because pathological processes are seldom of an all-or-none quality and because the peripheral nervous system is a very special part of the nervous system in that its units are capable of regeneration following injury.

The contents of mixed nerve trunks have been analyzed in great detail in regard to the relation of afferent and efferent function to fiber origins and terminations, fiber diameters, and specialized endings. Several generalizations are useful in the interpretation of clinical phenomena.

49

The largest myelinated afferents are from muscle and have powerful segmental reflex and cerebellar projections and a small, but definite projection to the cerebral cortex. Recent work suggests that they contribute something to proprioceptive sensation but certainly not much. Major proprioceptive sense derives from joint receptors, which have the next to the largest beta axons.

Response to a light mechanical disturbance, touch, derives from specialized endings in hair follicles and other cutaneous structures and probably from less specialized endings as well. Input comes via all but the largest myelinated fiber sizes, plus many unmyelinated fibers. In man, the unmyelinated fibers do not give rise to the sensation of touch. Touch projection upward in the spinal cord is in the dorsal column and probably bilaterally in the ventral and lateral columns. Thus, there is a large anatomical-physiological reserve for touch function in both peripheral nerves and sundry spinal pathways. As might be expected, clinical impairment of touch sensation is seldom seen except in well-advanced pathological processes.

Pain, the response to potentially injurious or nociceptive stimulation, derives from naked branched terminal endings and is represented only in the smallest myelinated delta fiber pool (pricking pain) and in upwards of one-half of the unmyelinated fibers (burning, aching pain). These small fibers enter the cord via the lateral division of the dorsal root into the dorsal gray; the larger fibers, serving other modalities, form the medial division, which sends axons into the dorsal column and segmental gray matter. In man, the second-order projection for pain decussates in the spinothalamic tract and has connections with the medial brain stem at several levels. Temperature sense is also represented in these small fiber groups. There is overlapping sensitivity for temperature and pain in some peripheral units and probably also in the central projection paths. Dissociation of sensory deficit for temperature and pain, however, is very rarely seen and then usually with slowly destructive spinal cord processes. Since temperature sensation is relatively difficult to test clinically, neurologists usually rely on the examination for pain sensation except in unusual cases.

The clinical manifestation of a muscle contraction in response to phasic muscle stretch, the tendon jerk, requires the functional integrity of at least six serial components. A reflex may be depressed or absent due to affection of any one factor or any combination. These are:

1. Fusimotor neurons and axons with tonic activity sufficient to maintain muscle spindle stretch receptor excitability. Depression of fusimotor activity in the state of spinal shock following cord transection is the critical factor in depression of the tendon jerk for many days.

2. Intact muscle spindle stretch receptors and afferent axons. Primary dorsal root neuropathy, as typified by the involvement in tabes dorsalis, depresses the tendon jerk.

3. Monosynaptic spinal cord connection to alpha motor neurons that are sufficiently excitable. Local spinal cord damage or metabolic insult as by anesthetic or hypoxia may block the reflex.

4. Functional alpha motor neurons, axons, and motor end-plates. Alpha motor neuron destruction, as in poliomyelitis or more chronic processes, will depress the reflex.

5. Normal end-plate synaptic transmission. In severe myasthenia gravis or botulism with paralysis, the reflex is depressed.

6. Normal muscle excitation-contraction coupling and contractile mechanism. The reflex may be depressed in a variety of primary myopathic disorders.

A complete nerve trunk lesion is a simple model to review first. Consider the result of traumatic transection of the sciatic nerve above the knee. Superficial sensory loss involves the textbook area of cutaneous distribution over the leg and foot for pain and touch. Position sense from joint receptors and vibration sense derived from rapidly adapting skin receptors and from deep Pacinian corpuscles are also absent. In clinical testing, one must pay attention to gradations of defective sensation related to overlapping innervation by neighboring nerves. Transection of the muscle spindle afferent fibers also abolishes the ankle jerk. On the efferent side, the lesion produces the paradigm of the lower motor neuron syndrome. This includes:

1. Flaccid paralysis of the leg and intrinsic foot muscles.

2. Absent ankle jerk.

3. Progressive muscle atrophy, beginning in a few days and becoming severe after several weeks.

4. Also developing over the course of 1 to 4 weeks is increased

irritability of denervated muscle fibers (especially to acetylcholine) manifested by fibrillation (spontaneous individual fiber contractions) as shown electromyographically and a brisk response to direct percussion in the clinical examination. (Fibrillation can be seen only where the affected muscle is thinly covered, as in the tongue and, rarely, in the hand.)

In addition the skin is dry and warm due to section of postganglionic sympathetic fibers to sweat glands and small arteries.

Immediately after an acute transection lesion, the distal stump of nerve remains electrically excitable up to 2 to 4 days, when the distal axons undergo histological degeneration with the destruction of myelin sheaths. Necrotic products of degeneration are then ingested and removed by macrophages over a course of weeks.

Axon regeneration is a unique phenomenon in cell biology because of the immense distances involved. For our illustrative lesion at the knee, this process must be sustained by cell body machinery almost a meter away in the spinal cord and dorsal root and sympathetic ganglia. Tiny unmyelinated sprouts grow out from the proximal stump and may even bridge gaps of several millimeters. At first they grow at random to form an enlargement called a neuroma, but those axons that do find their way to the old railroad tracks of the Schwann cell sheaths in the distal stump will progress at rates of 1 to 3 mm/day. The quality of ultimate function is best when proximal and distal stumps are well aligned so that axons grow back into their own channels. This is optimal when the original lesion is due to a crush. If the nerve is sectioned, it is obviously advantageous for the neurosurgeon to realign and suture the stumps together. When axons do grow into mistaken channels, the patient ends up with functional weakness and un-intended movement of muscles as well as poorly discriminative and poorly localized sensation.

The growing unmyelinated tips of regenerating axons are peculiarly hypersensitive to mechanical stimulation. This gives rise to a useful clinical phenomenon, a positive symptom called Tinel's sign. Light percussion over the nerve trunk results in a sensory experience, parasthesiae, referred by the patient to the distal sensory distribution of the injured nerve. If one regularly percusses from distal to proximal, one can thus locate the most advanced region of regenerating sensory axons when the paresthesiae suddenly appear. Repeated observations at regular intervals permit actual measure-

ment of the rate of regeneration down the nerve. Acute nerve transections are relatively rare in civilian practice, but Tinel's sign is
a more broadly useful sign of increased fiber irritability in many
chronic conditions where degeneration and regeneration are going
on continuously.

Motor axons may also be mechanically hypersensitive and may
discharge spontaneously and with increased activity following percussion. This is most commonly manifest with degeneration of
motor neurons in amyotrophic lateral sclerosis (motor neuron disease). Fasciculation, an individual spontaneous motor unit discharge seen as random twitches of fascicles, is exaggerated by light
percussion.

As axons that were originally myelinated grow back into the
distal nerve stump, the Schwann cells develop new myelin sheaths,
and the fibers grow to nearly their original diameters. When motor
axons finally reach the muscle end-plate regions and make new
connections, the muscle fibers become less hypersensitive, fibrillation disappears, and, soon, small, poorly synchronized motor unit
discharge can be recorded. Movement returns, and muscle fiber
diameter approaches normal, too. With time, some re-innervated
motor units may even reach supranormal amplitudes as the surviving nerve axons put out collaterals to neighboring denervated muscle fibers that were originally supplied from other anterior horn
cells. Such giant motor units and fasciculations are particularly
characteristic of motor neuron disease.

An understanding of neuropathies other than acute trauma requires consideration of the fine structure of peripheral nerve. All
nerve axons that conduct impulses have their cell bodies in the
spinal cord and ganglia. The unmyelinated fibers, usually in small
groups, are surrounded entirely by cytoplasmic processes of Schwann
cells. The insulating myelin sheaths that form the internodes of the
larger axons are specialized membrane layers derived from Schwann
cells. The uncovered nodal axon membrane is the locus of saltatory
conduction of the impulse by the sodium activation process of
Hodgkin.

CONDUCTION VELOCITY CORRELATIONS

The smallest detectable lesion visualized in biopsy specimens is
a change in nodal size. Widening of the nodal gap could result in

increased nodal activation time because of the decreased current density. The loss of the Schwann cell nodal processes and not the widening of the gap in the increased nodal area may be important. These processes contain large numbers of mitochondria and may support the nodal excitatory process metabolically. A decrease in conduction velocity is usually associated with such Schwann cell changes. Extension of the lesion, seen as segmental demyelination, is accompanied by a considerable decrease in conduction velocity and an inability to sustain high frequency discharge. When several adjacent segments are demyelinated, conduction may be interrupted. If axonal death occurs, beginning at the most distal processes, the conduction velocity will remain normal in the proximal segments still not affected. Distal slowing may be seen before axonal death occurs. Sensory and motor fibers may be disturbed to different degrees in the same nerve trunk.

Measurement of conduction velocity may be a guideline as to the type of pathological change. It is impossible, however, to infer from such measurements what the pathogenetic mechanism may be in any given case. The simplified concept of either segmental demyelination or "dying back" process does not necessarily apply to all cases (see below).

## Clinical aspects

SYMPTOMATOLOGY

Major symptoms of neuropathies include weakness and a variety of sensory complaints. Numbness may have a variety of meanings for the patient, and include both sensory loss and positive symptoms of spontaneous and exaggerated sensation. If it is not painful and if it is triggered by stimuli, the sensation is called dysesthesiae. When the experience occurs spontaneously, it is called paresthesiae. Loss of position sense may give rise to a symptom of instability or unsteadiness of walking, particularly in the dark. Tingling and other sustained sensations are attributable to lowered excitability of axons, with a tendency to fire repetitively.

Truly painful experience is commonplace and often out of proportion to the degree of pain deficit that can be demonstrated. One infers that there is increased irritability of the pain fibers still functioning. When a neuropathic process does impair the small myelinated delta fibers with relative sparing of unmyelinated C fibers, there is, of course, decreased pinprick perception. But when threshold for perception is reached, the patient may suffer a grossly exaggerated prolonged burning pain. It has been suggested that when C fiber input volleys are normally preceded by faster conducting delta fiber input into the same postsynaptic neuronal pool, there is occlusion, a less severe secondary discharge up the spinal cord; this is, therefore, a fairly tolerable experience. Another possibility is that delta fiber destruction produces a postsynaptic sensitization of the neurons still reached by the C fibers. Such mechanisms may occasion a painful syndrome, causalgia, due to incomplete traumatic nerve lesions. Dysalgesia may also occur with higher level lesions. In the thalamic syndrome, which is symptomatically similar, the lateral thalamic target of delta fibers is destroyed leaving the medial brain-stem C fiber target intact.

The C fibers are particularly important for the painful sensation of inflammation and for that peculiar variety of pain that we call itch. Dorsal root disease, typified by tabes dorsalis, may produce showers of very brief, shooting lightning pains into the lower extremities. Similar pain, usually triggered by innocuous stimuli, is characteristic of trigeminal neuralgia where the pathological basis is not clearly understood.

Almost all polyneuropathies are characterized by an earliest, most severe impairment in the largest and longest nerve fibers. Thus, when the pathogenesis involves a generalized disturbance, symptoms and signs are usually predominant in the lower extremities with a distal-proximal gradient like a stocking, and not in the distribution of nerve trunks or roots. Later involvement of upper extremities is similar. Although pain is a common symptom, earliest impairment is of large fiber functions: position and vibration sense and tendon jerks, with later and less impairment of touch and pain perception. Presumably, the largest and longest nerve cells are most susceptible to the metabolic failure that ultimately produces symptoms. In nerve compression conditions (entrapment syndromes), the lesser mechanical liability of small fibers is attributed to their relative resistance to collapse with compression.

PATHOGENESIS

Symptoms and signs of neuropathy can be attributed to any one or a combination of at least six pathogenetic mechanisms. These

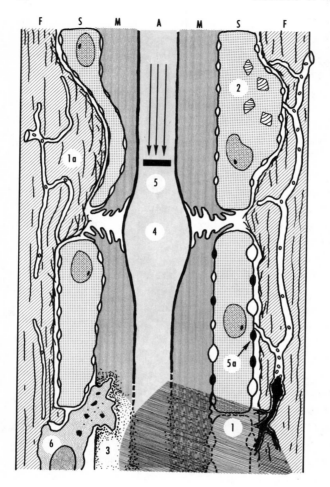

**Fig. 2-1** Schematic section of peripheral nerve. F, fibrous and collagen material; S, Schwann cell; M, myelin; A, axon. The following six pathogenetic mechanisms are shown in exaggerated fashion:

1. Obstruction of blood flow in capillaries resulting in diminished blood supply
1a. Proliferation of interstitial tissue leading to compression of blood vessels and displacement and compression of fibers and sheaths
2. Accumulation of debris within Schwann cell
3. Deficient maintenance of structure of myelin sheath
4. Osmotic pressure increase with axonal swelling
5. Longitudinal transport block
5a. Transverse transport block: occlusion or diminution of pores
6. Cellular invasion between Schwann cell and myelin

are schematically illustrated in Fig. 2-1. In descriptive terms, they include (1) ischemic processes, due to arteriosclerosis, accumulation of material in vascular endothelium, or compression of vessels (Fig. 2-1, mechanisms 1 and 1a); (2) accumulative-inhibitory processes, i.e., an accumulation, primarily in Schwann cells, of material that interferes with normal cell metabolism and function (Fig. 2-1, mechanism 2); (3) enzymatic deficit, cofactor deficiency, or enzymatic inhibition in the synthetic pathways of carbohydrates, lipids, or proteins needed to maintain the structure of the nerve fiber (Fig. 2-1, mechanism 3); (4) osmotic alterations in which accumulation of sugar alcohols, glycogen, or other materials change axonal properties (Fig. 2-1, mechanism 4); (5) transport mechanism alterations, either secondary to changes in basement or Schwann cell membrane properties or to interference with longitudinal transport (Fig. 2-1, mechanisms 5 and 5a); and (6) cellular invasion dislodging the Schwann cell from the axon (Fig. 2-1, mechanism 6).

*Ischemia.* Ischemia of the nerve does not usually occur as a result of damage to or occlusion of a single blood vessel, although it is so illustrated in the interest of simplicity. It has been shown that experimental ligation of major nutrient vessels does not produce ischemic lesions because of the rich anastomotic blood supply to the peripheral nerve. Collagen and amyloid neuropathies, with many small vessels involved, usually cause ischemic lesions. Multiple widespread endothelial and perithelial cell proliferation, associated with diabetes mellitus, may also cause focal ischemia. Other forms of multiple vascular dysfunctions include arteriolar participation in hypersensitization and antigen-antibody reactions.

External compression (i.e., that caused by habitual leg crossing) causes a local conduction block and the restricted loss of the myelin sheath over a small area. It appears that the first consequence of compression is obliteration of the luminal wall of perineural vessels with a subsequent development of proliferation of connective tissue and the creation of a region of focal ischemia. Nerves already damaged by other causes are especially susceptible to the effects of compressions (e.g., "Saturday night palsy" in a malnourished alcoholic).

*Accumulative-inhibitory processes.* Accumulation of phospholipid complexes in the cytoplasm of Schwann cells has been described in many neuropathies. Other lipids may also be present. It is not clear in many cases whether this accumulation represents the breakdown products of myelin destruction, or whether these lipids represent building blocks intended for the myelin sheath that due to transport difficulties or enzymatic deficiency were not used. Normal cellular mechanisms might then be pre-empted by the accumulation. This is an attractive explanation for the involvement of non-myelinated fibers, which are also embedded in a Schwann cell matrix, and this hypothesis might explain unmyelinated autonomic involvement as is common in diabetic neuropathy. Excess deposits in nerves are also seen in xanthomatous biliary cirrhosis and adiposis dolorosa. Disturbances of heat and pain perception in the mouth and extremities related to cholesterol deposits in peripheral nerves have been observed in cases of alpha-lipoprotein deficiency (Tangier disease). Complex lipoprotein accumulations are found in the Schwann cells in patients suffering from ataxia telangiectasia.

Whether reflecting an anabolic or catabolic deficiency, the accumulation of material in Schwann cells results from some metabolic disturbance. Once present, segmental dysfunction occurs but may be compensated for by remyelination with symptom development either late or not at all. At a later stage, the limit of tolerance of the peripheral nerve is exceeded, and symptoms, which may or may not be reversible, appear. The variations in the internodal length of biopsied single nerve fibers indicate that episodes of demyelination and remyelination may occur at varying times in the patient's life. We are, therefore, concerned with what first causes demyelination. The clue must lie in an interrelationship between the Schwann cell and its nerve segments. Facts about Schwann cells are scarce. There is a progressive decline of lipogenesis toward the distal end of the nerve, but we have no knowledge of other synthetic capabilities of the Schwann cell that might be helpful here. The interaction between Schwann cells and axons involves both ionic and energy metabolic factors and is poorly understood.

*Enzymatic deficiencies.* There is reasonable evidence that, in specific disorders, isolated enzymatic deficiencies occur. In diabetes, there is a deficiency in the activity of acetyl thiokinase and psychosine acetyl transferase enzymes in nerves from experimental diabetic animals and from human biopsies. In neither case does there appear to be competitive inhibition, but there is no explanation for the decrease in enzyme activity. It is difficult to reconcile the intermittent course of a neuropathy with an enzymatic deficiency, unless one can also show compensatory pathways and identify the processes by which these become activated. Among the better known cofactors, the absence of which may create disturbances in nerve function, are vitamins $B_1$ and $B_{12}$. Deficiency of either of these vitamins may produce a neuropathy, but the specific role of the vitamin in maintaining the nerve function is not known. Thiamine pyrophosphate probably plays a role in nerve conduction independent of its role as a cofactor.

Lipoproteins can act as enzyme cofactors or as intermediates in the synthesis of polysaccharides or proteins. A family has been described with hypobetalipoproteinemia (Bassen-Kornzweig disease) in which morphological disarrangement of the myelin sheath of the nerves was seen.

An example of enzyme inhibition is seen in patients with advanced chronic renal failure. Some toxic factor accumulates to inhibit transketolase activity; the inhibiting factor is dialyzable, but it is not an antithiamine because decreased transketolase activity cannot be compensated for by thiamine administration.

*Osmotic alterations.* Osmotic changes in association with the accumulation of sugar alcohols are part of an attractive theory supported by the model of galactosemic neuropathy. Sorbitol has been found to be located in the Schwann cell in diabetic neuropathy and in galactosemic neuropathy. Sorbitol is found in the axon and may increase the osmolality within the axon, as suggested by axonal swelling.

*Disturbed transport mechanisms.* Transport occurs both in the transverse and longitudinal direction (Fig. 2-1, mechanisms 5 and 5a). Vesicles are formed in the perikaryon and transported down the axon along microtubules. Interference with the transport mechanism or with release of material contained in the vesicles are two more potential sources of nerve dysfunction.

Ionic transport may be involved in the neuropathy of poisoning with DDT. Single nerve fibers display repetitive discharges accompanied by a prolonged negative afterpotential, believed to be due to modification of the closing of the sodium channels of the nerve membrane. Such alterations in sodium transport could either be related to changes in the structure of the axolemmal membrane or the nodal membrane; the latter is more likely, since there is an area surrounding the node that has an increased capacity for cation binding, particularly sodium and potassium. This is probably due to local concentration of nonsulfated mucopolysaccharides. Such accumulation of polysaccharides has been demonstrated in diabetic neuropathy.

Little is known about the micro-environment surrounding the axon, except that there is good evidence that the perineurium acts as a diffusional barrier between the extracellular and peri-axonal fluid. The effectiveness of this barrier has been estimated to be approximately one-tenth that of the blood-brain barrier for sodium and chloride, but it is three times more effective for potassium. Few data are available on the peri-axonal diffusion barriers in diseased nerves. Triorthocresylphosphate may produce a structural alteration of the surface membrane of the axon. This might lead to a collapse of the peri-axonal space, and this is often observed in such cases. Studies following the introduction of ischemia have led to the postulation that efflux of potassium from the intracellular compartment, which normally occurs under these circumstances, can be compensated for by increased leakage of potassium away from the axon through the peri-axonal diffusion barrier; therefore, conduction may continue. The peri-axonal space can thus act in a detrimental and a compensatory fashion in neuropathies.

*Cellular "invasion."* Neuropathy may take place without an apparent involvement of Schwann cells or axons. In experimental allergic neuritis, mononuclear leukocytes push their way between the Schwann cells without injury to the latter, and demyelination begins at the contact point. A similar mechanism may be operative in multiple myeloma.

### PATHOLOGICAL PICTURE

No neuropathy is really quite pure in the sense that it involves only one of the mechanisms described. The resulting pathological findings are complex. A normal myelinated axon is illustrated in Fig. 2-2, type A, contrasting with an axon that has disintegrated all along the course of the nerve in Fig. 2-2, type B to the best of our knowledge, at the same time and with equal speed, proximally and distally. Vinca alkaloids affect the nerve in this fashion, and nerves thus affected are among the rare examples of neuropathies that show this particular pattern.

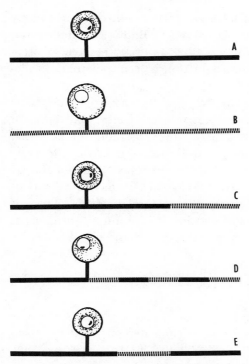

**Fig. 2-2** Dorsal ganglion neuron with attached axon showing different types of pathological lesions. (A) Normal state; (B) axonal degeneration—neuron diseased or damaged; (C) "dying back"—distal part of process nonfunctional; (D) segmental demyelination; (E) focal demyelination—distal portion may eventually undergo Wallerian degeneration.

In Fig. 2-2, type C, we see the disappearance of the axon (and, secondarily, the myelin) beginning at the extreme end of the nerve fiber and proceeding toward the neuron. This is what was originally called the "dying back" phenomenon. Several such neuropathies are known, and acute intermittent porphyric neuropathy is of particular interest. This neuropathy has certain features in common with isoniazid neuropathy, namely, that more motor than sensory fibers are involved and more long fibers than short, and that primary sensory fibers are selectively spared, with respect to muscle spindles. There is a decrease in available tissue pyridoxal phosphate in both neuropathies.

In segmental demyelination (Fig. 2-2, type D), some internodes along the course of the axon have lost their myelin. This is usually associated with disease of the Schwann cell. Both segmental demyelination and remyelination are visualized in teased nerve fiber preparations. "Pure" segmental demyelination is seen sometimes in diabetic and diphtheric neuropathy.

In "spot" demyelination (Fig. 2-2, type E), an area, of larger or greater extent, of the peripheral nerve lacks myelin, and the axon is partially destroyed. This is most always a result of ischemia. Sometimes function is remarkably well preserved within this area. For example, abnormal resistance to inactivation of conduction by ischemia is found in chronic liver disease and in diabetes. Fibers of different sizes are not affected equally by focal ischemia. There is ample evidence that vibratory sensation is resistant to ischemia in patients with diabetes. Whether this is due to the type of fiber or the result of compensatory mechanisms in the peri-axonal space, as referred to earlier, is not clear.

### General references

David, F. A. 1972. Impairment of repetitive impulse conduction in experimentally demyelinated and pressure-injured nerves. J. Neurol. Neurosurg. Psych. 35:537-544.

Erbsloh, F. and M. Abel. 1970. Deficiency neuropathies. In P. J. Vinken and G. W. Bruyn, eds. Handbook of clinical neurology. Vol. 7. North-Holland Publishing Co., Amsterdam.

Fessel, W. J. 1971. Fat disorders and peripheral neuropathy. Brain 94:531-540.

O'Leary, J. L., W. M. Landau, and J. E. Brooks. 1971. Electroencephalography and electromyography. Chapter 3 in A. B. Baker and L. H. Baker, eds. Clinical neurology. Vol. 1. Harper & Row, Hagerstown, Md.

Mayo Clinic, Department of Neurology. Electromyography and electric stimulation of peripheral nerves and muscle. Chapter 16 in Clinical examinations in neurology. W. B. Saunders, Philadelphia.

## DISORDERS OF NEUROMUSCULAR TRANSMISSION

JOHN E. BROOKS

There are only a few diseases in which a disorder of neuromuscular transmission occurs, and, except for myasthenia gravis, such disorders are rare. The pathophysiology of myasthenia gravis, the pseudomyasthenic syndrome of Eaton and Lambert, and botulism will be discussed in this chapter. Although disease only infrequently causes dysfunction of the myoneural junction, numerous pharmacologically active substances disturb neuromuscular transmission, to cause unwanted side effects or therapeutic muscle relaxation. The pharmacology of neuromuscular transmission will be described only as it relates to the diseases that disrupt transmission.

For a proper understanding of diseases of neuromuscular transmission, it is first necessary to understand the structure and function of the normal myoneural junction; thus, normal neuromuscular transmission will be reviewed briefly.

## The myoneural junction

The axon of the lower motor neuron sends a fine terminal branch to each muscle fiber in its motor unit. This axon branch, which is unmyelinated close to the muscle fiber, forms a single expanded terminal, which is closely applied to a specialized region of the muscle fiber membrane at a point roughly midway between the fiber's origin and insertion. The nerve terminal contains mitochondria and synaptic vesicles. There is good evidence to suggest that the synaptic vesicles contain acetylcholine (ACh), the neuro-transmitter, and that those vesicles situated close to or on the prejunctional membrane release ACh into the junctional cleft. The ACh is formed in the nerve terminal from choline acetylase and then incorporated into the synaptic vesicles, which move toward the prejunctional membrane to become available for release. The postjunctional membrane is a specialized region of the muscle fiber membrane folded into primary and secondary gutters so that the postjunctional area is ten times as large as the prejunctional area.

ACh is released both spontaneously and in response to a nerve action potential. The spontaneous release of ACh leads to brief depolarizations of the muscle fiber membrane, which are known as miniature end-plate potentials. When recorded *in vitro*, their rate of occurrence is one per second. From an analysis of their amplitude, it was discovered that the transmitter is released in fixed quantal amounts, each probably equal to the content of one synaptic vesicle. Similarly, in response to the invasion of the nerve terminal by an action potential, many quanta of ACh are released, each identical in amount to the ACh released spontaneously. The

ACh released into the junctional cleft attaches to receptor sites on the postjunctional membrane, leading to increased conductance of sodium and potassium ions and, thus, to formation of the end-plate potential. The end-plate potential amplitude is far in excess of that needed to induce an action potential in the muscle fiber, and its duration is limited by the almost immediate inactivation of the released ACh, which is broken down into choline and acetate by cholinesterase. The choline thus formed is taken up by the nerve terminal and used to synthesize the transmitter.

## Pathophysiology of myasthenia

Since the technique of intracellular recording by glass micropipettes inserted into the muscle fiber at the motor end-plate had proved so useful in revealing the character of normal neuromuscular transmission, it was utilized by Elmqvist to study myasthenic muscle. Small intercostal muscle nerve preparations were studied *in vitro*. It was discovered that the spontaneously occurring miniature end-plate potential had a normal frequency but that its amplitude was reduced to about one-fifth of normal. Similarly, when end-plate potentials were evoked by nerve stimulation, they were found to be of much reduced amplitude, and an analysis of their amplitude variation revealed that the number of quanta discharged was normal but that they were reduced in amount. There are two possible explanations for this reduction as measured by depolarization of the postjunctional membrane. The amount of ACh may be reduced, or the postjunctional membrane may be less than normally sensitive to transmitter action.

The second alternative, that is, reduced sensitivity of the postjunctional membrane, seems more likely in view of the observations of Grob, who demonstrated that the response of myasthenic muscle to intra-arterially injected ACh is less than the response of normal muscle; this suggests that myasthenic muscle is less sensitive to ACh or that the postjunctional membrane is desensitized to the transmitter. The sensitivity of the motor end-plates of the intercostal muscle nerve was tested by the iontophoretic injection of ACh and the application of transmitter analogues. These experiments, however, revealed a normally sensitive response to ACh, carbachol, and decamethonium. On the basis of these findings, Elmqvist proposed that the abnormality of neuromuscular transmission in myasthenia gravis is a presynaptic disorder involving failure in the packaging of a normal amount of ACh.

Obviously, Elmqvist's findings are crucial to our present understanding of the pathophysiological mechanism in myasthenia gravis. Unfortunately, the technique he used has two possible disadvantages: myasthenic muscle may not react the same way as normal muscle to the isolation procedure and miniature end-plate and end-plate potential quantal size may not be reduced *in vivo*. Furthermore, no correlation is possible with myasthenic weakness and degree of involvement, since the intercostal muscle is used. The intercostal muscles are rarely involved in the disease and then only in the final stages.

More recently, an attempt has been made to study miniature end-plate activity *in vivo*. When a fine metal electrode is inserted into the innervation zone of a muscle *in vivo*, small monophasic negative potentials, which have the duration and configuration of miniature end-plate potentials, may be seen. It has been demonstrated that the amplitude, duration, and frequency of the miniature end-plate potential as recorded by an extracellular electrode were the same in normal and myasthenic muscle. It was more difficult to find end-plate electrical activity. One of the striking differences between miniature end-plate potentials recorded *in vitro* and *in vivo* is the much higher frequency of discharge *in vivo;* rates were as high as 200/second after initial location of activity. The response of myasthenic muscle to intra-arterially injected ACh is a less marked increase of miniature end-plate potential amplitude and frequency than normal muscle. These findings were most consistent with the hypothesis of a reduced sensitivity of the postjunctional membrane to ACh. Before these findings, which are yet to be confirmed, are used as evidence of a postjunctional-membrane defect, the following points should be considered:

(1) One of the most important determinants of the amplitude of cellular activity, as recorded by extracellularly situated electrodes, is the distance between the site of activity and the position of the exploring electrode. (2) If an exploring electrode records from multiple motor end-plates and if myasthenic motor end-plates are difficult to find because they are dispersed rather than discretely located, then why is the frequency the same as in normal muscle? It

would seem reasonable to conclude that, with dispersal, fewer end-plates would be present at any given site. (3) If the motor end-plate in myasthenia gravis is relatively insensitive to transmitter, why are the amplitudes of the miniature end-plate potential the same as in normal muscle? (4) If the most marked effect of intra-arterially injected ACh is to increase the amplitude and frequency of the miniature end-plate potential, this suggests that its action is presynaptic. Its failure to produce an equally marked effect in myasthenic muscle has the same implication.

Many pharmacological agents can interfere with one or more steps in the transmission of activity from nerve to muscle, and models of myasthenia have been developed by using such agents. The initial use of physostigmine by Mary Walker in the treatment of myasthenia gravis was based on the known effect of this agent in counteracting the transmission failure caused by curare poisoning and the similarity that she saw between curare poisoning and myasthenia gravis.

One of the investigators in this field, Desmedt, has undertaken a detailed analysis of the effect of repetitive supramaximal nerve stimulation on normal and myasthenic human muscle. He has clearly defined the response of myasthenic muscle to repetitive stimulation at various rates. When a normal muscle is repetitively stimulated supramaximally through its nerve, the compound muscle action potential shows no decrement at physiological rates of stimulation, at least for the first few seconds. Myasthenic muscle, however, has a falling compound muscle action potential at all rates of stimulation greater than 2 or 3/second. This initial decline is followed by recovery. At higher rates of stimulation, or after tetanus occurs, there is a period of facilitation (post-tetanic facilitation) followed by a more prolonged compound muscle action potential decrement (post-tetanic exhaustion).

These changes in the response of myasthenic muscle, the initial decline and the period of tetanic or post-tetanic facilitation, derive from physiological events and may be seen in partially curarized normal muscle. The initial decline is thought to be due to a partial exhaustion of the most readily available transmitter, which, after the first few stimuli, is supplemented by mobilized ACh. The second phenomenon depends on an increasing action potential amplitude and, thus, upon transmitter release. Desmedt studied the effect on normal muscle of both hemicholinium and *d*-tubocurarine and compared normal muscle response to nerve stimulation with that of myasthenic muscle. The initial decline of the compound muscle action potential was evident in all three preparations. After tetanus there was also a period of facilitation in all three; only in the myasthenia and the hemicholinium model, however, was there a period of post-tetanic exhaustion. Desmedt concluded that the initial decline and post-tetanic facilitation were physiological phenomena unmasked by the loss of the safety margin of transmission, which is normally considerable, and that post-tetanic exhaustion was the characteristic disturbance in myasthenia gravis, the cause of the patient's myasthenic fatigue. *d*-Tubocurarine, which competitively blocks the ACh receptor sites, provided a model of postjunctional membrane defect; hemicholinium, by competitively blocking synthesis, provided a model of prejunctional defect. Since the hemicholinium model appeared to mimic myasthenia so closely, Desmedt suggested that myasthenia gravis is a presynaptic defect of transmitter synthesis.

The observations of Desmedt and Elmqvist et al. suggest a presynaptic disorder but differ in positing its exact nature. When hemicholinium is used to impair ACh synthesis, its competitive blocking action leads to a progressive decline in the quantal size during tetanic stimulation. Such alteration of quantal size was not observed by Elmqvist et al. when myasthenic muscle was repetitively stimulated, and this leads to the suggestion that the packaging rather than the synthesis of ACh is defective. This difference between the observations on acute hemicholinium poisoning and myasthenia gravis might be resolved if a more chronic form of hemicholinium block were studied.

In summary, the physiological evidence presently available suggests that the defect of neuromuscular transmission in myasthenia gravis resides in the prejunctional nerve terminal and is characterized by a reduced amount of ACh in each quantum and that post-tetanic exhaustion due to impairment of synthesis or mobilization is the cause of the patient's muscle fatigue.

## MORPHOLOGICAL OBSERVATIONS

Our discussion so far has not taken into account any structural change that may take place in myasthenic muscle. From time to time various changes have been reported, among them fiber atrophy secondary to denervation, myositis, and lymphorrhages. The systematic study by Coers and Woolf of the motor end-plate revealed such changes as terminal axon sprouting, beading, motor end-plate degeneration and/or elongation, and multiple end-plates on a single fiber. They also saw postjunctional end-plate areas devoid of nerve terminals. Of these changes, motor end-plate elongation with an increased area of synaptic contact was considered the most characteristic finding in myasthenia gravis, although in some cases the area of synaptic contact was shrunken rather than enlarged. More recently, Andrew Engel has demonstrated by electron microscopy that the nerve terminal of myasthenic muscle is reduced in size and that the postjunctional membrane is simplified, not having the usual complex array of primary and secondary folds. He noted, however, only a minor reduction in the ratio of prejunctional nerve terminal area to postjunctional membrane from myasthenic (1:8) to normal muscle (1:10).

Various explanations of the cause of these histological changes have been offered. At the present time it is impossible to know whether they are primary or secondary. Woolf has suggested that the dysplastic changes he saw might be due to a pre-existing disturbance on which the myasthenic process was superimposed. It is also conceivable that these changes reflect a disturbance of the impaired trophic influence of ACh secondary to impaired transmitter release. Probably the most reasonable hypothesis at present is that myasthenia gravis is accompanied, if not caused, by a process of nerve terminal degeneration and regeneration and that some of the physiological changes in neuromuscular transmission may reflect the activity of immature motor end-plates. Before histological changes, particularly those described by Woolf, are assigned an important role in the pathogenesis of myasthenia gravis, it should be remembered that there have been cases in which no histological changes were found.

## PATHOGENESIS

The etiology of myasthenia gravis is unknown, but various hypotheses have been proposed. The one that is now most widely accepted, and for which there appears to be the most evidence, is that myasthenia gravis is an autoimmune disorder. This theory was first proposed by Simpson because he noted that myasthenia gravis patients had an increased incidence of other such presumptive autoimmune diseases as rheumatoid arthritis and thyroid dysfunction. The long-noted association of thymoma and thymic hyperplasia with myasthenia is considered as further evidence of an autoimmune disturbance, particularly in view of the crucial role of the thymus in immune mechanisms. In an attempt to substantiate the pathogenetic import of antigen-antibody reactions, a search has been made for autoantibodies in myasthenic patients. Unfortunately, no antibodies to the myoneural junction have as yet been discovered. This theory of the pathogenesis of myasthenia gravis has led to a re-examination of the effect of ACTH and corticosteroid therapy, and it is now clear that partial or complete remission in many patients is possible through suppression of the immune mechanism by corticosteroids.

As an evanescent condition affecting the newborn children of myasthenic mothers, neonatal myasthenia has for many years been thought to involve a circulating substance that interferes with neuromuscular transmission. Hemodialysis helps myasthenic patients, and this is possibly further evidence of a circulating dialyzable substance. Recently, a normally present bioassayable substance has been demonstrated in increased amounts in the blood of myasthenic patients, and a thymic origin seems probable, since the substance disappears following thymectomy.

Research into the etiology of myasthenia gravis has been hampered by the absence of either frequent occurrence in animals or an experimental model of the disease. One particularly attractive animal model is the one proposed by Goldstein, who has postulated that animals develop a defect of neuromuscular transmission identical to that of human myasthenia following the injection of thymus and complete Freund's adjuvant. Changes in the animal's thymus are similar to those seen in the thymus of people with myasthenia gravis. It seems that this autoimmune thymitis releases two substances in excess, one, thymine, which causes the defect in neuromuscular transmission and another, thymotoxin, which produces myositis. In the experimental animals, autoantibodies to contractile protein of skeletal muscle fiber and also to myoid cells in the thymus are present. Analysis of the defect of neuromuscular transmission has revealed a mild reduction in quantal size and a normal output of ACh, suggesting that the site of the defect is the post-junctional membrane. Although this animal model is remarkably consistent with what is now known about human myasthenia, there has as yet been only a limited confirmation of the various phenomena described. Moreover, a number of investigators have been unable to repeat these experiments, and a few important differences exist between the experimental and the human disease.

## The pseudomyasthenic syndrome of Eaton and Lambert

This rare disturbance of neuromuscular transmission usually occurs as a complication of small, or oat cell carcinoma of the bronchus, but it may also appear in patients with other types of carcinoma and, even more rarely, in individuals without malignant disease. It is characterized by muscle weakness and diagnosed by the response of muscle to supramaximal repetitive nerve stimulation. The compound muscle action potential to single shocks is of markedly reduced amplitude, and a further decrement may occur when repeated shocks are applied at rates of less than 5/second. The most characteristic finding in this disorder is seen when shocks are applied at rates greater than 10/second; a marked increase in the compound muscle action potential is then evident. The diagnostic criterion is a facilitation greater than 200% of the initial compound muscle action potential.

Studies of the isolated muscle-nerve preparation have revealed characteristic changes in neuromuscular transmission. The miniature end-plate potential is of normal amplitude and, under conditions that are as close to physiological as can be achieved in the *in vitro* situation, spontaneous release is also normal. In response to nerve terminal stimulation, however, either by applying electrical shocks to the isolated nerve or increasing the external concentration of potassium, defective release of ACh occurs. This insufficient release of ACh has been suggested as the reason neuromuscular transmission fails in this syndrome. The marked facilitatory effect observed by recording the repetitively induced compound muscle action potential is due to post-tetanic potentiation, just as it is in normal, partially curarized muscle and in myasthenic muscle.

There is a considerable similarity between the pseudomyasthenic syndrome and the state induced by lowering the external calcium concentration or raising the external magnesium concentration. Certain antibiotics, for example, neomycin, are also thought to be capable of inducing an identical defect.

As might be expected, most people with the pseudomyasthenic syndrome are symptomatically improved by anticholinesterase drugs, but greater amelioration of weakness may be achieved with guanidine hydrochloride. This substance achieves its beneficial effect by enhancing the ACh-releasing mechanisms, both at rest and during activity.

## Botulism

*Clostridium botulinum* produces an exotoxin (botuline) that interferes with or blocks transmission at cholinergic nerve terminals. The exotoxin's portal of entry is almost always the gastrointestinal tract, being absorbed from the spoiled food in which it formed.

Because experimental models were available, botulism was the first of the diseases of neuromuscular transmission to be studied. By using intracellular microelectrodes with *in vitro* muscle-nerve preparations, it was discovered that botuline acts on the cholinergic nerve terminal to inhibit the release of ACh, both spontaneously and in response to a nerve action potential. Quantal size, however, is normal, suggesting that synthesis, packaging, and sensitivity of the postjunctional membrane are unimpaired. It has also been documented that a more prolonged blockade by botuline may lead to changes in the muscle fiber also seen in denervation, such as increased sensitivity of the postjunctional membrane to ACh. This transmission defect is similar to that of the pseudomyasthenic syndrome of Eaton and Lambert. As might be expected, the marked facilitatory response of the compound muscle action potential to fast repetitive volleys of supramaximal nerve stimulation are also found in botulism, reflecting the expression of a physiological post-tetanic potentiation.

Recent reports have demonstrated that guanidine hydrochloride has a beneficial effect in patients with botulism, another similarity to the pseudomyasthenic syndrome. Presumably, this is due to the increased release of ACh by guanidine.

## General references

Brooks, V. B. 1954. The action of botulinum toxin on motor-nerve fila-
    ments. J. Physiol. 123:501-515.
Cherington, M. and D. Ryan. 1968. Botulism and guanidine. New Eng. J.
    Med. 278:931.
Coers, C. and A. L. Woolf. 1959. Innervation of muscle. Blackwell Medical
    Publications, Oxford.
Desmedt, J. E. 1966. Presynaptic mechanisms in myasthenia gravis. Ann.
    N. Y. Acad. of Science 135:209.
Elmqvist, D. et al. 1964. An electrophysiological investigation of neuro-
    muscular transmission in myasthenia gravis. J. Physiol. 174:417.
Elmqvist, D. and E. H. Lambert. 1968. Detailed analysis of neuromuscular
    transmission in a patient with the myasthenic syndrome sometimes
    associated with bronchogenic carcinoma. Proc. of Mayo Clinic 43:689.
Engel, A. G. and T. Santa. 1971. Histometric analysis of the ultrastructure
    of the neuromuscular junction in myasthenia gravis and in the myas-
    thenic syndrome. Ann. N.Y. Acad. of Science 183:46.
Grob, D. 1971. Spontaneous end-plate activity in normal subjects and in
    patients with myasthenia gravis. Ann N.Y. Acad. of Science 183:248.
Grob, D. 1966. Alterations in reactivity to acetylcholine in myasthenia
    gravis and carcinomatous myopathy. Ann. N.Y. Acad. of Science 135:
    247.
Katz, B. 1966. Muscle, nerve and synapse. McGraw-Hill, New York.
Osserman, K. E. and G. Genkins. 1966. Studies in myasthenia gravis: Short-
    term massive corticotropin therapy. JAMA 198:699.
Otsuka, M. and M. Endo. 1960. The effect of guanidine on neuromuscular
    transmission. J. Pharmacol. Exp. Therapeutics 128:273.
Simpson, J. A. 1966. Myasthenia gravis as an autoimmune disease: Clinical
    aspects. Ann. N.Y. Acad. Science 135:506.

## PATHOPHYSIOLOGY OF DISEASE AFFECTING MUSCLE

JOHN E. BROOKS AND GEORGE H. KLINKERFUSS

### Normal muscle

Central to any discussion of the pathological anatomy of muscle
disease is the concept of the motor unit. Edströmm and Kugelberg
demonstrated that groups of fibers with identical physiological and
metabolic properties are innervated by a single anterior horn cell.
These fibers are scattered diffusely through a portion of a given
muscle, interlocking with other motor units of similar or markedly
dissimilar biochemical and physiological properties. Histochemical

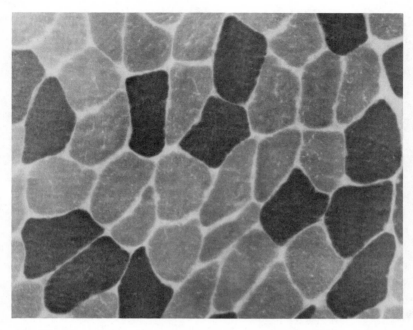

**Fig. 2-3** Normal muscle. Myofibrillar ATPase. Magnification 175 X. This section of male biceps muscle demonstrates the normal "checkerboard" appearance of histochemical reactions. The average fiber diameters of dark staining type II fibers range between 60-70 $\mu$ and for light-staining type I fibers approximately 50-60 $\mu$.

reactions of various intensity result in a "checkerboard" appearance of normal muscle in cross section regardless of the type of reaction used (Fig. 2-3). The careful handling of muscle at the time of biopsy and the subsequent histochemical techniques predicate any successful diagnosis obtained by histological methods; the general principles of interpretation, however, must dominate our present discussion. The myofibrillar ATPase reaction at pH 9.4 allows fibers to be divided into type I (light) and type II (dark) fibers and has generally been adopted for clinical classification because of its simple, clear-cut, and relatively constant results. Type II fibers can be subdivided, in turn, into type II a, II b, and II c fibers by manipulation of pH with preincubations, although the clinical value of this subclassification is limited at present. In terms of more biologically meaningful metabolic reactions, type I fibers usually are rich in oxidative enzymes (e.g., DPNH diaphorase) but weak in glycolytic enzymes (e.g., phosphorylase A and B). Conversely, type II fibers normally are rich in glycolytic enzymes and poor in oxidative enzymes. Intermediate fibers in oxidative-glycolytic metabolism, however, may be either type I or type II, and more complicated classifications of muscle fibers may be constructed for investigative purposes. Pathological changes in muscle will alter the histochemical reactions of oxidative and glycolytic enzymes; but the myofibrillar ATPase reaction appears to remain constant, unless changes in innervation occur.

### DETERMINATION OF FIBER TYPE

Many prestigious investigators believe that "trophic substances" transverse the axon and cross the neuromuscular junction to determine the metabolic composition of a given muscle cell as reflected in histochemical reactions. These substances to date have not been conclusively demonstrated. Several experiments in animals and man have indicated that fibers innervated by intact anterior horn cells markedly increase their oxidative enzyme content after repetitive, low-resistance exercise (running). This increase may reach levels sufficiently high to effect a "change in fiber type" when determined by appropriate stains, supporting a concept that staining reactions reflect the past metabolic demands placed upon muscle fibers by different firing patterns of individual anterior horn cells rather than the effects of hypothetical trophic or known neurotransmitter substances.

### FIBER SIZE

In order to measure fiber size, only cross sections of muscle may be considered, and the narrowest diameter is always used. Considerable variation in muscle fiber diameter can be seen in normal adult muscle biopsies, however; general guidelines are presented in the chart below.

|        |          | BICEPS    | QUADRICEPS |
|--------|----------|-----------|------------|
| Male   | Type I   | 60-65 $\mu$ | 50-60 $\mu$ |
|        | Type II  | 70-80 $\mu$ | 60-70 $\mu$ |
| Female | Type I   | 55-60 $\mu$ | 55-60 $\mu$ |
|        | Type II  | 40-50 $\mu$ | 40-45 $\mu$ |

It is apparent that type II fibers tend to be larger than type I fibers in males and smaller in females. Furthermore, variation with age and occupation will be reflected in muscle fiber diameter. Roughly, the more physical work against resistance, the greater the average fiber diameter. Physical activity against low resistance produces enzymatic changes in muscle fibers without a significant increase in diameter.

In the neonate, muscle fiber diameters are considerably smaller than in the adult and are the same for both fiber types and in both sexes. Up to 4 months of age, diameters from 12 to 20 $\mu$ are accepted as normal. By 6 years of age, diameters have reached approximately 30 $\mu$ and by 10 to 12 years of age, 40 $\mu$. Thereafter, adult sizes pertain. For a more detailed outline of muscle fiber size see Brooks and Engel (1969a, 1969b).

### OTHER STRUCTURES WITHIN MUSCLE TISSUE

Normal muscle biopsies frequently contain various-sized blood vessels and intramuscular nerves. Abnormalities in these structures may give valuable clues to the pathogenesis of muscle symptoms, but these are beyond the scope of this book. The absence or an apparent increase in number of nerves gives no clue to the disease process, due to the vagaries of random sampling.

Similarly, muscle spindles are occasionally noted within the fibrous tissue septa in biopsies, but these structures are rarely affected by disease processes, and their presence or absence is anecdotal.

Fibrous tissue septa interlace muscle fibers and divide groups of fibers into anatomical fascicles. (This term should not be confused with physiological fascicle, synonymous with motor unit.) Such groups usually contain ten to perhaps several hundred individual muscle fibers in the large somatic muscles, whereas they contain fewer fibers in extraocular, intrinsic hand, and intercostal muscles. Fibrous septa become much thicker and more frequent close to the tendon of origin or insertion, and thick septa are frequently encountered in normal deltoid and quadriceps.

Increased amounts of fibrous tissue are noted in almost all muscle diseases, and exact descriptions of patterns and quantities would be misleading and unreliable. In end-stage muscle disease of any type, there is an increase in fibrous tissue. The early stage of progressive muscular dystrophy (Duchenne) may show a marked increase in fibrous tissue around each individual muscle fiber so that the cross sections of muscle appear like the surface of a flagstone walk (Fig. 2-9). This characteristic alone does not allow an accurate diagnosis because similar patterns may result less commonly from scleroderma or other collagen-vascular disease involving muscle.

Fat cells contained within the confines of an anatomical fascicle are pathological and are a sign of a chronic or long-standing process. This finding is even less specific than an increase in fibrous tissue and is no help in specific diagnosis.

## Anterior horn cell disease

With the death of an anterior horn cell, those muscle fibers in the associated motor unit undergo a decrease in diameter by losing

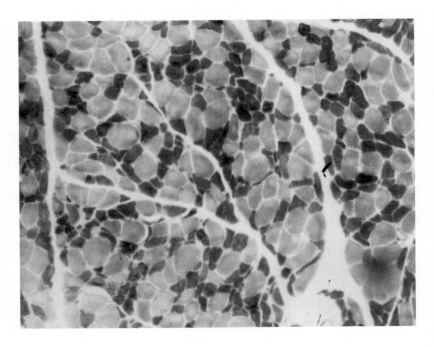

**Fig. 2-4** Type II atrophy of a severe degree. Myofibrillar ATPase reaction. Magnification 175 X. Type I and type II fibers are both abnormally small. The type II fibers are more severely affected than type I fibers and demonstrate angulation of their outline in many profiles. This specimen was obtained from a patient with an acute peripheral neuropathy.

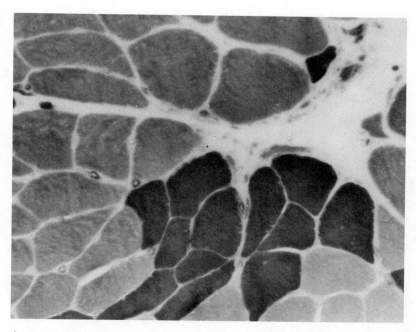

**Fig. 2-5** Type grouping. Myofibrillar ATPase reaction. Magnification 175 X. This muscle sample demonstrates the loss of the normal "checkerboard" pattern of muscle with grouping of type I and type II fibers. It is an adjacent section to Fig. 2-6 and was obtained from a patient who had a history of acute poliomyelitis 25 years before the biopsy was obtained.

contractile protein out of proportion to cytoplasm and nuclei. Type II fibers are particularly sensitive to denervation and atrophy at a faster rate than type I fibers; hence, early cases of anterior horn cell disease may exhibit only type II atrophy (Fig. 2-4). A picture may develop, in such instances, where many type II fibers are small but intensely reactive with incubations for oxidative enzymes due to the concentration of mitochondria after the loss of contractile proteins. With routine hematoxylin and eosin stains, the pattern of scattered large and small fibers can be, and frequently has been, confused with diseases usually thought to be "myopathic" in origin.

An unknown stimulus prompts the remaining axons and telodendria within the partially denervated muscle to arborize and re-innervate the neighboring fibers that have lost their nerve supply. The newly innervated fibers then change their metabolic composition to respond to the firing patterns of this second anterior horn cell. When repeated episodes of denervation and re-innervation occur, many fibers of the same histochemical pattern will be found side by side, and the normal "checkerboard" design of muscle is lost with resultant "type grouping" (Fig. 2-5). This is one of the most reliable signs of neurogenic involvement of muscle. A similar pattern may arise after such an acute illness as poliomyelitis. However, it is most frequently seen in motor system disease. In either condition, inadequate re-innervation gives a pattern of mixed groups of large and small fibers (Fig. 2-6), which is the time-honored hallmark of neurogenic atrophy. Infantile spinal muscular atrophy (Werdnig-Hoffman disease) presents an entirely different (and unexplainable) picture from neurogenic atrophy in adolescence or adulthood. In this condition the fibers are rounded, infrequently demonstrate type grouping, never have "targets" (see neuropathy),

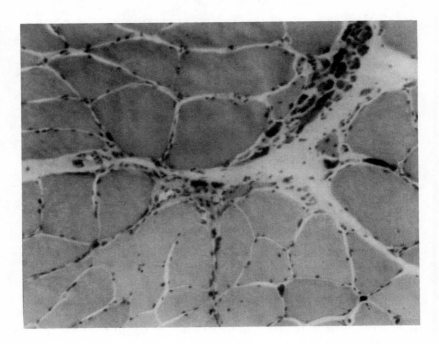

**Fig. 2-6** Mixed groups of large and small fibers. H & E stain. Magnification 175 X. The small size of the fibers in the picture demonstrates the typical features of anterior horn cell disease and can be seen in motor system disease as well.

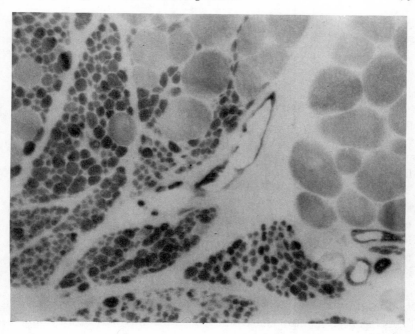

**Fig. 2-7** Werdnig-Hoffman disease. Myofibrillar ATPase reaction. Magnification 175 X. The preponderance of type I fibers in the largest and very smallest fibers in this section is apparent. Type II fibers are of intermediate size.

and demonstrate three populations of fiber size. The very smallest fibers are type I as are the large fibers, whereas fibers of intermediate size react strongly to myofibrillar ATPase and are type II (Fig. 2-7).

## Neuropathy

Almost all neuropathies can be traced to a "metabolic" abnormality of either the Schwann cell ("segmental") or axon ("dying back"), or both. (See page 61.) When such processes affect efferent axons, their hallmark is left upon muscle. The exact appearance of muscle in neuropathy is probably more dependent upon the rate of progression and universality of the process than upon its specific metabolic deficiency.

Hence, slowly progressive or healing neuropathies, whether caused by hereditary enzyme deficiencies, heavy metals, vitamin deficiencies, etc. will demonstrate identical features to anterior horn cell disease in some instances. In cases where peripheral sprouting of axons and subsequent re-innervation have not occurred, a pattern of mixed large and small fibers may suggest a primary myopathic process.

In acute neuropathies, where the majority of nerve fibers are simultaneously affected, type grouping does not occur, and all muscle fibers may lose mass rapidly resulting in uniformly small fibers. Type II fibers, however, usually lose substance at a more rapid rate than type I fibers. Only the fortuitous inclusion of intramuscular nerves within the specimen will reveal the true pathology of Wallerian degeneration, axonal loss, or the presence of fat-laden phagocytic cells. Such overwhelming good fortune rarely saves the pathologist from error!

### SPECIAL FEATURES OF DENERVATION

As has been mentioned earlier, type II atrophy may be an isolated early finding in many pathological entities, including denervation. Type grouping in muscles that are normally mixed, on the other hand, is almost pathonomonic of denervation and subsequent re-innervation.

*Target and targetoid fibers.* Single muscle fibers may also demonstrate changes that strongly reflect effects of denervation. Empirical observation has linked these peculiar fibers to denervation. Target fibers have a centrally placed core of altered contractile proteins, which appears almost homogenized and devoid of mitochondria by electron microscopy. Surrounding this central area, mitochondria (and sometimes other cytoplasmic constituents) are focally increased, whereas the remainder of the fiber contains normal amounts of mitochondria and essentially unaltered contractile protein. The appearance in cross section of three rings of different staining intensity (particularly with DPNH diaphorase) has prompted the analogy of a target (Fig. 2-8). If the ring of concentrated mitochondria is absent, the appearance becomes "targetoid." Fibers similar to "targets" are seen in biopsies of patients with the muscle disturbance called central core disease; in this condition, however, every fiber must be of uniform size and each must con-

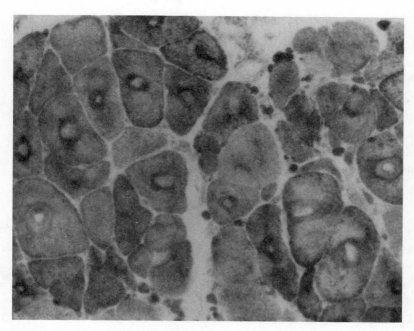

**Fig. 2-8** Chronic recurrent peripheral neuropathy. DPNH diaphorase reaction. Magnification 175 X. The marked abnormalities of internal architecture are apparent resulting in "targetoid" and "target" fibers. Scattered distribution of large and small fibers is reminiscent of the findings formerly thought to be classical for myopathy rather than neuropathy.

tain such a target; this is in contrast to neuropathy where relatively few fibers are so affected, and fiber size may vary.

"*Angulated fibers.*" Fibers with markedly reduced diameters and acute angles described by their sarcolemmae become compressed between more normal rounded fibers in the process of partial denervation. The internal architecture and enzymatic stains of these fibers remain normal. Angulated fibers do not contain basophilic cytoplasm or show increases in central and peripheral nuclei (Fig. 2-4). Since they occur interspersed among normal fibers, their characteristic outline can be attributed to compression of their semifluid cytoplasm by neighboring cells. Cells with a similar angulated outline can appear among regenerating muscle cells regardless of the stimulus responsible for the original damage. These cells contain increased ribosomes and embryonic-appearing myofibrillar components by electron microscopy and frequently are basophilic on hematoxylin and eosin staining.

## Myopathy

There is a large and diverse group of disorders of muscle, long considered to be the result of inherent metabolic abnormalities, that most strikingly affect skeletal muscle cells. Patients ordinarily present to the physician complaining of muscle weakness, and the muscles are indeed weak on direct testing. The metabolic abnormalities of most of these disorders have escaped detection (rare exceptions being hereditary myophosphorylase deficiency, phosphofructokinase deficiency, etc.), and recently some investigators have rehypothesized extra-muscular causes for some of these illnesses. Nonetheless, their histological characteristics can be discussed with some pragmatism at present, and the final pathogenesis deferred until more evidence is available.

### MUSCULAR DYSTROPHY

By definition, dystrophies are linked together because they are inherited disorders of muscle, and their histology theoretically could vary considerably from one type of dystrophy to another. In fact, their histologies are more similar than different, and the type of anatomical changes discovered depends more upon the muscle biopsied, the rate of progression of illness, and the stage to which the patient has progressed than the clinical subclass of dystrophy.

The time-honored "myopathic changes" are evident in biopsies from dystrophic patients. Not only will small fibers in the range of 5-15 $\mu$ be evident, but frequently giant fibers will range from 80-120 $\mu$ in a given specimen. There is no specificity for fiber type in either the large or small population, except in myotonic dystrophy, where type II fibers tend to be larger than the type I fibers. The internal architecture of individual fibers may be markedly deranged. When myofibrils are extensively destroyed and mitochondria and other cytoplasmic constituents lost, the cells appear "hyalinized" on hematoxylin and eosin stains and react faintly to histochemical reactions. Such cells may contain phagocytes within their sarcolemnal limits. Less severe internal abnormalities may be reflected by a pooling of oxidative enzymes or phosphorylase reac-

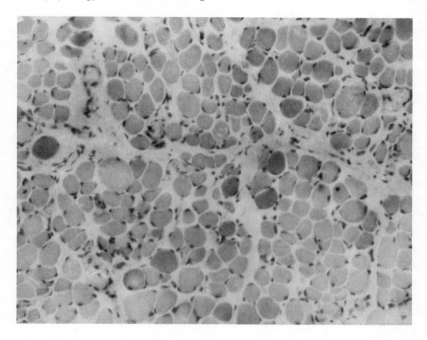

**Fig. 2-9** Duchenne dystrophy. H & E stain. Magnification 175 X. The very darkest staining fibers represent hyalin degeneration. One fiber, lower left, is undergoing vacuolar degeneration and phagocytosis, and, immediately above this fiber, a group of small fibers can be noted. There is a marked fibrosis around individual muscle fibers as well as an increase in fibrous tissue in the septa surrounding the "anatomical fascicles."

tions in other fibers. Other derangements of internal architecture include vacuolization, an increase in the number of nuclei (especially those located centrally in the fiber), and the presence of large pale or small dark nuclei (Fig. 2-9).

In addition to the change within individual fibers, small groups of two to four adjacent fibers may be simultaneously involved, and round cell infiltrates can surround as well as invade these cells. Usually these fibers are small in size and frequently are basophilic or display other internal abnormalities. Similar lesions are seen in experimental microembolization of muscle and have prompted renewed interest in a vascular etiology for some dystrophies.

As previously emphasized, fibrous tissue proliferates around each muscle fiber, as well as in major septa, and around blood vessels, spindles, and nerves. As time progresses, increasing numbers of fat cells are noted in the tissue. If there is a marked increase in fat and fibrous tissue in a muscle, it is reflected clinically as a large, relatively weak muscle. This is seen in the pseudohypertrophy characteristic of Duchenne dystrophy (Fig. 2-9).

In more slowly progressive cases of dystrophy (as exemplified by facio-scapulo-humeral dystrophy), biopsies may reveal unimpressive changes. Perhaps only a single fiber may be undergoing phagocytosis, or a modest increase in fibrous tissue is present to suggest a possible diagnosis.

The histopathology in myotonic dystrophy is sometimes quite distinctive. In the early stages of this disease, there appears to be a considerable increase in production of contractile protein with hypertrophy of fibers, formation of new fibers, and anatomical signs of activities usually only seen in regenerating or embryonic muscle fibers. These processes result in many fibers containing myofibril circumferential ringbands and cytoplasmic masses, which, coupled with long chains of central nuclei, are very indicative of this disease.

ACQUIRED MUSCLE DISEASE

Polymyositis may be acute, subacute, or chronic and, in the chronic form, mimics muscular dystrophy. A form of chronic polymyositis in middle-aged women has been termed menopausal muscular dystrophy. Polymyositis may occur at any age, and, although the major manifestation is a symmetrical weakness of trunk and proximal limb muscles, there is frequently an involvement of bulbar and neck muscles, an involvement not usually found in the metabolic myopathies. Muscle fatigue is rarely found in patients with myopathy and is usually a manifestation either of disorders of neuromuscular transmission or psychoneurosis. Individuals with polymyositis, however, may experience fatigue, although electrodiagnostic studies and pharmacological tests of neuromotor transmission are negative. The etiology of polymyositis is unknown. From its character, its association with other disease entities, and its response to immunosuppressive therapy, it seems possible that it is an autoimmune disorder. One interesting association with dermatomyositis in older patients is its frequent association with carcinoma, particularly bronchial carcinoma. It has been stated that in 75% of men over the age of 50 with dermatomyositis, a carcinoma will be found. In these individuals, dermatomyositis is considered to be a non-metastatic complication of carcinoma. Somewhat akin to polymyositis is focal nodular myopathy, in which focal collections of inflammatory cells are found within muscle. This condition is seen in systemic lupus erythematosus, rheumatoid arthritis, acute rheumatic fever, polyarteritis nodosa, and polymyalgia rheumatica.

The second major group of acquired muscle diseases are the metabolic myopathies. These disturbances are frequently associated with disease of the endocrine glands, particularly the thyroid. The thyroid gland has an interesting and complex relationship with muscle, causing muscle disorders in both hypo- and hyperthyroid states.

Hyperthyroidism may be associated both with an acute and a more chronic thyrotoxic myopathy. In recent years, the concept of acute thyrotoxic myopathy has fallen into disrepute. The much more common, chronic thyrotoxic myopathy is characterized by proximal muscle weakness, mainly involving limb-girdle muscles, with cramps and twitching of the muscles. Unlike hyperthyroidism, chronic thyrotoxic myopathy is more common in the male, tending to affect middle-aged men with what has been called "masked thyrotoxicosis." The electromyogram and muscle biopsy may be normal. This diagnosis rests on the diagnosis of thyrotoxicosis.

The muscle disorder most frequently associated with thyroid disease is exophthalmic ophthalmoplegia, which is also one of the most common causes of ocular myopathy. Exophthalmic ophthalmoplegia has a variable relationship with thyroid dysfunction or treatment, and, in some individuals, no thyroid dysfunction can be found. The condition may improve or worsen following treatment of thyrotoxicosis or may have its onset after successful treatment of the hyperthyroid state. All the ocular muscles are involved, with major affection of the levators and abductors. It is characterized by exophthalmos, orbital edema, and diplopia with or without ptosis. It may be complicated by papilledema, leading to optic atrophy and blindness. The treatment of this condition is difficult and often unsatisfactory. Thyroid hormone has been used to suppress pituitary function, and estrogens and corticosteroids are also used. When these regimes fail, surgical orbital decompression may be necessary.

Hypothyroidism is also associated with disease of muscle, and, in adults, Hoffman's syndrome is characterized by weak muscles, muscle cramps, and pseudohypertrophy of muscle. In children, the same disturbance is known as the Kocher-Debré-Semelaigne syndrome. In this particular syndrome, the muscles are often enlarged; the enlarged tongue of cretinism is thought to be part of this syndrome. The effect of thyroid hormone on the speed of muscle contraction, so that in hypothyroidism muscle contraction is slowed, is evidenced by the slowing of the ankle jerk, an almost pathognomonic sign of myxedema.

Corticosteroids also have an important effect on muscle, and a myopathic process can be seen in Cushing's syndrome. It may occur either spontaneously or as an iatrogenic complication of steroid medication. In the iatrogenic cases, treatment with corticosteroids containing a flourine atom more frequently led to this condition. A myopathy may also occur with Addison's disease, which may be complicated by contracture of fascia.

A further example of metabolic myopathy is the so-called dyscalcaemic myopathy. This condition is seen in osteomalacia but may also complicate hyperparathyroidism.

In most of the conditions so far considered, weakness has been associated with atrophy. Occasionally, however, hypertrophy, i.e., big muscles, which may or may not be weak, is seen as evidence of muscle pathology. Hypertrophy may be classified as either true or pseudohypertrophy. True hypertrophy may occur (1) in myotonia, and mainly in myotonia congenita; (2) as an early, but rare sign of muscular dystrophy; (3) in central nervous system disease due to overwork imposed by involuntary muscle activity, as in dystonia musculorum deformans; or (4) as a complication of an unnatural inclination for physical exercise. Pseudohypertrophy of muscle occurs (1) as a consequence of infiltration of muscles by fat and fibrous tissue, as is seen in Duchenne or pseudohypertrophic muscular dystrophy and less commonly in limb-girdle muscular dystrophy; (2) with myxedematous tissue in Hoffman's syndrome and the Kocher-Debré-Semelaigne syndrome; (3) with amyloid tissue in amyloidosis, particularly seen in the tongue; or (4) in sarcoidosis due to the presence of chronic granuloma within muscle.

One of the more interesting manifestations of muscle disease is myotonia. It is a condition characterized by the prolonged contraction of muscles and is due to the repetitive discharge of individual muscle fibers once an action potential has been induced either by voluntary or reflex activity or by electrical or mechanical stimulation of the muscle fiber. It is seen in myotonia congenita, dystrophia myotonia, paramyotonia congenita, hyperkalemic periodic paralysis, and the Schwartz-Jampel syndrome. Myotonia is recognized clinically by the patient's complaints of muscle stiffness and the demonstration of percussion myotonia. The diagnosis is confirmed by electromyography when the characteristic dive-bomber discharge occurs. Myotonia is made worse by external cold and rest and is relieved by exercise and alcohol. Occasionally, myotonia is made worse by activity, a condition termed paradoxical myotonia and said by some authors to be particularly characteristic of paramyotonia congenita.

Myotonia congenita (Thomsen's disease) is a familial condition transmitted by an autosomal dominant gene having variable expression, with some individuals being only mildly affected, whereas others are very severely affected. Myotonia is best seen in the hand (grip), in the eyelids, in the tongue, and following percussion of the thenar eminence. Affected individuals may have large hypertrophied muscles, which, despite their size, are surprisingly weak.

Dystrophia myotonica is transmitted as an autosomal dominant gene, also of variable expression. The onset can be as early as infancy, but usually patients present during the second or third decades. In infancy, a child may present as a "floppy" infant. The clinical features of adult dystrophia myotonica are (1) myotonia; (2) wasting and weakness of muscles, particularly affecting the face, sternocleidomastoids, temporalis, and the peripheral limb muscles (dystrophia myotonica being one of the conditions in which distal limb musculature may be affected preferentially); (3) cataracts; (4) frontal baldness; (5) gonadal atrophy, which in the female has apparently little effect and in the male may lead to infertility and impotence; (6) cardiac dystrophy with 90% of individuals having an abnormal electrocardiogram; (7) abnormalities of the skull, including a thick cranial vault, a small pituitary fossa, an abnormality of the sinus, and hyperostosis frontalis interna; (8) mental defect and early dementia with large cerebral ventricles (this change is an inconsistent finding in dystrophia myotonica); (9) pulmonary hypertension and hypoventilation; and (10) benign tumors of endocrine glands, particularly of the thyroid and pancreas, occasionally associated with myxedema. The condition is characterized by a wide progression and early death, usually after a period of some 15 to 20 years following recognition of the disease.

Most of the conditions so far considered have been those characterized by persisting weakness of muscle; there is a condition, however, in which weakness may occur intermittently, known as periodic paralysis. Two and possibly three varieties of periodic paralysis have been described.

The most common is familial periodic paralysis or hypokalemic periodic paralysis. This is a familial condition transmitted as an autosomal dominant gene in which attacks of flaccid paralysis are associated with a fall in serum potassium. Between attacks, the serum potassium is usually normal or in the lower part of the normal range. The attacks usually occur in the morning when the affected individual wakes from sleep, during rest after exercise, and after heavy meals containing large amounts of carbohydrate. Other precipitating factors noted are high salt intake and alcohol. The attacks are of acute onset, usually lasting several hours, of variable severity, with progression of weakness first affecting the proximal muscles, extending distally to involve all muscles except the extraocular muscles and, unless very severe, the bulbar muscles. When attacks are extremely severe, the muscles of respiration are also affected. Other features of the attack are the presence of excessive thirst, bradycardia, irritability, and sweating during recovery. The diagnosis depends upon determinations of the serum potassium during an observed attack and precipitation of an attack by glucose and insulin. Various theories have been proposed to explain the etiology of hypokalemic periodic paralysis. Some authors have suggested that it is a disturbance of glycogen metabolism, others a disturbance of aldosterone metabolism; the most probable explanation, however, is that there is a defect of the muscle fiber membrane with a disturbance of sodium permeability. The attacks usually occur less frequently and are less severe with advancing years, but some individuals are affected with a permanent weakness due to a vacuolar myopathy. The condition is a potentially serious disease, with a 10% mortality, usually due to cardiac involvement or involvement of the muscles of respiration during a severe attack.

The next most common variety of periodic paralysis is hyperkalemic periodic paralysis, also known as adynamia episodica hereditaria. This is also an autosomal dominant familial condition, in which attacks of flaccid paralysis, associated with a rise of the serum potassium, occur. These attacks also occur in the early morning and during periods of rest after exercise; but the attacks are briefer than those noted in hypokalemic periodic paralysis and are often less severe. The precipitating factors noted in this condition are exercise and alcohol. Myotonia is commonly seen, and is often induced by cold, and some authors have suggested the name myotonic periodic paralysis. Myotonia, however, has been described in hypokalemic periodic paralysis, although rarely, so the finding of myotonia may strongly suggest hyperkalemic periodic paralysis but should not be accepted as diagnostic. Myotonia congenita has been suggested by some authors to be identical to hyperkalemic periodic paralysis, but others see a distinct difference between the two conditions. The diagnosis depends on the recognition of an elevation of the serum potassium during either a spontaneous or an induced attack of muscle paralysis. Paralysis may be induced by potassium chloride or rest after exercise. The mechanism of this condition has not been finally settled, but it seems possible that there is an abnormality, either of the muscle fiber membrane or the sodium-potassium pump, with intermittent failure of pumping of sodium from the muscle fiber.

## Collagen-vascular disease of muscle

One must approach the histopathology of the so-called "non-suppurative inflammatory myopathies" with humility and optimism. Humility is necessary because changes may be varied and mimic features usually seen in other diseases and optimism because the findings may be quite obvious in a patient with an obscure clinical syndrome. Humility is also necessary in naming this (these) disorder(s). I have chosen the most general term, "collagen-vascular disease of muscle" because the anatomical findings in such disorders as lupus erythematosus, polymyositis, dermatomyositis, and "myopathy associated with malignancy" may have more features in common than they have for distinction. Other names are defendable on similar grounds.

ACUTE SYNDROMES

Patients who present with short histories of weakness, and perhaps pain and tenderness and swelling of muscle, usually have the most classical findings (Fig. 2-10). Individual muscle cells may exhibit simple necrosis and phagocytosis, vacuolization, or granular degeneration, or combinations of the above. Round cell infiltrates are present around blood vessels and muscle fibers to a varying degree and frequently in a spotty distribution. Basophilic fibers frequently are present; these fibers are usually of small diameter. Muscle fibers vary in size in a random distribution, but type II fibers almost always are smaller than type I fibers. Although there may be an increase in fibrous tissue, this may be absent or minimal. Banker and Victor described perifascicular atrophy of fibers in children as a frequent and reliable sign of "systemic angiopathy." In our experience this has been an unusual, but reliable sign in adults as well as children (Fig. 2-11).

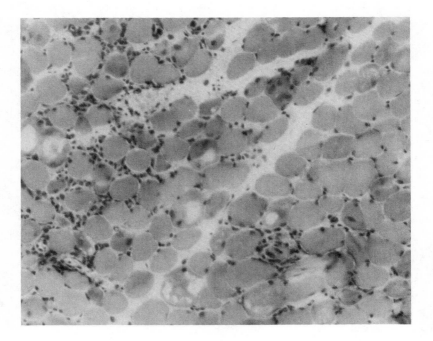

**Fig. 2-10** Acute collagen-vascular disease involving muscle. H & E stain. Magnification 175 X. Note the vacuolization of many fibers. The round cell infiltrate between muscle fibers and phagocytosis of several fibers scattered throughout the section is further evidence of the acute nature of this process.

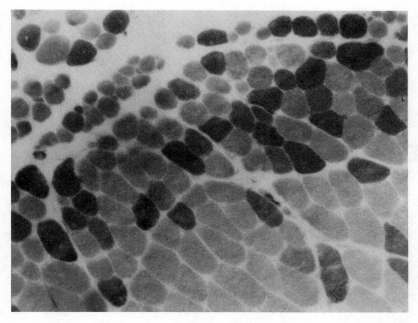

**Fig. 2-11** Chronic collagen-vascular disease of muscle. Myofibrillar ATPase reaction. Magnification 175 X. Although not apparent by this staining reaction, there is a slight increase in fibrous tissue in the muscle. The outstanding feature is the preponderance of small fibers surrounding the anatomical fascicles with relatively normal fiber size within the center of the fascicle, lower right.

### CHRONIC SYNDROMES

In unusual instances, "acute findings" will be present in a fortunate biopsy from a patient with a 5-year history of progressive weakness. More usually, the muscle will show only type II atrophy and increased fibrous tissue. One must, in these cases, settle for a "compatible with, but not diagnostic of" diagnosis.

### POSSIBLE PATHOGENESES

Although the mechanism of the various manifestations of muscle injury in collagen-vascular disease has not been fully characterized, an immune reaction has long been postulated from clinical and experimental observations. Recently, Johnson, Fink, and Ziff have demonstrated the liberation of a cytotoxic lymphotoxin from lymphocytes of ten out of ten patients with active polymyositis. Thus, the active lesions result from mechanisms of delayed hypersensitivity from specifically sensitized lymphocytes to muscle. The reason for the existence of these sensitized cells is not known. The observation of viruses in biopsies of muscle from patients with polymyositis and other collagen diseases has led to the speculation that the inciting event may be triggered by infection with "defective viruses."

## General references

Adams, R. D., D. Denny-Brown, and C. M. Pearson. 1954. Diseases of muscle. Hoeber, New York.

Baldwin, K. M., G. H. Klinkerfuss, R. L. Terjung, P. A. Molé, and J. O. Holloszy. 1972. Respiratory capacity of white, red and intermediate muscle: Adaptive response to exercise. Am. J. Physiol. 222:373.

Banker, B. Q. and M. Victor. 1966. Dermatomyositis (systemic angiopathy) of childhood. Medicine 45:261.

Brooke, M. H. and W. K. Engel. 1969a. The histographic analysis of human muscle biopsies with regard to fiber types. 1. Adult male and female. Neurology 19:221.

Brooke, M. H. and W. K. Engel. 1969b. The histographic analysis of human muscle biopsies with regard to fiber types. 4. Children's biopsies. Neurology 19:591.

Brooke, M. H. and K. K. Kaiser. 1970. Muscle fiber types: How many and what kind? Arch. Neurol. 23:369.

Chow, S. 1968. Myxovirus-like structures in chronic polymyositis. Arch. Path. 86:649.

Dubowitz, V. and M. H. Brooke. 1973. Muscle biopsy: A modern approach. Saunders, London.

Edström, L. and E. Kugelberg. 1968. Histochemical composition, distribution of fibers and fatigability of single motor units. J. Neurol. Neurosurg. Psychiat. 31:424-438.

Engel, W. K. 1967. Muscle biopsies in neuromuscular diseases. Ped. Cl. N.A. 14:963.

Greenfield, J. G., G. M. Shy, E. C. Alvord, Jr., and L. Berg. 1957. An atlas of muscle pathology in neuromuscular diseases. E. and S. Livingstone, Ltd., Edinburgh/London, 1957.

Johnson, R. L., C. W. Fink, and M. Ziff. 1972. Lymphotoxin formation by lymphocytes and muscle in polymyositis. J.C.I. 51:2435.

Klinkerfuss, G. H. 1967. An electron microscopic study of myotonic dystrophy. Arch. Neurol. 16:181.

Klinkerfuss, G. et al. 1967. A spectrum of myopathy associated with alcoholism. II. Light and electron microscopic observations. Am. Int. Med. 67:493.

Mendell, J. R. et al. 1971. Duchenne muscular dystrophy. Functional ischemia reproduces its characteristic lesions. Science 172:1143-45.

Romanul, F. C. A. 1964. Enzymes in muscle. I. Histochemical studies of enzymes in individual muscle fibers. Arch. Neurol. 11:355.

Thompson, S. W. 1966. Selected histochemical and histopathological methods. Charles C. Thomas, Springfield, Ill.

Varnauska, E., P. Björntorp, M. Fohlén, I. Prerovsky, and J. Stenberg. 1970. Effects of physical training on exercise blood flow and enzymatic activity in skeletal muscle. Cardiovasc. Res. 4:418.

"Z. D." 1973. Role of virus in collagen disease. JAMA 223:554.

*"Tropic Effects of Vertebrate Neurons"* Neurosciences Research Program Bulletin, Vol. 7: No. 1, 1969.

# 3
# Disturbances of Autonomic and Visceral Function

## THE AUTONOMIC NERVOUS SYSTEM

DARRYL C. DE VIVO

### Introduction

The autonomic nervous system is so named because of the involuntary manner in which it influences body function. This system has been alternatively called a visceral efferent system, since it innervates glandular structures, smooth muscle, and cardiac muscle. Denervation of these target organs, however, does not lead to their atrophy, as is the case in the peripheral nervous system subserving somatic tissues; rather, denervation results in asynchrony of the control of some body functions.

The parasympathetic and sympathetic systems are the two major divisions of the autonomic nervous system. Each division typically contains preganglionic cell bodies located within the central neuraxis. The axon traveling centrifugally from the cell body ultimately synapses upon a second cell body outside the central nervous system, which, in turn, gives rise to an axon innervating the specific target organ. These axons are accompanied by other fibers carrying sensory impulses from these visceral structures to the central nervous system. Such fibers, commonly called general visceral afferent fibers, should be viewed as the sensory limb of the autonomic nervous system.

94

Most of the innervated structures receive both parasympathetic and sympathetic nerves. This dual innervation is reciprocal in each case, with one division of the autonomic nervous system countering or antagonizing the effects of the other division. Exceptions include chromaffin tissue, piloerector muscles, and sweat glands, which are innervated solely by the sympathetic division. Whether there is a parasympathetic supply to blood vessels is still debated.

## Anatomy of the parasympathetic division

The cell bodies of the preganglionic portion of this division are located in the brain stem and the sacral region ($S_2$-$S_4$) of the spinal cord. This division is, therefore, called the craniosacral autonomic system. The general visceral efferent nuclei of the brain stem (Edinger-Westphal, superior salivatory, inferior salivatory, lacrimal, and dorsal motor nucleus) give rise to the preganglionic fibers. These fibers course through cranial nerves III, VII, IX, and X to

TABLE 3-1   *Principal Parasympathetic Pathways*

| PREGANGLIONIC CELL BODY | POSTGANGLIONIC CELL BODY | TISSUE INNERVATED | PHYSIOLOGICAL EFFECT |
|---|---|---|---|
| Edinger-Westphal nucleus via oculomotor nerve (III) | Ciliary ganglion | Pupillary sphincter and ciliary muscles | Meiosis and accommodation |
| Superior salivatory nucleus via facial nerve (VII) | Sphenopalatine ganglion Submaxillary ganglion | Lacrimal gland Submaxillary and sublingual glands | Tear formation Salivation (low sp. gr.) |
| Inferior salivatory nucleus via glossopharyngeal nerve (IX) | Otic ganglion | Parotid gland | Salivation (low sp. gr.) |
| Dorsal motor nucleus via vagus nerve (X) | Terminal ganglia | Cardiac, bronchopulmonary, gastric, myenteric, and submucosal plexuses | Bradycardia; bronchial constriction; acid secretion and peristalsis, sphincter relaxation |
| Sacral intermediolateral gray matter via anterior nerve roots | Terminal ganglia | Myenteric, submucosal, vesical, and ureteral plexuses; internal anal sphincter | Acid secretion and peristalsis; defecation and urination; penile erection |

synapse on terminal ganglia supplying viscera of the head and neck, thoracic cavity, and much of the abdominal cavity. Preganglionic fibers from the sacral portion of the parasympathetic division travel along the course of the pelvic nerves and subserve the descending colon and the pelvic organs. The preganglionic axon is usually quite long, traveling a substantial distance before terminating on the postganglionic cell body located in a terminal ganglion. The terminal ganglion, as the name implies, is situated in or near the wall of the viscus to be innervated and consequently gives rise to only a short postganglionic axon for innervation of the target viscus. The principal terminal ganglia, together with the effect on the innervated viscus, are listed in Table 3-1.

## Anatomy of the sympathetic division

The cell bodies giving rise to the preganglionic fibers in this division are distributed principally in the ventrolateral regions of the thoracolumbar segments of the spinal cord ($T_1$-$L_2$), the terms thoracolumbar division and sympathetic division being used interchangeably. Unlike the parasympathetic division, preganglionic fibers travel only a short distance to synapse principally on the paravertebral (chain) ganglia or on the prevertebral (collateral) ganglia. Cell bodies in these ganglia then give rise to long postganglionic fibers, which terminate within the viscus being innervated.

The sympathetic preganglionic fiber arises from a cell body in the spinal cord segments $T_1$-$L_2$ and courses through the ventral root and spinal nerve trunk before entering the white ramus connecting the nerve trunk to the paravertebral ganglion. The preganglionic fiber may terminate in a chain ganglion located at various segmental levels or pass beyond this point as a splanchnic nerve to synapse on a prevertebral ganglion cell. Postganglionic fibers may arise from cells in the paravertebral chain ganglia and return to the nerve trunk via the gray ramus to distribute peripherally with the spinal nerve, or they may arise from cells in the prevertebral ganglia and follow the course of blood vessels to innervate those structures being supplied by the vessels. Gray rami occur at all vertebral levels, whereas the white rami are restricted to the segments $T_1$-$L_2$.

The derivation of the postganglionic sympathetic fiber is, in part, regionally defined. Above the diaphragm, all viscera are innervated by postganglionic fibers whose cell bodies reside in the paravertebral chain ganglia. The major chain ganglia in this region are the superior cervical sympathetic and the stellate ganglia, usually derived from a fusion of the inferior cervical and first thoracic ganglia. Similar chain ganglia are distributed paravertebrally from the most rostral cervical region to the most caudal coccygeal region. Below the diaphragm, the preganglionic fibers usually pass through the chain ganglia to synapse on collateral ganglia before innervating the viscera in the abdominal and pelvic cavities. The major collateral ganglia are the celiac, the superior and inferior mesenteric, and the aortico-renal ganglia, and they are located just ventral to the abdominal aorta.

## Autonomic system pharmacology

Acetylcholine is the neuro-transmitter at the pre- and postganglionic synapses of the parasympathetic division and at the preganglionic synapses of the sympathetic division. Norepinephrine generally is the transmitter at the sympathetic postganglionic synapses. Certain exceptions include the sympathetic innervation of sweat glands, which require acetylcholine at both the pre- and postganglionic synapses, and the chromaffin tissues (e.g., the adrenal medulla), which are innervated directly by the preganglionic fibers. Pharmacologically, the sympathetic nervous system can be further subdivided according to the responses of its target organs to the transmitter substance. In this regard, two distinct effects of sympathetic nervous stimulation were characterized by Ahlquist in 1948 and arbitrarily named alpha-adrenergic receptor action and beta-adrenergic receptor action. Epinephrine is a stimulator of both receptor sites, but norepinephrine is the more potent stimulator of the alpha site and isoproteranol is the more potent stimulator of the beta site. Stimulation of beta adrenergic receptors produces tachycardia, a positive inotropic cardiac effect, relaxation or dilation of bronchial and skeletal muscle vessels, gastrointestinal hypomotility, and relaxation of the bladder detrusor. Alpha-adrenergic action produces constriction of cutaneous and splanchnic blood vessels, general body sweating, pilomotor erection, and dilation of the pupils.

As a rule, the preganglionic fibers of both divisions synapse on several postganglionic cell bodies, thereby producing a less discrete

TABLE 3-2   *Principal Sympathetic Pathways*

| PREGANGLIONIC CELL BODY SEGMENTAL LEVEL | POSTGANGLIONIC CELL BODY | TISSUE INNERVATED | PHYSIOLOGICAL EFFECT |
|---|---|---|---|
| $T_{1-2}$ | Superior cervical ganglion (paravertebral) | Pupillary dilator muscle; vessels and glands of head and neck | Mydriasis; vasoconstriction, pilo-erection, perspiration |
| $T_{2-4(1-7)}$ | Superior cervical and stellate ganglia | Thoracic viscera (heart, bronchi, lungs); upper extremities | Tachycardia; coronary artery and bronchial dilation; vasoconstriction, pilo-erection, perspiration |
| $T_{6-10(5-11)}$ | Celiac and superior mesenteric ganglia (prevertebral) | Abdominal viscera (digestive tract, pancreas) | Inhibition of secretion and peristalsis |
| | Paravertebral ganglia | Skin of trunk | Vasoconstriction, pilo-erection, perspiration |
| $T_{11}$-$L_2$ | Inferior mesenteric, hypogastric, renal, and other ganglia (prevertebral) | Abdominal and pelvic viscera  Adrenal gland | As above plus internal urethral sphincter constriction during ejaculation  Release of epinephrine |
| | Paravertebral ganglia | Lower extremities | Vasoconstriction, pilo-erection, perspiration |

response to stimulation than is seen in the somatic portion of the peripheral nervous system. The ratio of pre- to postganglionic fibers is lower in the parasympathetic division than in the sympathetic division, although this generalization is relatively inconstant within the divisions themselves. The principal sympathetic ganglia, together with the effect on the innervated viscus, are listed in Table 3-2.

The influence of the autonomic nervous system on the viscera can be modified by voluntary central nervous system mechanisms, emotions, and other poorly defined factors. Actions of the central portion of the autonomic nervous system, though less discretely defined, are enormously important in governing the activities of the whole system. These suprasegmental connections are diffuse and multi-synaptic with regional elements located in the cerebral cortex, diencephalon, brain stem, and spinal cord. Cortical systems project to the hypothalamus and mesencephalic tegmental nuclei, modulating the output of these centers, which, in turn, project caudally. Descending pathways from these two regions project upon reticular nuclei located within the brain stem, and these reticular nuclei, in turn, project locally to brain-stem motor nuclei (which give rise to visceral efferent projections) and to cells in the intermediolateral region of the thoracolumbar spinal cord segments. These latter cells give rise to the preganglionic visceral efferent fibers. The hypothalamus is the most critical region for effecting control over the peripheral tone of the autonomic nervous system. The hypothalamic region will be discussed later (p. 101ff).

Physiological experiments on animals have helped define the relative roles of the suprasegmental and segmental mechanisms in modulating the visceral efferent output at the spinal level. Experimental transections at the levels of thoracic cord, superior colliculi (decerebrate state), and cerebral cortex (decorticate state) produce different effects. The spinal transection interrupts all descending influences and initially results in a state of flaccidity and profound hypotension. This experimental state is analogous to the clinical condition of spinal shock that follows severe damage to the spinal cord. Subsequently, tone returns, normal blood pressure is re-established, and segmental reflex mechanisms predominate. For example, stroking of the skin in the perineal region may be followed by incomplete emptying of the small spastic bladder resulting from the cord transection. The dependent limb may become plethoric, reflecting poor vascular tone. This is not the case with selective mesencephalic sectioning or decortication, presumably because the aortic pressure receptors monitor the hemodynamic change, stimulate hypothalamic mechanisms, and enhance the suprasegmental descending influences projecting upon the segmental autonomic outflow.

## Diseases

Both diabetes mellitus and amyloidosis may selectively damage the peripheral nervous system, producing orthostatic hypotension, cardiac arrhythmias, disturbances in sweating, alterations in gastrointestinal motility, or difficulty with bladder contraction. Another disease involving the autonomic nervous system is syphilis, in which the autonomic innervation of the pupillary muscles is disturbed, and the pupil becomes small and nonreactive to light (the Argyll Robertson pupil). The site of the lesion is not known; but the mechanism could be explained by damage in the pre-tectal region of the mesencephalon, involving both the parasympathetic outflow from the pre-tectal nuclei and the principal descending sympathetic fiber tract from the hypothalamus (dorsal longitudinal fasciculus). Smallness of one or both pupils may result from injury to the sympathetic fibers innervating the facial region. Clinically, this injury, called a Horner's syndrome, is characterized by ipsilateral miosis, ptosis, enophthalmos, vasodilation of the face, and absence of sweating. A Horner's syndrome may be the consequence of a brachial plexus injury during delivery (Klumpke's palsy) or an apical lung tumor. Syringomyelia may also lead to autonomic disturbances, frequently at a specific segmental level in the spinal cord. Localized loss of sweating and vasodilation under these circumstances may help localize the level of the syrinx in the spinal cord. Disseminated degeneration of autonomic neurons occurs in the elderly, where it is often associated with the signs of parkinsonism (Shy-Drager syndrome). An autosomal recessive disease, presenting in infancy or childhood (familial dysautonomia), is also characterized by diffuse disturbances in autonomic regulation. The affected child in early infancy may have generalized hypotonia, psychomotor retardation, and feeding difficulties. Other clinical features that later become apparent and allow for accurate diagnosis include absence of tearing; orthostatic hypotension; marked elevations in blood pressure with anxiety; excessive sweating and salivation; blotchy skin lesions; striking swings in body temperature; a relative indifference to pain; decreased corneal sensation; and a reduction in the deep tendon reflexes. Pathological lesions involving the autonomic nervous system have been described in the diencephalon, brain stem, spinal cord, sympathetic ganglia, and myenteric plexus; and, recently, it has been suggested that synthesis of dopamine $\beta$-hydroxylase is disturbed in these patients.

## General references

Ahlquist, R. P. 1948. Study of adrenotropic receptors. Am. J. Physiol. 153: 586-600.

Appenzeller, O. 1970. The autonomic nervous system. American Elsevier Publishing Co., New York.

Pick, J. 1970. The autonomic nervous system. Lippincott, Philadelphia.

## SOME HYPOTHALAMIC DISTURBANCES

DARRYL C. DE VIVO

### Anatomical considerations

A knowledge of the hypothalamic nuclear groups and the contiguous neural structures is essential to appreciate the pathological effects of diseases affecting this general region of the central nervous system. The hypothalamus, in terms of volume, represents a small amount of cerebral tissue (3-4 gm), which is predominantly gray matter, located in the anterior region of the diencephalon.

Viewed in coronal section, the hypothalamus is symmetrically distributed on either side of the third ventricle and is divided into three zones: the periventricular zone, the middle zone, and the lateral zone. The periventricular zone may be subdivided into two regions: the preoptic periventricular nuclear complex and the posterior periventricular nuclear complex. The preoptic periventricular complex surrounds the anterior wall of the third ventricle and includes the preoptic periventricular nucleus and the suprachiasmatic nucleus. This region is important in controlling the dissipation of body heat, principally through the parasympathetic portion of the autonomic nervous system. The posterior periventricular nuclear complex is adjacent to the caudal portion of the third ventricle and is represented by the paraventricular nucleus, infundibular (arcuate) nucleus, and the posterior hypothalamic nucleus. The paraventricular nucleus is involved in body fluid homeostasis, but its principal importance is probably as the site for synthesis of oxytocin. The arcuate nucleus is involved in gonadotropin function and the posterior hypothalamic nucleus with mechanisms of thermoregulation. The middle zone includes the medial preoptic nucleus, anterior hypothalamic nucleus, ventromedial and dorsomedial nuclei, and the premamillary nucleus. The lateral zone includes the lateral preoptic nucleus, the tuberomamillary nucleus, and the supraoptic nucleus. The supraoptic nucleus is most important in body fluid homeostasis and is the site for synthesis of vasopressin [antidiuretic hormone (ADH)].

In the sagittal plane, nuclear groups have again been designated by their location in the anterior, middle, and posterior portions of the hypothalamus. The supraoptic and paraventricular nuclei are the best understood cell collections in the anterior group. The dorsomedial and ventromedial nuclei, tuberal nuclei, and the lateral hypothalamic nuclei have received particular attention in the middle nuclear group. The posterior group include the medial and lateral mamillary nuclei and the posterior hypothalamic nuclei. The arcuate nucleus, which is in the periventricular zone (as visualized by coronal section), is the medial portion of the tuberal nuclear complex. This arcuate-periventricular nucleus, often called the infundibular nucleus, is located on either side of the midline of the floor of the third ventricle. The median eminence corresponds to the infundibulum of the neurohypophysis.

The hypothalamus is richly supplied by terminal branches of the internal carotid and basilar arteries and by vessels originating from the arterial structures forming the circle of Willis. Clinically, significant vascular occlusive syndromes to this region are very rare because of the abundant blood supply.

The hypophysis is vascularized by the superior hypophyseal artery, inferior hypophyseal artery, and the portal venous system. The median eminence is perfused by the superior hypophyseal artery, which, in turn, drains into the portal venous system. This venous plexus then runs ventrally through the anterior pituitary gland, subsequently converging and emptying into the major venous channels draining the head and neck region. Conditions resulting in a transection of the pituitary stalk disrupt the portal venous plexus, but the inferior hypophyseal artery will maintain the anterior pituitary gland, ensuring its viability. Studies in animals have also demonstrated regenerative abilities of the proximal portion of the portal venous system after surgical transection of the pituitary stalk to eventually re-establish vascular continuity between the median eminence of the hypothalamus and the adenohypophysis.

From the above comments, it is clear that the hypothalamus, despite its small mass, contains a large number of nuclear groups that control many aspects of body function. The histological complexity of these nuclei extends also to the diffuse multisynaptic afferent and efferent systems that link the hypothalamus to other areas of the central nervous system. Fiber tracts connect the hypothalamus to the cerebral cortex, the thalamus, the mesencephalic periaqueductal gray matter, the superior colliculi, and the tegmental nuclei in the midbrain. The mamillothalamic tract of Vicq d'Azyr is particularly prominent, connecting the medial mammillary regions with the anterior thalamic nuclei, which in turn project to the cingulate cortex. The mamillotegmental tract connects the tegmental reticular structures with the medial mamillary nuclei. The more complicated periventricular fiber tract passes caudally through the periventricular gray matter from the supraoptic, posterior, and tuberal nuclei. This system projects onto the dorsomedial thalamus and midbrain tegmental reticular nuclei, constituting the principal input to the dorsal longitudinal fasciculus. This latter fasciculus probably represents the major hypothalamic outflow to the parasympathetic cranial nerve nuclei and the sympathetic preganglionic cell bodies located in the thoraco-lumbar segments of the spinal cord. Major afferent systems carrying impulses into the hypothalamic region include the fornix, connecting the hippocampus to the mamillary bodies; the medial forebrain bundle, connecting the lateral hypothalamic nuclei, mamillary nuclei, and preoptic region to the ventromedial areas of the rhinencephalon; and the stria terminalis, linking the amygdaloid nuclei with the anterior hypothalamic nuclear regions.

In addition, there are very important connections between the hypothalamus and the hypophysis or pituitary gland. The pituitary gland is classically divided into an anterior lobe derived from the epithelium of the primitive pharynx and a posterior lobe derived from the neural tube. The posterior hypophysis comprises the median eminence of the tuber cinereum, the infundibular stalk, and the posterior lobe of the pituitary gland. The supraoptic-hypophyseal tract is comprised of the axons from cell bodies located in the supraoptic and paraventricular nuclei. This tract terminates on cells located in the posterior lobe of the pituitary. Vasopressin synthesized in the supraoptic nucleus and oxytocin synthesized in the paraventricular nucleus are transported along the supraopticohypophyseal tract and are deposited in the storage cells located in the posterior lobe, from which they are secreted into the bloodstream as dictated by physiological circumstances. Vasopressin release is principally responsive to alterations in body osmolality and hydration. A rise in the serum osmolality or a reduction in the circulating vascular volume promotes a release of vasopressin, resulting in increased renal absorption of water. The principal action of oxytocin is to stimulate uterine contractions and to produce contraction of the muscle cells around the mammary gland alveoli leading to the secretion of milk.

The anatomical relation between the anterior pituitary lobe and the hypothalamus is based on a different mechanism. No direct neural connections between the hypothalamus and the anterior pituitary gland have been demonstrated. Rather, short axonal processes derived from cells in the hypothalamus terminate on a network of capillaries at the base of the hypothalamus. This capillary network was originally defined by Popa and Fielding in 1930 and later named the portal venous system. Five years later, Houssay and associates correctly observed that the flow of blood in this system was directed from the hypothalamus to the anterior pituitary region. Subsequent investigations have demonstrated that releasing factors derived from cells in the hypothalamus pass into the portal venous system and either stimulate or inhibit the release of pituitary hormones synthesized in the anterior lobe.

## Physiology

Several hypothalamic releasing factors have now been identified and partially characterized. There appear to be three mechanisms by which the hypothalamus controls the secretory activity of the anterior pituitary gland. Certain releasing factors appear to be stimulatory, including corticotropin-releasing factor (CRF), thyrotropin-releasing factor (TRF), leuteinizing hormone-releasing factor (LHRF), and follicle-stimulating hormone-releasing factor (FSH-RF). In the case of prolactin secretion, there appears to be a specific inhibiting factor (PIF) in the hypothalamus, which tonically inhibits the prolactin-synthesizing cells in the pituitary gland. The release of the pituitary gland from the tonic hypothalamic inhibition is exemplified by the development of galactorrhea following infundibular stalk section. Finally, certain pituitary hormones appear to be under a dual mechanism of stimulation and inhibition. Growth hormone releasing factor (GHRF), growth hormone inhibiting factor (GHIF), melanocyte stimulating hormone-releasing factor (MSH-RF), and melanocyte stimulating hormone-inhibitory factor (MSH-IF) are examples of the titrated effect between release and inhibition of a pituitary hormone. The hypothalamic releasing factors are chemically defined as polypeptides, certain of which have now been synthesized. The precise hypothalamic regional location of the cells that synthesize each of the releasing factors has not been discovered; there seems to be a diffuseness in the location of these cells throughout the hypothalamic regions, as measured by the responses to electrical stimulation. The cells involved in the synthesis of the hypothalamic-releasing factors are probably specifically responsive to one of the neuro-transmitter substances (acetylcholine, norepinephrine, serotonin, and dopamine). The recent evidence demonstrating the release of growth hormone from the pituitary gland after the oral ingestion of L-dopa would suggest that this particular mechanism is under a dopaminergic influence.

The regulation of body temperature is also under the direct control of the hypothalamus. The mechanisms controlling conservation or dissipation of body heat are clearly complex but involve an interaction between the autonomic nervous system and the neuroendocrine system. Ablation and stimulation studies have demonstrated a regional predisposition in the hypothalamus as it relates to the maintenance of body temperature. Bilateral destruction of the anterior hypothalamus in animals, particularly laterally in the chiasmatic region, results in insensitivity to elevated body temperatures. These animals usually die from hyperthermia when placed in a heated environment. Conversely, when a bilateral destructive lesion is created in the posterior hypothalamus dorsolateral to the mamillary bodies, the animal is rendered incapable of maintaining its body temperature and is inclined toward a poikilothermic state. Cold exposure under these circumstances fails to elicit the normal peripheral responses of cutaneous vasoconstriction, shivering, and piloerection and the release of epinephrine. These adaptive mechanisms that are designed to maintain the body temperature reflect increased activity along descending hypothalamic efferent pathways to the peripheral sympathetic nervous system. The direct sympathetic innervation of the adrenal medulla allows a rapid hormonal response to cooling of the organism.

Other experimental studies have been designed to study the effects of local tissue alterations in core temperature. Elevation of the core temperature in the anterior hypothalamic region by a fraction of a degree centigrade will result in cutaneous vasodilation and sweating even when the skin temperature is reduced. Similarly, if the local temperature of the posterior hypothalamus is reduced by a fraction of a degree centigrade, violent shivering, peripheral vaso-constriction, piloerection, and epinephrine release will follow, rendering the whole organism hyperthermic. These studies demonstrate that the thermoregulatory mechanisms are more responsive to changes in body core temperature than body peripheral temperature.

The neuroendocrine system is also responsive to changes in body temperature. Body cooling will result in increased circulating levels of thyroxin, accelerating the metabolic rate. It appears that the hypothalamic neurons involved in the synthesis of TRF are under noradrenergic influences. The direct instillation of norepinephrine into the third ventricle in certain species produces a rise in body temperature. Furthermore, instillation of this neuro-transmitter into the lateral hypothalamic area leads to increased food consumption. Such observations have led to the suggestion that the hypothalamus acts as an integrating mechanism for thermal homeostasis by its action on the autonomic nervous system, body metabolic rate, and phagic drives.

Hypothalamic mechanisms involved in feeding and water balance have also been defined. The phagic center appears to be located in the lateral hypothalamic nuclear group. The satiety mechanisms are associated with ventromedial nuclear groups. Destruction of the more medially placed hypothalamic nuclei leads to massive obesity, whereas laterally placed ablations produce a picture of emaciation. Teitelbaum and Ebstein, evaluating the pattern of recovery in rats after bilateral destruction of the lateral hypothalamic regions, identified four stages of recovery: (1) adipsia and aphagia—the acute stage when both food and water must be given by gavage feedings; (2) adipsia and anorexia—the subacute stage when animals will consume extremely palatable wet foods but refuse dry pellets and water; (3) adipsia with secondary dehydration and aphagia—a subsequent stage when the rat consumes a liquid diet but still refuses water. The animal can be trained to "eat" a saccharin solution and will consume more of this solution when food is denied but will not do so when dehydrated; (4) a late stage of recovery is finally reached by many rats who will drink water but only in relation to food intake, a condition referred to as "prandial drinking."

Stimulation studies demonstrate that the lateral hypothalamic nuclei can be inhibited by ventromedial nucleus stimulation. Ventromedial nuclei respond to gastric distention, elevations of the blood glucose concentration, and increases in body temperature by inhibiting the lateral phagic centers. The feeding drives located in the far lateral hypothalamic regions appear to be under the control of an adrenergic mechanism, as stated earlier, whereas drinking seems to be mediated by a cholinergic mechanism.

## Pathophysiology

Many pathological entities may produce alterations in hypothalamic function. The lesions are often diffuse, involving several different hypothalamic functions, although one functional disturbance may dominate the clinical picture. Various hypothalamic syndromes result from discrete vascular insults, particularly hemorrhages, from strategically located tumors, and from such inflammatory diseases as viral encephalitis, tuberculosis, and sarcoidosis. Head trauma may also produce disturbances in hypothalamic function. In certain instances, the shearing effects from cranio-cerebral trauma may interrupt the continuity of the infundibular stalk. As noted earlier, an understanding of the anatomical relationships of the hypothalamus to surrounding structures permits one to conceive of several different pathological phenomena that would produce damage in the hypothalamic region. For example, hydrocephalus producing third ventricular dilation and compression of the periventricular tissue may result in loss of anterior pituitary function and thirst perception; tumors involving the optic chiasm or optic tract might result in compression of the surrounding hypothalamic tissue and/or direct invasion by the malignant process producing disturbances in body growth, eating patterns, electrolyte balance, and thermoregulation. Tumors located in the pituitary gland or in the suprasellar regions, for example, a craniopharyngioma or a suprasellar meningioma, might lead to similar disturbances of hypothalamic function. Occasionally, a tumor may arise directly in the hypothalamus, an astrocytoma, for example, leading to hypothalamic destruction and death. Surgical removal of such tumors is frequently incomplete, and, post-operatively, many patients develop diabetes insipidus resulting from an insufficiency of antidiuretic hormone. Also, some children may experience a massive increase in body weight during the months after surgery, presumably related to damage of the ventromedial hypothalamic nuclear groups.

Clinically, certain pathological lesions involving the hypothalamus may be characterized as anterior, middle, or posterior hypothalamic syndromes. As noted earlier, anterior hypothalamic syndromes may be expected to involve the supraoptic nuclei and lead to diabetes insipidus. Middle (or lateral) hypothalamic syndromes are characterized principally by disturbances of growth, and posterior (or inferior) hypothalamic syndromes may lead to precocious puberty or other disturbances in gonadotropin function. Histiocytosis X (Hand-Schuller-Christian disease) frequently involves the anterior hypothalamus, producing diabetes insipidus and disturbances in the regulation of body temperature. The middle hypothalamic syndrome is perhaps best exemplified by the group of profoundly emaciated infants originally described in 1951 by Russell. The term diencephalic syndrome was introduced to describe these patients who were suffering from hypothalamic astrocytomas. More recently, it has also been demonstrated that tumors arising from the optic chiasm produce this clinical picture of failure to gain weight. The phagic mechanisms based in the lateral hypothalamic nuclear complexes are presumably involved early in the course of these lesions, accounting for the clinically emaciated appearance of the patient. Other clinical findings, including vomiting, nystagmus, and pallor of the optic discs, may coexist or develop subsequently. The posterior hypothalamic syndrome is less clinically striking, although it may produce disturbances of body temperature and of sexual maturation. Precocious puberty has been identified with hamartomas of the tuber cinereum. The postulated mechanism for precocious puberty under these conditions is the excessive production of hypothalamic-releasing factors, specifically LHRF, which, in turn, promotes the release of pituitary gonadotropins into the circulation. Either precocious puberty or delayed sexual maturation may result from tumors of the pineal gland, presumably depending on whether the glandular function is destroyed or enhanced by the neoplastic tissue. Hydrocephalus usually results from such posterior third ventricular masses consequent upon blockage of cerebrospinal fluid flow through the cerebral aqueduct. Dilation of the posterior region of the third ventricle, as seen in aqueductal stenosis, may also lead to impairment of vertical gaze and pupillary dilation, presumably due to pressure exerted against the midbrain tectum.

Finally, certain inflammatory conditions, including bacterial meningitis, may lead to a lowering of the serum osmolality. Urine osmolality, under these circumstances, exceeds serum osmolality, supporting the contention that antidiuretic hormone is being released inappropriately. Fluid restriction is necessary until the condition corrects itself; otherwise, volume expansion, cardiac failure, and/or cerebral edema may be expected.

## General references

Astwood, E. B. 1972. Recent progress in hormone research. Vol. 28, Academic Press, New York.

Bell, W. E. and W. F. McCormick. 1972. Parapituitary, pituitary, and hypothalamic tumors. *In* Increased intracranial pressure in children. Saunders, Philadelphia.

Burgus, R. and R. Guillemin. 1970. Hypothalamic releasing factors. Ann. Rev. Biochem. 39:499.

Gellhorn, E. 1957. Autonomic imbalance and the hypothalamus. University of Minnesota Press, Minneapolis.

Haymaker, W., E. Anderson, and W. J. H. Nauta. 1969. The hypothalamus. Charles C. Thomas, Springfield, Ill.

McCann, S. M. and J. C. Porter. 1969. Hypothalamic pituitary stimulating and inhibiting hormones. Physiol. Rev. 49:240.

Popa, G. and U. Fielding. 1930. A portal circulation from the pituitary to the hypothalamic region. J. Anat. 65:88-91.

Russell, A. A. 1951. A diencephalic syndrome of emaciation in infancy and childhood. Arch. Dis. Childhood 26:274.

Teitelbaum, P. and A. N. Epstein. 1962. The lateral hypothalamic syndrome. Psychol. Reviews 69:74-90.

## PATHOPHYSIOLOGY OF THE BLADDER

SAUL BOYARSKY

## Introduction

The bladder stores an adequate volume of urine and periodically expels it by a contraction of the detrusor muscle coordinated with relaxation and shaping of the outflow passages. Micturition is a volitional act of the individual organism like defecation, walking, or swallowing.

## Bladder innervation and pharmacology

The autonomic innervation of the bladder smooth muscle is both cholinergic and adrenergic, derived from the thoraco-lumbar sympathetic outflow and the sacral parasympathetic outflow through the hypogastric and pelvic nerves, respectively. The pelvic floor and urethral sphincter have a somatic (voluntary) motor innervation through the pudendal nerve and its branches arising from the second, third, and fourth segments of the sacral cord. Histochemically, the cholinergic and adrenergic innervation is dual throughout the detrusor and trigone, but the cholinergic innervation predominates in some areas. The pelvic parasympathetic supply is the chief motor supply of the bladder. The hypogastric nerves have been described variously as having a relaxing function, a vascular function, no function, or as supplying the internal sphincter, i.e., the bladder neck, during ejaculation. The adrenergic nerve fibers distribute to the bladder smooth muscle and blood vessels. Experimentally and pharmacologically, the sympathetic function has been demonstrated to be both contractor and relaxor, both alpha adrenergic and beta adrenergic. Histochemical evidence suggests that the two divisions of the autonomic nervous system are joined together by communicating fibers at a preganglionic and postganglionic level; they also innervate the effector cell dually. Hence, there is a possibility that sympathetic and parasympathetic autonomic functions are coordinated at a peripheral as well as a central level. The sensory fibers accompanying the parasympathetic pelvic nerves transmit pain, proprioception, and the desire to void. Those fibers accompanying the sympathetic hypogastric nerves transmit proprioception and pain. The afferent fibers in the pudendal nerves apparently transmit no conscious sensations.

The sacral cord, at levels $S_2$, $S_3$, and $S_4$, contains the micturition center in its intermediate gray matter. Tracts dealing with bladder sensation ascend in the dorsal and lateral spinal columns and in the paramedian superficial layer of the cord terminating on the para-alar nucleus of the medulla. Another group of fibers decussate in the lumbosacral cord and ascend in the cerebral column to terminate on other medullary nuclei. Descending (motor) spinal tracts include the lateral reticulospinal, ventro-reticulospinal, and medial reticulospinal systems.

## Physiology of bladder function

Bladder function is best described as a reflex contraction, modulated by vesical constrictor and relaxor centers at successively higher levels, including the medulla, pons, mesencephalon, and cerebral cortex. Usually, neurogenic bladder dysfunction is classified as either upper or lower motor neuron, but it is well to remember that normal micturition is regulated by a complex interaction of inhibitory and excitatory centers at successively higher levels of the neural axis to which upper and lower motor neuron functions cannot be attributed without qualification.

Physiologically, micturition is divided into three phases: (1) initiation, (2) continuation, and (3) cessation. Reflexes relating to the initiation of micturition include (1) spinal detrusor reflex, (2) vesico-urethral reflex, (3) bulbar vesico-detrusor reflex, (4) pelvico-abdomino-perineal reflex, and (5) bulbar relaxer-inhibiting reflex. Reflexes relating to the continuation of micturition are (1) pontine detrusor-detrusor reflex, (2) relaxer-inhibiting reflex, (3) pontine urethral-detrusor reflex, and (4) spinal urethral-detrusor reflex. Reflexes related to the cessation of micturition involve the bulbar vesical relaxer center and pontine center for the external sphincter and the sacral vesico-inhibitor center. Each of the three phases of micturition has entirely different dynamics and involves different anatomical components of the bladder, urethra, and accessory muscles of micturition.

Many reflexes that describe phases of the bladder's responses to stimulation have been identified. The biological elegance of bladder function depends upon the integrity of these reflexes. These include (1) vesical contraction following distention of the bladder; (2) vesical contraction evoked by urethral flow; (3) vesical contraction evoked by proximal urethral distention; (4) relaxation of the urethra resulting in relaxation of the external sphincter; (5) relaxation of the proximal urethral smooth muscle by distention of the bladder; and (6) vesical contraction related to running liquid through the urethra. Reflexes involved in urine storage include (1) storage reflex, (2) continence reflex, and (3) guarding reflex.

Still other reflexes link the bladder to different systems. For example, distention of the bladder causes a rise in blood pressure and a fall in renal blood flow and glomerular filtration rate. Bladder distention will inhibit uterine activity and produce changes in cardiac rate and rhythm, respiratory rate, and blood pressure. Urinary retention may be associated with painful anal and perianal conditions. Bladder contraction has been evoked by stimulation of the anal region, the thighs, the abdominal skin, and other areas, as well as by distention, cold stimuli, and electrostimulation within the lumen. Proximal urethral stimulation and genitosexual associations have also been suggested as initiating stimuli for micturition. Monitoring of the sensory input along the pelvic nerve of the cat shows greatly diminished activity when the bladder is empty rather than full. The bladder muscle shows denervation-sensitivity to acetylcholine and responds to sympathomimetic, sympatholytic, catecholamine-blocking, and catecholamine-potentiating drugs as if it contained both alpha adrenergic and beta adrenergic receptors.

In order to understand the regulation of bladder functions, one must use modern physiological concepts and not just concepts based on the cystometrogram. Both bladder storage and expulsion require coordinated activity of the detrusor and the sphincteric region together with modulation of the tone of the accessory muscles of micturition, the diaphragm, the abdominal wall, and the pelvic floor. The cystometrogram used alone is a meaningless gauge of bladder function, unless muscular relaxation of the outflow passages and pelvic floor is also measured. Also important is an assessment of the sensory integrity of the bladder and the modulating influences or interferences from the central nervous system centers rostral to the sacral micturition center.

Since the bladder fills slowly, the intraluminal pressure rises almost imperceptibly until the capacity is approached. At this point, the pressure rises more steeply, and micturition is initiated. With the initiation of micturition, the urethra opens, the bladder neck and proximal urethra form a facilitating funnel, intra-urethral pressure falls below intravesical pressure, and flow starts. As the bladder contracts, the intraluminal pressure levels off and then falls as the bladder empties. The differential pressure gradient reverses itself, and, as the urethral pressure exceeds the bladder pressure, flow stops. Urodynamically, these pressure gradients can be measured by multiple monitoring techniques and by electromyography of the pelvic floor, showing levator ani, external sphincter, and associated muscle relaxation during the flow of the normal stream. The urethral resistance is calculated from the flow rate (uroflometry) and intraluminal pressure, or it is measured by direct sphincterometry. Urinary stream cast distance and measurements of energy and exit pressures and flows serve to relate detrusor force and outflow resistance. Urethral caliber is estimated either by radiological visualization or by direct inspection and calibration.

## Pathophysiology

With a sensory-deprived or deafferented bladder, as can occur in tabes dorsalis or diabetes mellitus, there is a flattened detrusor pressure curve, a large capacity, little or no awareness of filling, and little urge to void. This results in muscular overdistention and further loss of tone. The sphincters do not relax, and incontinence is rare. Immediately after spinal injury, spinal shock produces a hypotonic, unresponsive bladder. Upon recovery from spinal shock, a reflex or upper motor neuron type of neurogenic bladder appears with a steep pressure curve and premature emptying. The upper motor neuron (reflex) bladder, however, also shows dyssynergia between detrusor and sphincters, so that the outflow passages fail to open properly or fail to maintain their funneled position. It becomes trabeculated, overly active, and continues to empty poorly. The uninhibited neurogenic bladder responds inappropriately to incomplete filling due to poor central nervous system control of the primitive micturition reflex. In cystitis and other irritable bladder wall conditions, the bladder is hypersensitive and tends to contract prematurely, abnormally, and forcefully. The overdistended bladder, due to obstructive lesions of the urethra, shows a hypotonic urodynamic picture much like that of the tabetic bladder. Vesicourethral reflux may have either a neuropathological or an inflammatory etiology. The valvular function of the ureterovesical junction is lost, and bladder urine is regurgitated into the ureter. This damages the ureter and the kidney, particularly in the presence of urinary infection. In autonomic hyperreflexia, bouts of headache, sweating, flushing, palpitation, hypertension, and various subjective sensations can be induced by bladder distention, emphasizing the close relationship between the autonomic fibers that mediate bladder function and the remainder of the autonomic nervous system.

## General references

Bors, Ernest and A. E. Comar. 1971. Neurological urology. University Park Press, Baltimore, Md.

Boyarsky, S. ed. 1967. The neurogenic bladder. Williams & Wilkins, Baltimore.

Boyarsky, S. and H. Ruskin, 1970. Physiology of the bladder. Chapter IV *in* M. F. Campbell and J. H. Harrison, eds. Urology. Saunders, Philadelphia.

Hinman, F., Jr., S. Boyarsky, J. Pierce, Jr., and N. Zinner, eds. 1968. The hydrodynamics of micturition. Charles C. Thomas, Springfield, Ill.

# PATHOPHYSIOLOGY OF THE BOWEL

DARRYL C. DE VIVO

## Innervation

Like other viscera, the gastrointestinal tract has a dual autonomic innervation. The parasympathetic innervation of the digestive tract is divided into two parts. The stomach, the small intestine, and the large intestine, to the level of the descending colon, derive their parasympathetic innervation from the vagus nerve. The descending colon, sigmoid colon, rectum, and internal anal sphincter are innervated by the sacral parasympathetic outflow. The preganglionic parasympathetic fibers terminate in the myenteric plexus (Auerbach's plexus) located between the smooth muscle layers and in the submucosal plexus (Meissner's plexus). The myenteric plexus then sends a short postganglionic axon to innervate the smooth muscle of the intestinal wall. Short postganglionic fibers derived from the submucosal plexus innervate the intestinal glands. Stimulation of the vagus nerve enhances gastrointestinal peristalsis and increases secretion of hydrochloric acid and pepsin. Conversely, sectioning of the vagal nerve leads to atony of the stomach, contraction of the pyloric sphincter, and reduction in the secretion of hydrochloric acid. Because of the effects of vagal denervation, a vagotomy combined with a pyloroplasty is frequently employed in the treatment of peptic ulcer disease. The wisdom behind the use of belladonna alkaloids (anticholinergic in action) for the treatment of gastric irritation and hyperacidity may be appreciated when one considers the role of the vagus nerve (a cholinergic structure) in bowel motility and secretion of hydrochloric acid.

The sympathetic innervation of the bowel is derived from cells located in the intermediolateral aspects of the thoracolumbar segments. Preganglionic fibers from these cells course to prevertebral ganglia before synapsing on the postganglionic cell. The postganglionic fibers travel along the course of the major abdominal arteries, innervating the smooth muscle of the gastrointestinal wall. Increased sympathetic activity is accompanied by decreased gastrointestinal motility and contraction of the internal sphincters. In patients who have been subjected to sympathectomy as a treatment for hypertension, a net increase in gastrointestinal peristalsis may be demonstrated. Visceral afferent nerves also carry sensory stimuli from the bowel wall and travel with the parasympathetic and sympathetic efferent fibers.

## Disease states

Disturbances in bowel motility may result from the diseases of the peripheral nervous system that also affect the autonomic components. Gastric dilation and ileus may be seen in diabetes mellitus and amyloidosis; and it is acute in the Landry-Guillain-Barré syndrome (postinfectious polyneuritis). Diabetes mellitus may also be complicated by chronic diarrhea, frequently nocturnal in character. The precise site of pathology in the autonomic nervous system is not clear. Damage to the spinal cord, particularly if acute, may lead to profound depression in gastrointestinal motility resulting in ileus. This is a common accompaniment of traumatic spinal cord transection, producing the clinical picture of spinal shock. A gradual return of intrinsic peristaltic activity is the rule under these circumstances, although voluntary control over defecation will be permanently lost.

Deafferentation of the bowel is a poorly understood phenomenon and consequently has no distinct clinical correlate.

Embryological disturbances in neural tube closure (e.g., myelomeningocele) may permanently impair large bowel function. Damage to the sacral portion of the spinal cord, as seen with tumors of the conus medullaris or injury to the sacral nerve roots in diseases affecting the cauda equina, may interrupt the somatic innervation of the external anal sphincter ($S_4$) as well as the autonomic innervation of the internal anal sphincter and the bowel wall. Such lesions frequently damage the visceral afferent fibers from these same regions. Distention of the rectal ampulla by feces can no longer be monitored because of the deafferentation. Patients with such lesions, therefore, suffer from fecal incontinence, particularly when the stool is soft, but they may also be prone to fecal impaction, if fecal material is allowed to accumulate in the colon and rectum.

Congenital aganglionic megacolon (Hirschspring's disease) results from the congenital absence of the myenteric (and submucosal) plexuses in a segment of the colonic wall. The aganglionic segment of tissue is usually located in the rectum or rectosigmoid region, resulting in a constricted portion of intestinal tract devoid of peristaltic activity. The normal intestine proximal to the aganglionic segment gradually becomes massively dilated with hypertrophy of the muscular layer of the intestinal wall. The young infant develops lower gastrointestinal obstruction with abdominal distention and, subsequently, vomiting. A rectal biopsy that fails to demonstrate intramural nerve plexuses is an aid in the diagnosis of this condition. A similar clinical picture may arise in patients suffering from Chagas' disease. Megaesophagus and megacolon in an adult with cardiomegaly suggests this diagnosis. Toxic destruction of the neurons in the myenteric plexus by *Trypanosoma cruzi* results in this gastrointestinal disturbance.

### General references

Bingham, J. R., F. J. Ingelfinger, and R. H. Smithwick. 1951. Effect of combined sympathectomy and vagectomy on the gastrointestinal tract. JAMA 146:1406-1408.

Garrett, J. R., E. R. Howard, and N. H. Nixon. 1969. Autonomic nerves in rectum and colon in Hirschsprung's disease: A cholinesterase and catecholamine histochemical study. Arch. Dis. Child. 44:406-417.

Pick, Joseph. 1970. The autonomic nervous system: Morphological, comparative, clinical and surgical aspects. Lippincott, Philadelphia.

# 4
# Disorders of Movement

## THE UPPER MOTOR NEURON SYNDROME

WILLIAM M. LANDAU

### General principles and history

All planned experiments concerning the organization of movement by higher levels of the central nervous system are derived from three primary analytical strategies:

1. The behavioral effects of ablation of critical structures.
2. The behavioral effects of excessive activation of critical structures.
3. The time-locked correlation of activity in undamaged neural elements to normal behavior.

Of these strategies, the third obviously permits the least experimental and inferential distortion. I shall return to this approach later. For clinicians, the study of the physiology of movement is practically restricted to strategies 1 and 2, the observation of behavioral changes resulting from disease.

A century ago, basing his conclusions upon careful clinical and pathological studies of patients, Hughlings Jackson generalized that symptoms in any central nervous system impairment should be considered to be specific combinations of negative and positive components. Jackson used the pathophysiological phenomena of the upper motor neuron system (which he called the middle level of the

117

motor system) as a paradigm of his analytical approach. He started with the simple premise that dead or depressed neurons cannot be directly responsible for behavior. A common-sense corollary is that a behavioral deficit, a negative symptom, is a direct result of this lack of action by damaged tissue. It follows that residual behavior after a lesion, in particular, distorted behavior or positive symptoms, must be the result of secondary changes of excitability and functional organization in surviving neurons. Positive symptoms may imply apparently spontaneous neuronal hyperactivity as in the epileptic focus or fasciculating spinal motor unit, or increased reactivity as in a hyperactive knee jerk, or both, as in a sensory-induced seizure. An increased level of neuronal baseline activity and a decreased response threshold may have similar or different physiological mechanisms at the cellular level. At the outset, it is useful to distinguish a change in the steady state from a change in reactivity.

Jackson's inferences about upper neuron function were based upon the relationship between patterns of negative symptoms due to destructive lesions of forebrain and its descending projections (strategy 1) and patterns of movement due to excessive discharge in the same system during focal motor cortical seizures (strategy 2). The middle level, he emphasized, is organized in terms of movements, not individual muscle activity, unlike the situation for lower motor neuron disease (lowest level) where individual muscle weakness is directly correlated to the degree of neuronal loss. Considering the nervous system in terms of both evolutionary phylogenesis and the levels of organization of behavior in an individual, he generalized, "the more gray matter, the more movements." By this he meant that the capacity for highly adaptive and varied motor performance increases with increasing involvement of larger, and more interrelated brain regions.

Thus, the earliest negative symptom of upper motor neuron impairment is loss of distal, highly developed, learned motor behavior. This comprises "the least automatic movements." With progression of the lesion, the repertory of adaptive movement is constricted to the limited, stereotyped synergies of severe hemiparesis. Strength for any movement may ultimately be affected, but the disability is already severe at a level of weakness that is readily compensated for in subjects with lower motor neuron or muscle disease.

In focal seizures, predominant activity is manifest in the same distal foci: the corner of the mouth, the thumb, and the hallux. These are also most impaired transiently in the postconvulsive depression or inhibition of function known as Todd's paralysis. The negative symptoms of Todd's paralysis are exactly like those due to structural lesions.

Jackson held that the organization of movement at the lowest level, the spinal segment, is "released" by the loss of control from higher levels of the neuraxis. He preferred to use the general term "control" rather than imply only the loss of an inhibitory action, for descending paths obviously have predominantly excitatory action in normal behavior. Recent observations on motor organization can be correlated with the framework of Jackson's concepts.

## Anatomical premises

First, what structures are involved? By consensus, the structure of the upper motor neuron complex includes at least the pyramidal tract and the electrically excitable precentral motor cortex. In the monkey and in man, the pyramidal tract, defined by the fasciculus at the base of the medulla, is synonymous with the corticospinal tract. The origin of the tract has been well documented in the monkey and is far from synonymous with Brodman area 4 of the motor cortex; 30% of the fibers, including all of the largest ones, do derive from the precentral area 4. Another 30% come from the frontal cortex anterior to area 4, including area 6; 40% are derived from the parietal lobe. There is a similar widespread origin of pyramidal fibers from a large region surrounding the central sulcus in man.

The pyramidal tract is poorly designed for instantaneous action, even though it has the great advantage of direct access to spinal neurons. Of the million fibers in the human tract, less than 2% are larger than 10 $\mu$ (40 to 60 m/second conduction velocity), 40% are 4 to 1 $\mu$ (4 to 25 m/second), and 50% are less than 1 $\mu$ (0.5 to 3 m/second).

The somatotopic pattern noted in the cerebral cortex is already indistinct at the level of the internal capsule because face and extremity projections overlap. When these fibers reach the upper medulla, the projections to the extremities are completely mixed. Upper extremity fibers do deviate medially toward their terminations in the lower cervical cord, but there is no anatomical basis in the brain-stem pyramidal tract for monoparesis or for the alleged decussation syndrome of alternating limb paresis.

Furthermore, it is clear that the pyramidal tract is more than a pure pathway to anterior horn cells. Pyramidal fibers also project toward fusimotor neurons and the sympathetic system. There are also facilitatory effects upon afferent transmission through the dorsal column nuclei in the medulla and more complicated actions upon afferent relays in the spinal dorsal horn. Such sensory modulation probably relates to the predominant dorsal horn projection from parietal lobe pyramidal fibers.

In an operational sense, the upper neuron system also includes the complex gray matter masses and tracts of the basal forebrain. These include cerebello-thalamocortical, somatosensory, and other thalamocortical projections, and the basal ganglia with their reciprocal and nonreciprocal connections, all of which ultimately project upstream to the sensorimotor cortex. There are also pertinent downstream projections from the cortex to brain-stem relays parallel to the pyramidal tract.

In summary, the upper motor neuron syndrome, as it commonly occurs, is related primarily to the function of the sensorimotor cortex centered about the central sulcus and to its major projections, the pyramidal tract and parallel pathways in the brain stem.

## Abnormally increased neural activity (strategy 2)

The fact that repetitive electrical shocks applied to regions of animal cerebral cortex evoke various localized and complex movements was shown during Jackson's lifetime by Hitzig, Ferrier, and, most carefully, by Sherrington. Plots on diagrams of the cortical surface of the mosaic of loci (the motor cortex) that give rise to different local movements demonstrate an anatomically distorted somatotopic pattern of the body musculature (almost entirely contralateral). More recently, Woolsey's somatotopic motor maps for many species provide detailed anatomical information about the location and number of neuronal connections. Similar physiological observations by Penfield in man were artistically integrated in his famous homunculus caricature of the representation of body areas in the motor cortex. It is obvious that such lightning strokes of the cortical meshwork do not result in movements that stimulate those seen normally. Yet variations of the evoked movement with stimulus intensity, anesthesia, repeated stimulation, other associated stimuli, and the passage of time indicate that the stimulating current is not simply short circuiting a rigid wiring system. For example, the response of a limb to cortical stimulation varies, depending upon the posture of the limb at the time of stimulation. By applying the artificial stimulus directly to medullary pyramidal tract, it has been shown that much of this modulation is intraspinal, since similar variations still occur. The pyramidal tract is not the only pertinent cortical output channel, for Lewis and Brindley showed the persistence of a higher threshold, less variable somatotopic pattern after the pyramidal tract was severed in the baboon.

Although the excitable motor cortex in the monkey closely fits histological area 4, this is not so for man in whose brain the excitable region is larger. The excitable field mapped by Penfield and Boldrey is much larger than area 4. Motor excitability probably represents the lower threshold of the largest cortical neurons, where they are sufficiently close together, both at the cortex and the spinal termination, to provide enough spatial and temporal summation to fire the final common path to muscle. Local neuronal unit recording during such stimulation shows the effective stimulus field to have a diameter of a centimeter or more. Not only do neurons immediately adjacent to the stimulating electrode respond directly, but they also, along with stimulated cortical afferent axons, synaptically activate indirect responses in nearby neurons. Repeated stimuli build up a synaptic barrage to evoke mini-seizures with high frequency discharge of individual corticofugal pyramidal neurons.

Thus, the movement that follows repetitive cortical stimulation is a complex result of the anatomical projection pattern, expanded intracortical excitation, high frequency efferent discharge to internuncial and motor neurons of the spinal cord or brain stem, and interactions with the spinal reflex mechanisms.

In 1951, Phillips began to explore the effect upon movement of single, relatively long duration electrical pulses to the motor cortex. The results were quite different from the "mosaic" somatotopic map of the body musculature. Over wide cortical fields representing the lower extremity, the upper extremity, or the face, the invariant response was a simple flick movement of the distal portion of the appropriate extremity or of the lower face. The higher the stimulus intensity, the broader was the field. This threshold pattern is thus precisely that which Jackson had described for the onset of clinical focal motor seizures.

A decade of investigation has provided a clear explanation of this phenomenon. A single anodal pulse stimulus evokes only a single response in the neurons of the excited field, thus eliminating the complexities introduced by intracortically relayed, repetitive excitation. These highly synchronized, pyramidal volleys in the primate impinge directly upon motor neurons. When the motor cortex is stimulated in this manner, direct activation of spinal motor neurons as a result of spatial summation of impulses is greatest for intrinsic hand and forearm motor neurons and much less or absent for proximal and axial muscles, indicating that the motor cortex has its densest direct influence upon the "leading" parts of the limb most involved in finely adjusted, adaptive movements.

It seems fair to conclude that studies of gross stimulation of the motor cortex tell us more about anatomical connectivity than about organized, normal movement. Study of the responses of single neurons in the course of normal motor behavior, however, has increased our understanding of cerebral control of movement.

## Correlation of neural activity and behavior (strategy 3)

Evarts developed the technique of recording from single motor cortex neurons in the waking monkey. By antidromic stimulation of the corticospinal tract in the medulla, each neuron was identified as to whether or not it had a tract axon. For a food reward, the animals were conditioned to perform highly stereotyped, repetitive motor tasks, thus permitting the reliable correlation of individual neuron activity with a specific behavior. For technical reasons, all recorded pyramidal tract units were necessarily very large cells and axons, but even within this group certain patterns were clear. The largest cells tended to be silent at rest and phasically active before the pertinent muscle contracted. Smaller cells were often tonically active and might increase or decrease their firing rates before and during movement. The behavior-locked activity of non-pyramidal tract cells had generally similar characteristics.

In other experiments, the monkeys were conditioned to produce posture-holding movements of the wrist. By varying the end position of the wrist joint and the external load upon the forearm muscles, it was shown that the rate of pyramidal cell discharge correlated most consistently with the force of the related movement, independent of joint position or hand displacement. A significant minority of neurons behaved in a different and less consistent manner, possibly because their strongest linkage was with muscles other than the prime movers under direct study. These data are the first distinct evidence that a major function of pyramidal tract control is control of graded force.

By a different microphysiological approach, intracortical stimulation with fine electrodes and minimal microampere tetanic volleys, Asanuma determined which muscles were activated from a given locus at the lowest electrical threshold. The somatosensory input to the same locus in the brain was found to originate in the deep and superficial structures of the same limb in the direction toward which the electrical stimulus moved it. This is direct evidence at the cellular level that we are dealing with a closely linked sensorimotor cortex.

Goldring has been able to study motor cortex units in conscious human subjects. Such unit activity consistently preceded a purposeful movement, as in Evarts's monkeys. These units usually responded strongly to passive joint movement, and they often displayed bilateral sensory and motor correlation. Superficial somatic and auditory inputs were ineffective in producing neuronal discharge. Goldring infers that, in man, compared with lower species, motor cortex cells are less capable of multisensory integration and are functionally farther downstream toward the final output path.

## Effects of destructive lesions (strategy 1)

Most of the clinical and experimental literature concerning the effects of upper neuron system lesions is based upon studies of acute processes. A typical acute hemispheral lesion in man produces maximal negative symptoms (depression of movement) at the outset. Proximal movement and strength are recovered first; later, movement in distal parts may reappear. If recovery is sufficient, dexterity develops. Stretch reflexes may be depressed at the outset, presumably due to sudden removal of major tonic excitatory pathways. They recover in a day or so and increase as spasticity evolves and movement returns. With maximal recovery of movement, reflex hyper-activity resolves to varying degrees. In spinal shock due to an acute cord lesion, all reflexes and even fusimotor tone are greatly de-pressed and require weeks to recover.

It is also well known that hyper-reflexia (a positive reflex release effect) evolves *pari passu* with negative symptoms when the patho-logical process moves slowly. In general, the very nature of negative and positive symptoms and the fact that they have different time courses and degrees of severity in relation to the nature and rate of the pathological process support Jackson's view that separate mech-anisms are involved.

In prolonged experiments on monkeys with acute lesions, Denny Brown, and Botterell showed that the amount of motor cortex re-moved and its proximity to the central sulcus correlated directly with the degree of initial movement disability and inversely with the rate and degree of recovery. They also emphasized the important relationship of motivation and performance. Hyper-reflexia devel-oped and disappeared more rapidly with smaller lesions. With the conspicuous exception of that work, the experimental ablation stud-ies of the last generation give inadequate attention to the param-eter of time. Many unsuccessful efforts were devoted to defining separate cortical loci and tracts to explain the positive and negative symptoms that are more influenced by time than by locus. Demon-stration of a "suppressor area" was shown to be an experimental artifact, and careful ablation in the monkey of the "supplementary motor cortex" was shown to be without effect.

## Negative symptoms

The recent, painstakingly detailed experiments by Lawrence and Kuypers do focus more helpfully upon the structural basis of nega-tive symptoms. With primary emphasis upon long-term tests of capacity for skilled motor performance in the monkey, these investi-gators produced carefully controlled lesions of the pyramidal tract and other descending pathways. They state that "In the absence of the corticospinal pathways, the descending subcortical spinal path-ways are capable of guiding the range of activity which includes independent limb movement in addition to total body-limb ac-tivity. The corticospinal pathways superimpose speed and agility upon these subcortical mechanisms, and, in addition, provide the capacity for a high degree of fractionation of movements as exemplified by individual finger movements."

In another series of experiments, lesions of the ventromedial or lateral regions of the brain stem or spinal cord were superposed in animals that had survived bilateral pyramidotomy. Both of these paths terminate with spinal internuncial neurons, but the lateral system has more direct access to limb musculature and the medial to axial muscles. They conclude: "Interruption of the lateral brain stem pathways produced an impairment of independent distal extremity and hand movements and an impaired capacity to flex the extended limb. Total limb movements and combined movements of body and limbs were relatively unaffected. In contrast, interruption of the ventromedial pathways resulted in a flexion bias of trunk and limbs and a severe impairment of axial and of proximal extremity movements. At the same time, independent distal extremity movements were relatively unaffected."

The pyramidal tract, too, has predominant connections with spinal interneurons, even though there are some direct motor neuron synapses. Furthermore, there are ample cortical relay projections to the brain-stem gray origins of those non-pyramidal pathways. The importance of the non-pyramidal projections is also attested by Lewis and Brindley's description of somatotopic responses to cortical stimulation after corticospinal tract section and by Evarts and Goldring's observations of behavior of non-pyramidal tract cortical neurons. I conclude that the negative upper motor neuron syndrome can best be attributed to lesions of direct and pauci-synaptic (few neuronal relays) projections, especially those to distal muscle motor neurons.

Although this may be a reasonable hypothesis of the anatomical basis of negative symptoms, it still fails to explain the pathophysiology of the qualitative movement deficit in the upper neuron syndrome. For this, we are largely reduced to theory. It seems reasonable to presume that the finely adjusted discharge of each lower motor neuron contributing to a special movement is attained by its combined temporal and spatial integration of multiple excitatory and inhibitory inputs. If a major input channel is blocked, it seems obvious that more impulses per unit time in surviving inputs will be needed to fire the motor neuron. But the maximal firing rates of the upper neuron elements have finite limits. Recalling the normally graded levels of activity found by Evarts in pyramidal neurons, one can see that any motor neuron activity and movement may require near maximal activity in surviving input units. The normal dynamic range of activity in the input channels would be lost, and the motor neuron population would be forced to operate in a restricted, nearly all-or-none fashion.

This view of the deranged system might account for the clinical observation that an enlarging upper neuron lesion correlates first with loss of fine adjustment and later with increasing weakness. The idea of higher level neurons working to a maximal degree also offers insight into the commonplace symptom of fatigability associated with upper motor neuron disease.

But why do negative symptoms lessen following acute destructive lesions? Although we postulate that some neurons are restored from what was only functional impairment associated with a lesion, there is no viable evidence that surviving brain cells actually improve their functional connections. Related questions are raised by the greater tolerance of young organisms to a given lesion and by the impressive degree of adaptation to very slowly evolving lesions (at any age), for example, some intramedullary spinal cord processes. Although these naturally favorable phenomena have obvious therapeutic implications, they are presently unexplained.

## Positive signs and symptoms

Babinski's sign (the extensor plantar reflex) is the most subtle and reliable index of impairment of the upper motor neuron system. Applying the usual sharp moving stimulus to the lateral aspect of the plantar surface of the foot, Clare and Landau analyzed the electromyographic response of normal flexor and of extensor plantar reflexes. Although the flexor response is characterized by some variability of muscle contraction patterns and the extensor by lower threshold and wider afferent field, they share the following features: specific activation by pain endings and nerve fibers, minimal threshold in the $S_1$ segment, and high effectiveness of temporal and spatial summation. The central latencies are identical, indicating a multiple polysynaptic segmental linkage, and the motor focus of contraction is in the short flexor muscles of the hallux, with associated flexion at ankle, knee, and hip.

The unique feature of the extensor reflex is the low threshold for recruitment of the extensor hallucis longus into contraction with its near neighbors, the tibialis anticus and extensor digitorum longus. The three muscles share in the reflex action of dorsiflexing the ankle. Peroneal nerve block of the hallux extensor does not abolish the plantar reflex but permits the flexors to dominate. Thus, in the extensor response, there is an actual mechanical competition between the hallux flexors and the extensor hallucis longus. The extensor reflex is not a different reaction from the flexor, but rather a hyperactive flexor response in which the extensor of the great toe is included almost by accident in the radiation of normal reflex activity. The neural mechanism of this polysynaptic hyperexcitability is unknown.

Two other superficial polysynaptic reflexes that also depend upon slow, small diameter afferent fibers, and a large component of nociception, behave quite differently. Both the abdominal reflex and the corneal reflex have latencies too short to provide for relay beyond the local segment of afferent supply. But both these reflexes are depressed by upper neuron lesions. This suggests a normal dependence upon tonic excitation from above for response by the reflex pathway to a transient stimulus input.

SPASTICITY

The term spasticity is used vaguely in the literature, almost always without definition, but usually with a connotation of exaggerated proprioceptive reflexes. We define spasticity in this text narrowly as a specific pattern of increasing muscular resistance to continuous passive stretch, up to the point of a relatively sudden decrease in resistance, the so-called claspknife reaction. An important generalization is that spasticity is a phenomenon of increased reactivity. In contrast to rigid and dystonic states, the main muscle is flaccid and electrically silent at rest.

The muscle spindle proprioceptive stretch reflexes are predominantly monosynaptic. The motor neurons of normal muscles can be brought to the reflex firing level only by highly synchronized volleys in many afferent fibers, as in the temporal summation of the tendon jerk. The asynchronous spindle afferent activity generated by slower passive stretch produces no consistent reaction in the normal muscle. Thus, the earliest evidence of proprioceptive hyperreactivity is exaggeration of the tendon jerk. Fully developed spasticity seldom appears suddenly but usually evolves from the state of increased tendon jerks through increasing and variable plastic resistance to stretch, often without a distinct phase of decreased resistance. The release phase of the claspknife reaction probably represents several factors, among which are (1) the relative decrease of input from spindle sense organs (mechanically in parallel with main muscle) due to a degree of unloading by contraction of the main muscle; (2) activation of the Golgi afferent sense organs (in mechanical series with the muscle) whose activity increases with stretch to inhibit the muscle stretched; and (3) for extensor muscles, inhibition by small secondary spindle stretch receptors, which excite flexor muscles.

The simplest proximate explanation for spasticity is that it represents a lower threshold for synaptic excitation at the anterior horn cell level. There is an increased population response to a synchronized excitation and a lack of normal adaptation to a less intense tonic excitation. The most direct proof of this in man is the observation that the maximal response to direct electrical stimulation of the spindle afferent fibers, the H reflex, is increased on the involved side in hemiplegia. There are so many theories for the mechanism of this reflex release that it seems certain none is adequate. Long-term changes have been attributed to sprouting of additional primary afferent neuron collaterals to form new synaptic endings on anterior horn cells and to post-synaptic sensitization, as predicted by Cannon's Law of Denervation. Long-term changes could theoretically be based upon almost any conceivable change in the presynaptic terminal, transmitter agent or the post-synaptic membrane, including both excitatory and inhibitory mechanisms. Short-term changes occurring in minutes, for example, after transection of the cat's spinal cord, must be attributed to a change in the total synaptic impingement upon the test system.

The relationship of the fusimotor system to spasticity has been debated. A fraction of these specialized small motor neurons are tonically active at rest, causing contraction of the intrafusal muscle fibers and keeping the stretch receptors taut and sensitive to external stretch. Since the small fibers are more sensitive to local anesthetic agents, it is possible in the normal subject to desensitize the stretch receptors and grossly depress the stretch reflexes without affecting main muscle strength. A diffuse anesthesia by spinal or epidural block in man produces remarkably little functional disability, only a peculiar feeling of looseness similar to what may be noted after sitting in one position for a long time. Similar treatment of spastic patients will abolish spasticity along with the hyperactive tendon jerks, but impaired motor performance (the negative symptom) does not improve and may be worse. This proves only that sensitive muscle spindles are necessary for spasticity to occur. Recent reflex experiments by Dietrichson do indicate also that the stretch receptors in human spasticity have increased sensitivity. That increased alpha motoneuron excitability and increased fusimotor neuron activity go together is compatible with animal and human experiments that indicate that both types of anterior horn cells are usually activated together in normal movement behavior. It is not true, however, that spasticity is entirely or even largely due to increased fusimotor tone.

Clonus, often associated with spasticity, is a series of rhythmic phasic stretch reflex contractions interrupted by silent periods. Physiologically, it is the negative of the phasic stretch reflex (tendon jerk). The first sudden passive stretch to the tested muscle produces a reflex contraction strong enough to unload the muscle spindles (in parallel). The resulting transient cessation of excitatory input to the spinal cord depresses alpha motoneuron excitability and results in the silent period. Reapplication of continued stretch then renews the cycle.

It is important to emphasize that, for the patient, spasticity is not an important symptom. Indeed, it may be a functional asset; for example, the hemiparetic patient whose knee tends to buckle finds that the spasticity provides a useful bracing action. To be sure, clonus can be an annoying symptom, and adductor spasticity in young patients may lead to a scissor gait, but, for most patients, proprioceptive release phenomena are of no symptomatic significance. This conclusion can be validly based upon simple clinical observation and is confirmed by the experiments cited above where abolition of spasticity by fusimotor blockade did not improve motor function.

The greatly exaggerated release phenomena of severe paraparesis and paraplegia are probably, in large part, an exaggeration of the polysynaptic, sustained patterns of the flexion reflex minimally represented by Babinski's sign. Undoubtedly intermixed are secondary exaggerated proprioceptive responses. Most characteristic of these mass responses is their capacity to be triggered by weak superficial stimuli. Therapeutic approaches with depressant drugs have not been rewarding, but several approaches to destruction of dorsal root triggering input pathways may be.

### THE DECEREBRATE STATE

Another state of maximal positive symptom release is associated with gross insult to the upper brain stem. The glib clinical terms "decerebrate rigidity" and "decorticate rigidity" mask a treasure trove of misinformation. Decorticate rigidity is supposed to be a condition of hyperreflexia, with stable flexion of the upper limb and extension of the lower due to lesions at the highest level of the upper motor neuron. An extensive review of the literature shows clearly that there are neither experimental nor clinico-pathological data to support the idea.

Decerebrate rigidity in man is also supposed to be a stable state and to include even more extension of the lower extremities plus inversion and extension of the upper limbs. This phenomenon certainly exists in patients with upper brain-stem impairment, but decerebrate posturing most often must be induced by a stimulus, usually noxious. When the posturing is spontaneous and persistent, the patient is usually moribund.

Feldman prepared a series of monkeys with intercollicular brain-stem transection and managed to keep them alive for a day or more. These animals had unfixed flaccid posture with subtle intermittent claspknife spasticity in both flexors and extensors, along with brisk tendon jerks. Extensor posturing (reactive extensor postural synergy) was manifest only as a response to nociceptive stimulation of face or trunk, passive neck extension, or hypoxia. Thus, decerebrate extensor responses are indeed released by upper brain-stem lesions, but they are not stable passive postures. They must be reflexly driven or they must be triggered by brain-stem metabolic insult (e.g., hypoxia).

The extensor synergy is present to a minor degree in normal subjects. With a forceful voluntary extension of the neck, there is an associated contraction of triceps and biceps (more in the former), a pattern quite similar to that in the monkeys. In hemiparetic subjects, these responses are significantly exaggerated on the affected side. Thus, just as in the case of plantar reflex and proprioceptive reflex, an upper neuron lesion also releases an exaggerated reflex, which is most distinctive in the upper extremities.

## General references

Denny-Brown, D. and E. H. Botterell. 1948. The motor functions of the agranular frontal cortex. Res. Publ. Assn. Res. Nerv. Ment. Dis. 27: 235-345.

Dietrichson, P. 1971. Phasic ankle reflex in spasticity and parkinsonian rigidity. The role of the fusimotor system. Acta Neurol. Scandinav. 47: 22-51.

Evarts, E. V. 1968. Relation of pyramidal tract activity to force exerted during voluntary movement. J. Neurophysiol. 31:14-27.

Feldman, M. H. 1971. The decerebrate state in the primate. Arch. Neurol. 25:501-525.

Goldring, S. and R. Ratcheson. 1972. Human motor cortex: Sensory input data from single neuron recordings. Science 175:1493-1495.

Landau, W. M. and M. H. Clare. 1964. Fusimotor function. Part VI. H-reflex, tendon jerk and reinforcement in hemiplegia. Arch. Neurol. 10: 128-134.

Landau, W. M. and M. H. Clare. 1959. The plantar reflex in man. Brain 82:321-355.

Landau, W. M., R. A. Weaver, and T. F. Hornbein. 1960. Fusimotor nerve function in man. Differential nerve block studies in normal subjects and in spasticity and rigidity. Arch. Neurol. 3:10-23.

Lawrence, D. G. and H. G. Kuypers. 1968. The functional organization of the motor system in the monkey. Brain 91:1-36.

Lewis, R. and G. S. Brindley. 1965. The extrapyramidal cortical motor map. Brain 88:397-406.

Phillips, C. G. 1967. Corticomotoneuronal organization. Arch. Neurol. 17: 188-195.

Phillips, C. G. 1969. The Ferrier Lecture, 1968. Motor apparatus of the baboon's hand. Proc. Roy. Soc. B. 173:141-174.

Phillips, C. G. 1973. The Hughlings Jackson Lecture, 1973. Cortical localization and 'sensorimotor processes' at the 'middle level' in primates. Proc. Roy. Soc. Med. 66:41-56.

Porter, R. 1973. Function of the mammalian cerebral cortex in movement. Prog. Neurobiol. 1:1-51.

Russell, J. R. and W. DeMyer. 1961. The quantitative cortical origin of pyramidal axons of *Macaca rhesus*. Neurol. 11:96-108, 1961.

Taylor, J. ed. 1958. Selected writings of John Hughlings Jackson. Basic Books, New York, 2 vols.

Twitchell, T. E. 1951. The restoration of motor function following hemiplegia in man. Brain 74:443-480.

Walshe, F. M. R. 1961. Contributions of John Hughlings Jackson to neurology. A brief introduction to his teachings. Arch. Neurol. 5:119-131.

Wiesendanger, M. 1969. The pyramidal tract. Recent investigations on its morphology and function. Ergebn. Physiol. 61:72-136.

## MOVEMENT DISORDERS

WILLIAM M. LANDAU

## Introduction

When neurologists use the generic term movement disorders, they are usually referring to conditions characterized by purposeless or involuntary muscle contraction implicitly related largely to cerebral disease, excluding cerebellar system disturbances.

## Parkinsonism—Clinical physiology

Parkinsonism is a common and complex syndrome, with many known (genetic, toxic, viral, vascular) and more unknown etiologies, and with consequently varying clinical presentations and time courses. Neurochemical aspects of basal ganglia function are described in Chapter 4.

The primary features of the syndrome are (1) the positive symptom of constant innervated contraction of most of the musculature when the patient is relaxed and at rest and (2) the associated negative symptom of generalized weakness and particular difficulty in starting movements (hypokinesia). These are manifest to varying degrees in individual patients. In many patients, the baseline muscle activity may break up into rhythmic resting tremor, which was classically named paralysis agitans. Although patients may fatigue rapidly, have trouble starting to move, and be handicapped by severe tremor, fine movements are relatively well preserved.

The increase in baseline tone is persistent throughout the range of passive movement of an extremity. Careful observation, manipulation, and cajolery can often produce electrical silence in the electromyogram that lasts for brief periods in selected muscles. Nevertheless, it is obvious that the threshold for involuntary sustained muscle contraction is abnormally low, and, typically, there is palpable and visible muscle contraction during subjective relaxation.

The passive resistance encountered in parkinsonian rigidity is of about the same degree throughout joint excursion. Its cogwheel character is produced by rhythmic interruption at a frequency of about 5 to 10 cycles/second (5 cycles/second is the usual rate range of resting tremor, contraction bursts alternating in antagonist muscles at the double frequency). Since the pattern of muscle contraction is changed by passive stretch, it is obvious that there is a reflex component in rigidity. It seems equally certain that there must be some related central mechanism to account for the augmented tone.

Students of parkinsonism are divided into two groups; one group believes that rigidity and tremor are separate phenomena, and the other group (led by Hughlings Jackson) believes that they are only different aspects of one phenomenon—that rigidity represents tremor run together or that tremor represents interrupted rigidity. Jackson's view is supported by electromyographic observations in parkinsonian patients at rest and during passive and active movements. In a patient remaining as quiet as the tremor permits, individual motor units and groups of units are not perfectly locked into the tremor bursts. Even slight passive movements may break up rhythmic contractions into relatively tonic activity. With more extensive passive movements, several variations in both stretched and shortened muscles are seen. These include conversion of tonic activity to tremor and of tremor to tonic activity, as well as the doubling of tremor frequency in one muscle so that it also tends to follow the frequency of its antagonist.

In parkinsonian patients with a vigorous alternating tremor, one may sometimes see suppression of tremor bursts with passive flexion or extension. Such records suggest that a disturbance of the beat in alternating neuronal groups suppresses the reciprocal bursts in both flexor and extensor neurons, regardless of which muscle is stretched and which is shortened. One forms the impression, which is also acquired in clinical observations, that a given muscle combination has an optimal posture for the development of reciprocal tremor. Clearly, reciprocal innervation in alternating tremor, as in normal movement, is not a simple all-or-none phenomenon.

Usually the frequency of alternating tremor bursts in antagonistic muscles of the same resting limb is constant, but variation of frequency between limbs, or even in different portions of the same limb, is often seen. Rarely, the frequencies in antagonistic muscles are slightly different so that the antagonist periodically comes into synchrony.

In patients with parkinsonism, the typical electromyogram pattern during purposeful movement shows unit activity filling the gaps between tremor bursts in the prime mover and some decrease of tremor burst amplitude in the antagonist muscle. Thus, the resting tremor tends to disappear during activity. A doubling of frequency, reciprocal or synchronous, is commonly seen, and overflow excitation to the antagonist muscle may take on a rhythmic or nonrhythmic form. In some patients, absence of tremor is assignable to synchronous rhythmic or tonic activity occurring in antagonistic muscles when the patient is at rest.

In normal persons, rhythmic alternating tremor, including at times the frequency doubling effect of synchronous contraction in agonist or antagonist, can be induced by strong muscular effort. Reaction to passive stretch varies in the resting state from none to contractions in both stretched and shortened muscles, just as in parkinsonian patients. These patterns of response to passive movement are exaggerated by epinephrine injection or by chilling to the point of shivering; both mechanisms are presumed only to provoke involuntary tonic descending neural activity toward the final common path for movement. It may be added that a variety of animal and human studies indicate an optimal frequency for synchronous muscle contraction at about 10/second. This appears to be an intrinsic rhythm of the neurophysiological excitability pattern in the mammalian spinal cord.

Rhythmic tremor and rhythmic clonus obviously have some of the features related to the behavior of proprioceptors and the intrinsic physiology of the spinal segment in common. Thus, the monosynaptic motoneuron reflex (H reflex) excitability curve shows an increase above normal in patients with parkinsonism, an increase quite similar to that found in spasticity. Also rigidity, like spasticity, is diminished with the phasic stretch reflex by fusimotor nerve block. Detectable baseline activity in the electromyogram in rigidity may persist, and tremor also remains. The blocking experiments certainly exclude the theory that rigidity is due to hypofunction of fusimotor neurons. Hyperfunction seems improbable simply because the phasic stretch reflexes are not increased in parkinsonism, whereas, in animals, the amplitude of the stretch reflex is a function of experimental variation of fusimotor activity.

In summary, muscles have a low threshold for tonic motor unit discharge in patients with Parkinson's disease. Variations in the threshold at rest, with postural change and with active movement, indicate that individual units may spontaneously or reflexly enter and leave the group that is firing. These observations suggest that many motoneurons are near the tonic firing level. Their tendency to fire synchronously in rhythmic bursts seems to be characteristic of the organization of spinal neurons at high levels of excitation. Rhythmic activity in muscle antagonists is typically alternating at about 5/second, but doubling of frequency may be seen at rest and during active and passive movements. There often is a favorite posture for maximal tone and tremor. In purposeful movement, overflow excitation beyond muscles that are prime movers is commonplace.

Efforts to put these data together require a review of the observations of both the clinician and the pathologist. First, the patient with parkinsonism tends to have a continuous level of muscle contraction. Second, when the test muscles are silent, the phasic muscle stretch reflexes are ordinarily within normal limits. Third, the only pathological abnormalities yet found in Parkinson's disease are in the forebrain. A simple conclusion is that forebrain lesions somehow result in the release of sustained excitation at the spinal cord level that is in itself physiologically normal. In contrast to spasticity, the primary abnormality is one of elevation of the spontaneous tonic activity level at the spinal segment; the released neuronal hyperactivity must be upstream from the motoneuron involving spinal and possibly brain-stem interneurons.

## PATHOLOGICAL CORRELATIONS

The specific pathology of the parkinsonian syndrome is not clear cut. Certainly, in most cases, there is some degeneration of the substantia nigra, and many authors have emphasized that additional damage to the pallidum and to the cortical connections with the pallidum occurs. Although tremor is a major symptom in only a

minority of cases, there is no question that this symptom is the one
most impressively ameliorated by surgical lesions in the globus pallidus or ventralis lateralis nucleus of the thalamus. While preparing
for the production of thalamic lesions, surgeons have recorded from
single neural units in patients (and also in monkeys who present a
near model of parkinsonism when lesions are made in the brain
stem near the substantia nigra). Units whose firing rhythm is similar
to that of a tremorous muscle in the conscious patient have been
seen. The theory that tremor is driven by rhythmic discharge of
masses of forebrain neurons, however, is contradicted by the fact
that gross ganglionic rhythms representing many neurons have not
been recorded at tremor rate. Whether the few neurons in the
thalamus are primary pace setters, or whether the pace is set by the
spinal reflex loop or by intrinsic ganglionic rhythms in the spinal
cord has not yet been determined. The abnormal rhythmic activity
does provide a way to test correlations, but neither all neurons nor
all muscles can be sampled, so that the issue of which comes first
remains uncertain. For patients without active tremor, there is no
ready way to provide temporal correlation. Experiments with local
electrical stimulation in the forebrain gray matter have not clarified
the matter.

## Other basal ganglia syndromes

### HEPATOLENTICULAR DEGENERATION

Somewhat similar to the symptoms of parkinsonism are those of
hepatolenticular degeneration (Wilson's disease). Lesions due to
toxic copper accumulation are most prominent in the putamen. A
peculiar silly smile and a wing-beating tremor of the wrist on posture-holding are characteristic. There may also be features of rigidity, resting tremor, and ataxia. The genetic metabolic disturbance is
discussed in Chapter 1. This illness is exceedingly rare, the most
likely differential diagnostic probability in a young person with
something like parkinsonism being phenothiazine toxicity.

### CHOREA

The second most common movement disorder is chorea, a name
derived from the Greek word for dance. Involuntary movements at
rest are irregular, jerky, and highly varied; a finger or hand may

twitch or flick in any direction. Often minor movements are concealed by the patient beneath some quasi-purposeful movement like scratching. Irregular twitching movements of the tongue, the face, and the lower extremities are common. In advanced cases, the movements involve whole extremities, and the patient may be bedridden.

### HEREDITARY CHOREA

In hereditary chorea (Huntington's chorea), there is progressive degeneration of the striatum, especially the caudate, and of the cerebral cortex. Occasionally, occlusive or small hemorrhagic vascular lesions in the striatum can produce a contralateral hemichorea syndrome. The anatomical basis of the self-limited, presumably vascular condition in chorea associated with rheumatic fever (Sydenham's chorea) is unknown.

It is clear that there is some relationship between the parkinsonian and the choreic syndromes, although they are dramatically different in appearance. In some rare diseases, there may be spontaneous evolution from one type of symptom to another. Several drugs useful in the treatment of chorea (haloperidol or phenothiazine) tend to produce parkinsonism. Phenothiazine may also produce toxic symptoms of chorea as well as of parkinsonism in patients previously not afflicted with either motor disorder.

### BALLISM

A more violent species of chorea is called ballism. The patient is afflicted with gross flinging movements of the extremities, particularly the arms. This symptom is usually unilateral following a contralateral lesion in or near the subthalamic nucleus of Luys. The syndrome can be simulated by experimental lesions in the monkey, and, as in man, it can be relieved by a secondary lesion in the pallidum, thalamus, or upper motor neuron system.

### ATHETOSIS

The term athetosis is generally applied to a condition with bizarre twisting distortions of purposeful body and limb movements affecting, especially, the hands, distal limb segments, and face. When the patient is quiet, there is no resistance to passive movement in affected extremities. The abnormal movements are usually irregular and tend to be stereotyped, i.e., hyperextension of the

fingers with hyperflexion at the wrist. Lesions are predominantly
of the striatum. Usually the symptoms are present from birth, although they may develop progressively. Athetotic movements may
be associated with chorea.

DYSTONIA

The term dystonia refers to a type of rigidity involving peculiar
disturbances of posture. Strictly speaking, it may be considered
analogous to the rigidity of parkinsonism in that there is a steady-
state muscular contraction when the patient is at rest. The term is
usually used to describe the condition of (or resembling) dystonia
musculorum deformans, in which a child develops progressively
severe tonic distortions of posture and movement, most conspicu-
ously affecting trunk, neck, and proximal limb musculature. There
are no consistent pathological findings. Some authors have suggested that dystonia is a proximal version of athetosis. In some patients, there are arrhythmic spasms of affected limbs, which may be
exaggerated by a particular posture. It seems probably that the
increased motor neuron activity level represents a release effect at
internuncial levels of the spinal cord or brain stem, as in parkinsonism, rather than at the final common path, as in spasticity.

## Other types of disturbed movement

ACTION MYOCLONUS

Action myoclonus is a descriptive term for vigorous jerking movements that occur only when the patient attempts voluntary movement. Myoclonic movements are sometimes associated with what
would otherwise be called cerebellar ataxia. In some cases, they
are associated with paroxysmal electroencephalogram findings and
suggest a relationship to epilepsy. Myoclonus is seen in several varieties of widely diffuse neuronal disease. Both the pathology and
pathophysiology are obscure.

PALATAL MYOCLONUS

Myoclonus of the palate is a regular elevation of the palate at a
frequency of 1 to 2/second, persisting even during sleep in many
cases. Concomitant synchronous movements may occur in facial, extraocular, and respiratory muscles, and there seems to be a common

central pacemaker. The precise mechanism is not known, and an experimental model has not been produced. Lesions are always found in the brain-stem region bounded by the inferior olivary nucleus, the dentate nucleus, and the red nucleus.

### OCULOGYRIC CRISES

Oculogyric crises are involuntary tonic upward movements of the eyes, which may last minutes to hours. They are seen with brain-stem involvement in encephalitis and may be triggered in normal patients by drugs that produce parkinsonism. The mechanism is not understood.

### THE STIFF-MAN SYNDROME

A rare condition called the stiff-man syndrome consists essentially of continuous involuntary generalized motor unit discharge. This condition has been likened to chronic tetanus. It may be dramatically relieved by diazepam. It has been suggested that there is a spinal cord disturbance. Chronic destructive processes within the spinal cord may also be associated with continuous motor neuron discharge.

### MYOTONIA

Myotonia is a common condition of repetitive discharge of muscle fibers once triggered by neural excitation or percussion. Thus, it is manifest as an involuntary maintenance of contraction after the cessation of voluntary effort. A patient may have trouble undoing a handshake, for example. Myotonia occurs in several varieties of hereditary myopathy, it seems to be related to a disturbance of ionic transport in muscle fibers, and it can be produced artificially by the administration of a cholesterol-like substance, desmosterol, which presumably affects the excitable muscle membrane.

### OTHER MOVEMENT DISORDERS

A condition originally described by Isaacs manifests itself as continuous muscle fiber activity localized by clinical experiments with nerve block and curare to the muscle-end plate region, which seems to continuously discharge transmitter substance. There is evidence of peripheral nerve conduction slowing in some cases, along with depressed tendon jerks. Patients often respond well to Dilantin.

Lower level causes of persistent muscle contraction include hypocalcemia (tetany) and tetanus. In both cases, there is peripheral neuromuscular hyperexcitability and some hyperexcitability in the spinal cord.

For most of the movement disorders, the serious gaps in understanding of pathophysiology relate to the lack of adequate experimental models, the rarity of the clinical conditions, and the inaccessibility of the involved structures.

## General references

Carpenter, M. B. 1961. Brain stem and infratentorial neuraxis in experimental dyskinesia. Arch. Neurol. 5:504-524.

Denny-Brown, D. E. 1962. The basal ganglia and their relation to disorders of movement. Oxford University Press, London.

Landau, W. M., A. Struppler, and O. Mehl. 1966. A comparative study of the reactions to passive movement in parkinsonism and in normal subjects. Neurology 16:34-48.

Landau, W. M. and J. L. O'Leary. 1970. Disturbances of movement. Pages 692-711 in C. M. MacBryde, ed. Signs and symptoms: Applied pathologic physiology and clinical interpretation. 5th ed., Lippincott, Philadelphia.

Landau, W. M. 1969. Spasticity and rigidity. Pages 2-32 in F. Plum, ed. Contemporary neurology, Series 6, Recent advances in neurology. F. A. Davis, Philadelphia.

## PHARMACOLOGY AND CHEMISTRY OF MOVEMENT DISORDER

JAMES FERRENDELLI AND GEORGE H. KLINKERFUSS

During the last few decades, neurological research has produced important new knowledge concerning the biochemistry, pharmacology, and physiology of the basal ganglia. This section will review some of the biochemical and pharmacological observations that have led to a better understanding of the pathophysiology of some of the extrapyramidal motor system disorders associated with diseases of the basal ganglia, and it will outline the pharmacological principles underlying the rational medical therapy of these disorders.

To our knowledge, all intercellular communication responsible for the multiple functions of the central nervous system is mediated by chemical agents. Of the several substances implicated as neuro-transmitters, dopamine and acetylcholine (ACh) appear to be particularly important in extrapyramidal system function. Dopamine is a precursor of norepinephrine and epinephrine. These catecholamines, in turn, are metabolites of tyrosine, which has been converted to 3,4-dihydroxyphenylalanine (dopa). The enzyme responsible for this conversion, tyrosine hydroxylase, requires a pteridine cofactor and is the rate-limiting step in the pathway. Conversion of dopa to dopamine is mediated by the enzyme dopa decarboxylase, which requires pyridoxal phosphate as a coenzyme. In some areas of the central nervous system, and in all parts of the sympathetic nervous system, dopamine is further metabolized to norepinephrine by dopamine $\beta$-oxidase. Degradation of dopamine occurs rapidly, and several products are formed during its catabolism, the major ones being 3-O-methyldopamine, 3,4-dihydroxyphenylacetic acid (DO-PAC), and homovanillic acid (HVA). These products result from the actions of catechol-O-methyl-transferase and the mitochondrial enzyme, monoamine oxidase, on dopamine. In the brain, most of the dopamine is apparently metabolized to HVA, since little of the other metabolites are found.

Both dopamine and HVA seem to be unequally distributed in the central nervous system. For example, relatively high concentrations of both are found in the striatum, the substantia nigra, and the globus pallidus, whereas very little dopamine or HVA is found in the cerebral cortex or the white matter. Of considerable importance to our present discussion is the localization of dopamine in the substantia nigra and striatum. It appears that large pigmented cells, e.g., those in the pars compacta of the substantia nigra, contain large amounts of dopamine. In the striatum, most of the dopamine appears to be in small nerve endings and not in cell bodies, themselves, and proof of this derives from the observation that much of the dopamine in the striatum disappears after the substantia nigra is destroyed or after disruption of fibers leading from the substantia nigra to the striatum; this would indicate that a large portion of the dopamine in the striatum is localized in endings of nerves originating in the substantia nigra.

The concentration of ACh and choline and the activities of choline acetylase and acetylcholine esterase (the enzymes that synthesize and degrade ACh) are all high in the striatum. As with dopamine, much of the ACh in the striatum seems to be localized in presynaptic nerve endings. The origin of the nerve cells of these endings, however, has not been conclusively established. Although indisputable evidence concerning the physiological actions of dopamine and ACh is difficult to obtain, it appears that the major action of dopamine on striatal neurons is to reduce their firing rates (inhibition), whereas the action of ACh is excitation. Consequently, the action of the two neuro-transmitters may be that of maintaining an appropriate balance of excitation-inhibition functions among striatal neurons.

## Parkinson's disease

The necessity of ACh and dopamine in extrapyramidal motor system function is best understood from studies of Parkinson's disease. Dopamine and HVA concentrations are reduced in the substantia nigra and striatum of patients with Parkinson's disease. The degree of reduction of dopamine in both regions appears to correlate with the estimated per cent loss of nerve cells lost in the substantia nigra as well as with the severity of the clinical signs and symptoms. The correlation between parkinsonism and striatal dopamine deficiency has been observed in patients with postencephalitic and idiopathic parkinsonism and the parkinsonism that results from manganese poisoning. These observations, as well as those in experimental animals, have led to the generally accepted conclusion that the signs and symptoms of parkinsonism result from a relative deficiency of striatal dopamine.

The concept of relative striatal dopamine deficiency requires further deliberation. Although Parsinson's disease per se is associated with an absolute decrease in striatal dopamine levels, parkinsonism due to some known causes is not. For example, the symptoms and signs of the parkinsonism that frequently accompanies therapy with phenothiazines or butyrophenones probably are not associated with an absolute deficiency of striatal dopamine. Instead, these psychopharmacological agents probably competitively block post-synaptic dopamine receptor sites to reduce the influence of dopamine on striatal neurons. Parkinsonism of almost any etiology is frequently improved by such centrally acting anticholinergic agents as atropine, which would be expected to block cholinergic receptor sites and inhibit the actions of ACh in neurons in striatum as well as in other regions of the central nervous system. This suggests that the cholinergic influence on the striatum, and perhaps other areas of brain, is an important factor in the etiology of parkinsonism. In summary, therefore, parkinsonism may be considered to be a result of a relative deficiency of the dopaminergic influence on the striatum in relation to the cholinergic influence.

There are several lines of evidence indicating that dopaminergic and cholinergic mechanisms also play a role in the production of dyskinesias. In patients with parkinsonism treated with L-dopa, frequent dose-related side effects are dyskinesias or chorea. Reserpine, phenothiazines, butyrophenones, and other agents that reduce dopaminergic influence in the central nervous system have been shown to alleviate the abnormal movements in patients with Huntington's and Sydenham's chorea, whereas L-dopa makes the choreic movements worse in patients with Huntington's chorea. Physostigmine, an anticholinesterase able to penetrate into the central nervous system, diminishes choreic movements in patients with Huntington's chorea. These observations have led to the tentative hypothesis that chorea is the result of an increase in the dopaminergic influence relative to the cholinergic influence in the striatum.

Abnormalities in other putative neuro-transmitter systems, especially serotonin and norepinephrine, have been implicated in the production of parkinsonism and chorea, but at the present time there is no convincing evidence that these substances have any major role.

Although the use of L-dopa for the treatment of Parkinson's disease is an excellent example of the development of a rational therapy based on anatomical and biochemical observations, it is well to remember that it was possible to improve the function of many patients with movement disorders prior to our current understanding of their possible biochemical basis. In many instances, the use of these drugs was purely empirical and it was by investigating the effects of the pharmacological agent that the underlying pathophysiology of the disorder was clarified. Even now, no scientific formula can be constructed for the successful treatment of all patients with movement disorders, and therapy is generally individualized. Many drugs must be used in combinations to achieve the best therapeutic response for the individual patient. Furthermore, the desired therapeutic effect must be balanced against untoward side effects. This may necessitate frequent dosage changes and make careful follow-up of the patient mandatory.

Historically, the first successful drugs used for the treatment of Parkinson's disease were anticholinergic. The use of these drugs was widespread, and their effects unequivocal, despite the fact that at that time no theories existed regarding the relationship of movement disorders to a balance between cholinergic and dopaminergic neurons. The institution of L-dopa therapy for this disorder was a great advance, and it is certainly at present the most effective drug for the treatment of Parkinson's disease. As indicated, its use was based on biochemical information. L-Dopa is the immediate precursor of dopamine, and, unlike dopamine, it is capable of entering the central nervous system when administered systemically. It can be converted into dopamine in the striatim, thus increasing striatal dopamine levels, which presumably is the basis for the beneficial effects of the medication. Unfortunately, L-dopa can also be converted into dopamine in other areas of the nervous system, as well as other organs of the body. Thus, there are numerous side effects such as cardiac irregularities, postural hypotension, nausea and vomiting, depressive reactions, and, after a longer period of time, dyskinesias. Such adverse reactions require that the drug be increased slowly over a period of weeks until a satisfactory clinical response is obtained.

Amantadine hydrochloride is a second medication, which has recently been introduced and which is extremely helpful in the therapy of Parkinson's disease. Although amantadine does possess some anticholinergic activity and has been shown to increase dopamine release in animal brain, its exact mechanism of action in parkinsonian patients is not known.

## Huntington's chorea

The drug therapy of Huntington's chorea remains entirely unsatisfactory as far as deterioration of intellectual function and personality are concerned. There are now drugs that can reduce the choreic movements early in the course of the disease. The most effective drugs are phenothiazines or butyrophenones, which, as was indicated previously, competitively block post-synaptic dopamine receptor sites. As the disease progresses, these drugs become less effective.

The rigidity frequently associated with Huntington's chorea is not appreciably influenced by the currently available medications.

## General references

Barbeau, A. and F. H. McDowell, eds. 1970. L-Dopa and parkinsonism. F. A. Davis, Philadelphia.

Klawans, H. L. 1970. A pharmacologic analysis of Huntington's chorea. Europ. Neurol. 4:148-163.

McDowell, F. H. and C. H. Markham, eds. 1971. Recent advances in Parkinson's disease. F. A. Davis, Philadelphia.

McDowell, F. H., ed. 1972. Symposium on levodopa in Parkinson's disease. Neurology 22 (5) Part 2.

# 5
# Disorders of Cortical Function

## PATHOPHYSIOLOGY OF CLINICAL EPILEPSY

WILLIAM B. HARDIN, JR.

### Introduction

Epilepsy is a reflection of an altered physiological state of the central nervous system. Virtually any disordered function of the body that is capable of changing the ionic milieu, metabolism, or structure of a nerve cell within the central nervous system may provoke a clinical seizure. On the other hand, not all nerve cells within the central nervous system can produce the clinical features of epilepsy. For example, neurons of the cerebellum, lower brain stem, and spinal cord, although capable in many instances of extremely rapid firing rates, are not believed to be in the critical anatomical positions that trigger an epileptic attack.

Clinically, epilepsy is characterized by brief recurrent episodes of convulsions or other stereotyped motor behavior in association with disordered perception and impairment or actual loss of consciousness. Electrophysiologically the epileptic seizure begins with either a local, paroxysmal, high frequency neuronal discharge or else a lower frequency, higher voltage discharge, which then proceeds to induce central nervous system dysfunction either locally or at a distance by spreading along neural pathways.

The clinical signs of an epileptic seizure depend upon the region

146

of the brain where functions are being impaired by seizure activity. Thus, consciousness is lost when the seizure discharge invades the upper brain stem and thalamus. Contractions of the somatic musculature occur when the discharge involves the frontal motor areas. Peripheral autonomic discharge occurs when the excitatory activity extends to the hypothalamus. Various sensory experiences may result when the activity reaches parietal and occipital structures before it involves centers of consciousness. Epilepsy associated with loss of consciousness can be grouped into three basic types: grand mal, petit mal, and psychomotor.

Once a cluster of neurons has been triggered into an abnormal, hyperexcitable state of activity, there are three possible consequences: (1) the discharge may remain localized to that cluster of neurons and eventually cease its activity; (2) the discharge may spread a variable distance through nervous structures without involving the entire brain, meet "resistance," and then cease altogether; or (3) the discharge may spread through the entire central nervous system before terminating. In the first two cases, the seizure

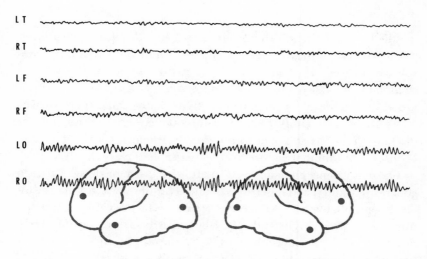

**Fig. 5-1** Normal adult electroencephalogram. LT, left temporal; RT, right temporal; LF, left frontal; RF, right frontal; LO, left occipital; RO, right occipital scalp leads. Heavy horizontal line, 1 second of recording time; small vertical line, equivalent to 50 μV amplitude. Note: The basic resting occipital frequency is approximately 10 ± 2 cycles/second in adults, and alpha rhythms are not prominent in the frontal and anterior temporal leads. The approximate recording sites are indicated on the small right and left hemispheres (insert).

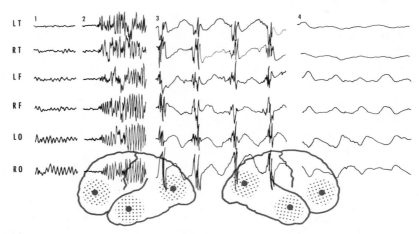

**Fig. 5-2** Brief excerpts from an electroencephalogram during a grand mal seizure. (1) Normal record preceding the attack; (2) onset of the attack; (3) clonic phase of the attack; (4) post-ictal period of coma and subsequent recovery. The horizontal and vertical lines have magnitudes equivalent to those in Fig. 5-1. Dotted areas around the recording sites on the hemisphere diagrams indicate electrically active regions picked up by the scalp electrodes

is called *partial;* in the third case, it is *generalized.* In generalized seizures, consciousness is always impaired, and both cerebral hemispheres as well as their connections with the subcortical nuclei (thalamus, basal ganglia, upper brain stem, and limbic structures) are always involved in the seizure activity at the same time. In partial seizures, consciousness is usually preserved when the seizure discharge remains confined to one cerebral hemisphere, but it may be lost when limbic structures or the diencephalon are involved.

The electroencephalogram is useful in distinguishing between generalized and partial seizures. Figure 5-1 shows a normal adult electroencephalogram. Notice the symmetry of wave forms and frequencies between right and left. Generalized seizures can be recognized on the electroencephalogram by the appearance of synchronously distributed spikes [Fig. 5-2(A)], spikes and waves [Figs. 5-2 (C) and 5-3], or asynchronously distributed spikes and waves over both hemispheres (Fig. 5-4). Partial or focal seizures may be identified by the sporadic appearance of spikes or spike and wave combinations confined to a small area of brain (Fig. 5-5). Brief "seizure bursts," such as those identified in Fig. 5-5, often occur without any

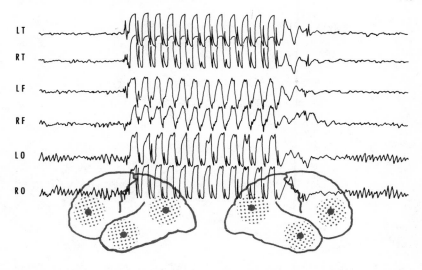

**Fig. 5-3** A 4-second episode of a 3 cycles/second single spike and wave burst characteristic of a petit mal discharge. The burst appears from out of a normal appearing background and disappears abruptly back into the normal pattern. Time and voltage markers are equivalent to those in Fig. 5-1. Hemispheres indicate that electrical activity is diffuse.

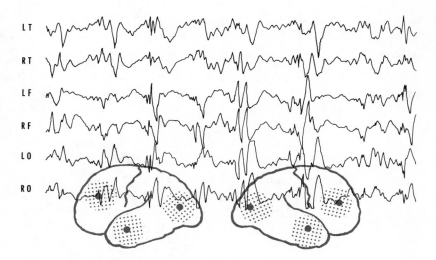

**Fig. 5-4** Hypsarrhythmia in the electroencephalographic recording of a child. There is diffuse irregular spiking and high amplitude slow waves without a clearly focal or lateralizing trend. Time and voltage markers are equivalent to those in Fig. 5-1.

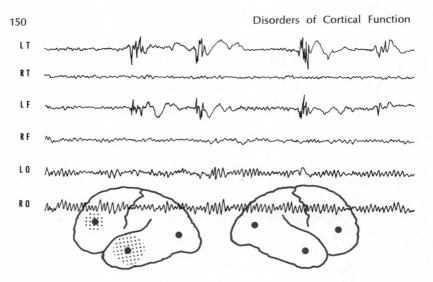

**Fig. 5-5** Electroencephalogram characteristic of partial epilepsy shows a multiple spike and slow wave focus on the left side near the temporal and frontal recording electrodes. Time and voltage markers are equivalent to those of Fig. 5-1.

concurrent subjective sensations or observable changes in the patient.

### Grand mal

Characteristically, a grand mal attack begins with an immediate loss of consciousness because the epileptogenic focus lies either within, or else projects very quickly to, the brain's alerting centers. Excitatory discharges then set up positive feedback oscillating circuits between the cerebral cortex and the thalamus, with eventual excitatory discharges descending to the lower motor centers of the brain stem and spinal motor centers. With millions of neurons firing at rates often exceeding 500 to 100 Hz, these lower motor centers discharge continuously into the somatic and visceral musculature. Therefore, all somatic musculature contracts strongly. The limbs, trunk, and neck stiffen in rigid extensor postures, since extensor muscles tend to be more powerful than flexors. The pupils dilate, respiration ceases, the heart rate slows, and salivation, micturition, and defecation may occur. This so-called initial tonic phase of the convulsion lasts from 30 to 90 seconds. The tonic phase corresponds to the electroencephalographic pattern illustrated in Fig. 5-2(B). It is gradually succeeded by a brief period (10-15 seconds) of tremulousness, which, in turn, is followed by generalized bilaterally synchronous muscle jerks alternating with periods of relaxation corresponding to a pattern of periodic bilaterally synchronous spikes and waves [Fig. 5-2(C)]. Clinically, this is termed the clonic phase. The generalized seizure ends with the patient in a deep coma for 3 to 10 minutes, and, during this period, high voltage slow waves, without spikes, predominate in the electroencephalogram [Fig. 5-2 (C)]. The patient arouses confused and tired, and then he generally falls into a normal sleep. Upon awakening some 2 to 10 hours later, he is usually back to his pre-seizure level of behavior. The electroencephalogram, however, may take 24 to 48 hours to recover its pre-seizure pattern.

Any epileptic seizure, including grand mal, begins when biochemical and physiological events trigger excitatory discharges of high energy from a susceptible nerve cell or cluster of nerve cells. As we noted earlier, we can only speculate about the nature of these events. The seizure ends when "resistance" to the central excitatory state builds up, but, again, the exact nature of this resistance is not clearly understood (see p. 163). Undoubtedly, hyperpolarization in the surrounding neuropil and inhibitory input to the excitable neurons, as well as exhaustion of nutritive substances and withdrawal of potassium ion from the excitable regions by gial cells, act to stop the seizure.

## Petit mal

Petit mal epilepsy begins with a quasi-electrical disturbance in or near the centers of consciousness. The electroencephalographic pattern characteristic of a petit mal seizure (Fig. 5-3) differs from that of grand mal, since each excitatory discharge (single spike) is immediately followed by a longer-lasting, high-voltage, hyperpolarizing, inhibitory discharge (slow wave). The spike-wave pattern is repeated at a rate of 3/second for periods of 5 to 20 seconds. Clinically, the patient is rendered unaware of his environment almost immediately. He abruptly stops his normal activity during the seizure (ictus) and stares vacantly into space. There may be a generalized, but slight, increase in muscle tone and a few bilaterally synchronous muscle jerks or eye blinks at the frequency of 3/second. Then the clinical seizure and the series of single spike and wave discharges end together as abruptly as they began.

## Psychomotor

Psychomotor seizures have their triggering events within structures of the temporal lobes. The electroencephalographic pattern characteristic of some psychomotor seizures is one of 4-6 Hz, 50-100 microvolt, flat-topped waves from all regions of the cerebral cortex. In other seizures, the discharges are limited to the deep lying limbic system and may not be seen in the routine electroencephalogram, which is recorded from the surface. The interictal electroencephalographic pattern, unlike that of generalized grand mal and petit mal, is usually normal (Fig. 5-1) and often indicates a focus of epileptogenic activity in one temporal lobe (Fig. 5-5). Clinically, psychomotor seizures differ from both grand mal and petit mal attacks. Although consciousness is impaired and memory for the duration of the attack obliterated, there continues to be automatic, stereotyped, semi–purposeful, well-coordinated movement. As a rule, the seizure is a 1- to 4-minute period of masticatory (licking or mouthing) movements and rhythmic body rocking accompanied by rubbing, picking, or patting movements of the hands and feet, the face otherwise remaining expressionless and dull. Psychomotor seizures, however, may become more complex and prolonged. The individual may amble about the room interacting with various objects (including people) in strange, inappropriate, and ineffective ways. Some such habitual acts as brushing the teeth, dressing and undressing, and even driving a car can be performed during a psychomotor seizure, but complex actions requiring learning, judgment, propositional speech, and socially responsible behavior cannot. The "psycho" portion of the term psychomotor epilepsy derives from the observation that patients during a seizure may display wild-eyed excitement, fear, or other emotions and interact with persons and objects as though they had some highly charged psychological significance.

## Generalized seizures

Some generalized seizures present clinically as intermittent, symmetrical, myoclonic flexor jerks of the trunk, neck, and proximal extremities in infants and young children (infantile spasms). The electroencephalogram correlate of this is a diffuse pattern of high voltage slow waves, single and multiple spikes that occur synchronously (Fig. 5-4, arrows) and asynchronously or multifocally (hypsarrythmia). The entire record is in a continuous state of epileptiform activity, and the child, correspondingly, is dull and incompletely aware of the world about him. He appears, and often is, mentally retarded.

## Partial seizures

Partial seizures, which begin and end without significantly blocking the patient's consciousness or memory for the seizure events, are of two types: focal motor (jacksonian seizures) and focal sensory. Focal motor attacks begin with a slow repetitive jerking of some body part, e.g., one thumb or a corner of the mouth, which jerks faster and more strongly over a period of 5 to 15 seconds before the spasm spreads to adjacent body parts contralateral to the hemisphere containing the epilectic focus. The seizure ends uneventfully with a gradual slowing down of the clonic jerking. The victim of such a jacksonian motor "march" has no control over the limbs affected by the seizure.

Focal sensory seizures originate with hyperexcitable neurons in or near cortical areas responsible for sensory experience. As a rule, the experience is wholly subjective and remains confined to a primary sensory modality (somesthetic, visual, auditory vestibular, or olfactory), but, occasionally, the experience is complex enough to elicit emotional feelings and long-forgotten memories of past events. In the case of partial seizures limited to special somatosensory receiving or association regions, the experiences are perceived on the side of the body or in the spatial field opposite the involved cerebral hemisphere. Emotional experiences and memories associated with epileptiform discharges have no spatial reference, that is, they do not evoke specifically localized sensory experiences.

Experimental counterparts to focal seizures in humans have been provided by the studies of Wilder Penfield and his neurosurgical colleagues at the Montreal Neurological Institute. Penfield was able to reproduce sensory experiences and involuntary movements in awake, conscious epileptic subjects simply by electrically stimulating discrete cortical areas during surgery. Similar reports from different patients over the years led Penfield to construct a composite "map" of the human cerebral cortex in which cortical location (structure) correlated with experience or movement (function.) Before some epileptics have their generalized seizure they have brief experiences similar to those of Wilder Penfield's electrically simulated ones. The epileptic, in these instances, receives a warning that he is about to have a seizure shortly before he loses consciousness. The warning, sometimes called an aura, after the Latin word for breeze, tends to be specific for the individual epileptic and can be readily identified by him from among the thousands of other sensations that crowd his consciousness daily. It is not unusual for the patient with generalized grand mal or psychomotor epilepsy to experience his aura and yet not have a generalized seizure. This form of partial seizure is termed abortive epilepsy.

The clinical phenomena of focal epilepsy cannot be adequately described by grouping them into motor, sensory, partial, or abortive types because reverberating excitatory discharges within the central nervous system are capable of producing behavioral disturbances that cannot be easily linked to a particular region of the brain. Poggio and others have described four main cortical-subcortical circuits within which oscillatory discharging seizure activity can be produced. They are (1) the frontal granular cortex to the caudate nucleus and dorsomedial thalamic nucleus; (2) the peri-Rolandic cortex to the putamen and the lateral nuclear mass of the thalamus; (3) the temporal cortex to the amygdala, the hippocampus, and the septum; and (4) the visual striate cortex to the pulvinar and lateral geniculate nucleus of the dorsal thalamus. It is probable that temporary episodes of aphasia, paralysis, apraxia, agnosia, and disorientation, as well as experiences of displacement in time or place, paranoia, or depression, may be associated with epileptic activity in one or more of these circuits.

## Summary

All epilepsy is essentially the same electrophysiological process, which can be triggered by a wide variety of insults including glial scars, tumors, nutritional distrubances, and metabolic disorders. Some seizures are clinically stereotyped, such as grand mal and petit mal, but most seizures may present more varied clinical as well as electroencephalographic patterns depending upon their site of origin and mode of spread within the brain. The discovery of a potential location for the physiological triggering events by means of a spike and wave focus on the electroencephalogram or the patient's description of an aura helps in making an accurate diagnosis among the innumerable clinical presentations of epilepsy.

## General references

Boshes, L. D. and F. A. Gibbs. 1972. Epilepsy handbook, 2nd ed. Charles C. Thomas, Springfield, Ill., 196 pp.

Jasper, H. H., A. A. Ward, and A. Pope, eds. 1969. Basic mechanisms of the epilepsies. Little, Brown, Boston, 835 pp.

Lennox, W. G. and M. A. Lennox. 1960. Epilepsy and related disorders. Vols. I and II. Little, Brown, Boston, 1168 pp.

Livingstone, S. 1972. Comprehensive management of epilepsy in infancy, childhood, and adolescence. Charles C. Thomas, Springfield, Ill., 657 pp.

Penfield, W. and T. C. Erickson. 1941. Epilepsy and cerebral localization. Charles C. Thomas, Springfield, Ill., 623 pp.

Poggio, G. F., A. E. Walker, and O. J. Andy. 1956. The propagation of cortical after-discharge through subcortical structures. Arch. Neurol. Psychiat. 75:350-361.

Rodin, E. A. 1968. The prognosis of patients with epilepsy. Charles C. Thomas, Springfield, Ill., 454 pp.

Schmidt, R. P. and B. J. Wilder. 1968. Epilepsy. Contemporary neurology Series No. 2, F. A. Davis, Philadelphia, 220 pp.

Sutherland, J. M. and H. Tait. 1969. The epilepsies: Modern diagnosis and treatment. E. and S. Livingstone, London, 128 pp.

## PATHOPHYSIOLOGY OF EPILEPTIC DISCHARGE

SIDNEY GOLDRING

## Introduction

Figure 5-6 shows an electroencephalogram made during a seizure that occurred spontaneously in a patient with idiopathic epilepsy. The same wave pattern could appear with seizures caused by a brain tumor, anoxia, hypoglycemia, disturbances of blood electrolyte composition, convulsant drugs (Metrazol), electric shock, etc. suggesting that a common pathophysiology underlies many different seizure

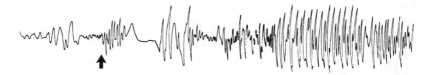

**Fig. 5-6** Electroencephalogram showing the onset (arrow) of a spontaneous seizure in an epileptic patient.

states. Recently, many studies have examined the behavior of single cells during the development of experimentally induced seizures with brain wave patterns similar to those shown in Fig. 5-6. The data accumulating from these studies are beginning to identify mechanisms that lead to and sustain seizure discharge in cellular aggregates, and it is with this aspect of epilepsy that this section deals.

## Normal neuronal function basic to the understanding of seizure mechanism

*Membrane potential.* The neuronal membrane is leaky with respect to the principal ions that inhabit the extra- and intracellular fluid. Thus, $Na^+$, $K^+$, and $Cl^-$, which are all distributed unequally in the intra- and extracellular compartments, move across the cell membrane. Being more abundant extracellularly, $Na^+$ and $Cl^-$ leak in, while $K^+$, which is more concentrated intracellularly, leaks out. The movement is one of passive diffusion, which requires no energy to sustain it. The consequences of such ionic diffusion will be demonstrated by using $K^+$ as an example. As this ion moves downhill along its concentration gradient, the membrane's capacitance (think of the membrane as a condenser) becomes electrically charged. The potential at which this electrostatic charge comes to oppose any further ionic movement is the equilibrium potential for $K^+$. Each ion has a different equilibrium potential, and membrane permeability to a specific ion is determined by the state of neuronal activity. Thus, at any one moment, the membrane potential is the equilibrium potential for the ion or ions to which the membrane is permeable at that time. For example, at rest, when the neuronal membrane is much more permeable (50-75 times) to $K^+$ and $Cl^-$

than to $Na^+$, the membrane potential is largely determined by these ions (mainly $K^+$). Actually, the resting membrane potential is about —70 mV, which is considerably less than the equilibrium potential for $K^+$ (i.e., the $E_k$ is around —90 mV).* This probably relates to the fact that we can only gather data concerning membrane potential by impaling cells with microelectrodes, and such injury very likely leads to an underestimation of all recorded membrane potentials. That is, under experimental conditions neurons in the resting state are partially depolarized. Furthermore, since the resting membrane is slightly permeable to $Na^+$, there is a steady, albeit small, intracellular leakage of this ion, which also tends to depolarize the cell.

*The sodium pump.* At this junction, it is convenient to review another cellular mechanism that will bear on our discussion of the epileptic discharge. Obviously, if $Na^+$ leakage continues unchecked, the unequal distribution of $Na^+$, which we know exists across the resting membrane, could not be maintained; some mechanism must operate to expel $Na^+$ outwardly against its concentration gradient. This has been shown to be an active process, which uses metabolic energy derived from phosphorus-rich compounds, that is, adenosine triphosphate (ATP)—the sodium pump. Actually, it is a Na/K coupled pump, and, until recently, it was thought to be an electrically neutral one, neutrality being maintained by one $K^+$ moving inward for every $Na^+$ pumped out. There is now good evidence, however, that the pump is electrogenic, especially during intense neuronal activity, when it appears to cause an unequal exchange of ions with 2 $K^+$ being taken in for every 3 $Na^+$ that are expelled. Such unequal pumping hyperpolarizes the membrane, and, as will be seen later, this mechanism of altering membrane potential may play an important role in terminating seizure discharge.

*Synaptic transmission.* During synaptic transmission, the post-synaptic membrane becomes selectively permeable to a specific ion or ions. The release of transmitter substance by the pre-synaptic terminal evokes the permeability change, but specialization of the post-synaptic junction determines whether the induced permeability change will have an excitatory or inhibitory influence. For ex-

* The polarity of the potential refers to the cell's interior, the inside (as measured with the microelectrode) being negative to a large extracellular reference electrode.

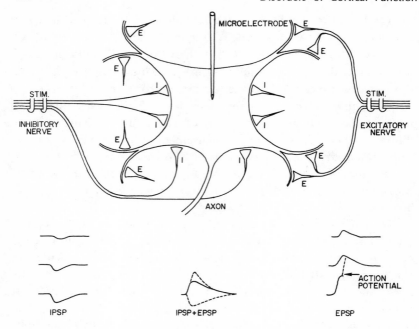

**Fig. 5-7** A diagram of excitatory (E) and inhibitory (I) synapses converging on a neuron. Stim, stimulating electrodes. These records of inhibitory and excitatory post-synaptic potentials are responses to stimuli of increasing intensity, stimulus intensity increasing from top to bottom. The excitatory post-synaptic potential (EPSP) to strongest stimulus is of sufficient magnitude to generate an action potential, the rising limb of which is shown. The stimulus used to evoke this response will not generate an action potential if it is applied simultaneously with a stimulus to the inhibitory nerve, since the canceling effect of the inhibitory post-synaptic potential (IPSP) generated prevents the excitatory post-synaptic potential from reaching the firing level (middle).

ample, acetylcholine released at the nerve-muscle junction produces excitation, whereas its release by vagal terminals at the pacemaker region of the heart inhibits that organ's action. It is important to our discussion that the two different states (excitation and inhibition) relate indirectly to the specific ion or ions to which the membrane is made transiently permeable and more directly to the change in membrane potential caused by that altered ionic permeability.

In the central nervous system, the excitatory transmitter opens channels in the post-synaptic membrane to both $Na^+$ ($E_k = + 60$

mV) and $K^+$ ($E_k = -90$ mV). The net effect is an equilibrium potential that approaches zero and depolarization of the membrane by the excitatory post-synaptic potential. Release of the inhibitory transmitter has the opposite effect, stabilizing the membrane at its resting level or hyperpolarizing it. Selective permeability to Cl (and perhaps also $K^+$) accounts for the inhibitory post-synaptic potential. In any one neuron, both of these competing influences (depolarization and hyperpolarization) interact to modulate the resting membrane potential because synaptic drives from many nerve cells, some excitatory and others inhibitory, usually converge on the membrane of a single neuron.

The potentials generated at each of the many synapses summate so that the greater the number of synapses brought into play, the larger the synaptic potential that one measures with a microelectrode. That is, the membrane responds in graded fashion to increasing intensities of activation. When the balance of synaptic drive favors excitation, the membrane depolarizes; and, if the depolarization reaches $-15$ to $-20$ mV, an explosive and huge additional depolarization occurs (the membrane potential not merely goes to zero but reverses to $+60$ mV), signaling the sudden development of $Na^+$ permeability. This is the all-or-none action potential or nerve impulse. In contrast to synaptic potentials, it is propagated along the axon and, upon reaching the axon terminal, it causes a quantal release of transmitter that alters the membrane potential of a neighboring cell (Fig. 5-7).

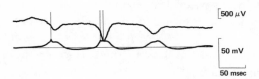

$\lceil$ 500 μV

50 mV

50 msec

**Fig. 5-8** Simultaneous recordings (cat) of spontaneous activity from the cortical surface (electroencephalogram) and a single neuron impaled in the cortex directly underlying the surface electrode. The top trace is an electroencephalogram; the bottom an intracellular record. In the intracellular record, the first two excitatory post-synaptic potentials generate an action potential; the last does not; each potential corresponds to a deflection of similar configuration in the surface record. In this, and Figs. 5-8 through 5-14, negative is downward in the surface record; in the intracellular trace, upward excursion signifies depolarization. (From Goldring, unpublished data.)

Synaptic potentials last much longer (some 20 times) than action potentials, but, for our purposes, it is more important to know that the electrical records made from the scalp or brain's surface reflect synaptic potentials and not the propagated nerve impulse (Fig. 5-8). Examining the membrane potential changes that correspond to changes in the electroencephalogram as an epileptic discharge develops has revealed some important aspects of seizure pathophysiology. Most of our information derives from studies in the cerebral cortex and hippocampus of the cat and monkey, and the most common methods for producing epileptic discharge have been strong electrical stimulation and convulsant drugs administered topically or systemically. In general, neuronal activity in all of these experimental settings undergoes a similar transition as normal cortex is made to behave paroxysmally. Depending upon the experimental animals, however, the region of brain, the convulsant stimulus, and the specific question being explored, one or another aspect of the seizure mechanism is emphasized. We draw on several of the many recently published studies to answer, tentatively, some common questions.

**Why does a seizure begin?**

In most experimental models of epilepsy, excessive depolarization of the neuronal membrane is the necessary prelude to the appearance of seizure activity. To illustrate this point we will describe the effect of electrical stimulation applied to the brain's surface. Such stimulation, if of sufficient intensity, evokes seizure activity in the electrocorticogram recorded in the immediate surroundings of the site of stimulation.

A single strong electrical stimulus applied to the surface of the cat cerebral cortex will cause a cortical neuron located directly beneath the stimulating electrode to discharge. The resulting nerve impulse is followed by a prolonged membrane hyperpolarization (about 200 msec; probably an inhibitory post-synaptic potential), during which all spontaneous discharge stops (Fig. 5-9). If the stimulus is applied repetitively (i.e., 20/second), the second stimulus may not generate a nerve impulse, only an excitatory post-synaptic potential because this potential is produced during membrane hyperpolarization, and the net change in membrane potential is not

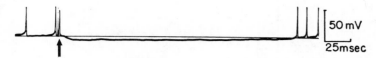

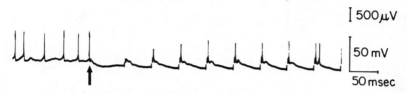

**Fig. 5-9.** Neuronal intracellular responses to electrical stimulation of the surface of the cat's cerebral cortex. *Upper:* Arrow indicates the response to a single stimulus interrupting spontaneous discharge. Note the prolonged hyperpolarization (inhibitory post-synaptic potential) that follows the evoked action potential. *Lower:* Arrow indicates the onset of repetitive electrical stimulation The excitatory post-synaptic potential evoked by the second stimulus does not generate a nerve impulse, the last gives rise to repetitive firing. See text for explanation.

sufficiently depolarizing to generate a nerve impulse. As repetitive stimulation continues, the hyperpolarization is replaced by depolarization, which grows progressively in amplitude, and the cell begins to fire repetitively, rather than singly, to each of the sequential stimuli (Fig. 5-9). Thus, the main effect of the epileptogenic stimulus is a depolarizing excitation, which overcomes the protective hyperpolarizing action of the cell's inhibitory mechanism. At the stimulus intensity used in Fig. 5-9, the cell returns to its pre-stimulatory state almost immediately after the electrical stimulation ceases. If stimulus strength is increased, however, the recurring and growing excitatory post-synaptic potentials summate and fuse into a sustained membrane depolarization, and the cell begins to fire at an abnormally high frequency (500/second rather than 60-80/second) [Fig. 5-10(A)]. Now, upon turning off the stimulus current, the cell does not resume its normal pre-stimulatory firing pattern as it did when stimulation is less intense. Rather, the membrane remains depolarized, and the membrane potential begins to oscillate [Fig. 5-10(B and C)]. The oscillations are recurring de-

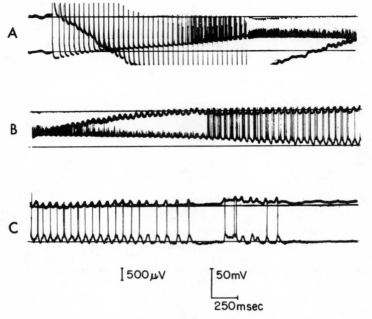

**Fig. 5-10** Changes in intracellular potential incident to a strong repetitive stimulus that leads to seizure discharge. (A), (B), and (C) are continuous. The straight horizontal lines are baselines from which potential changes are read. The lower trace of each pair is the intracellular record. In (A), the surface and the intracellular record cross so that the intracellular record becomes the upper one. The stimulus period is identified by shock artifacts in (A). (From Sugaya, Goldring, and O'Leary, 1964.) The baseline swing in the surface record indicates that the cortical surface becomes negative with the onset of seizure activity. At its onset, it roughly mirrors the sustained depolarization shown in the intracellular record. Such dc shifts are not observed in the electroencephalographic records because electroencephalographs employ capacity-coupled amplifiers, which block direct current.

polarizations (excitatory post-synaptic potentials?) and appear at approximately the same time that seizure activity appears in the surface record. Each surface deflection (convulsive "spike" in electroencephalographic terminology) mirrors a depolarizing oscillation, and this strongly suggests that the electroencephalographic seizure activity is the field potential generated by membrane potential oscillations occurring synchronously in thousands of neurons.

Similar correlations between surface and intracellular recordings are seen following intravenous injection of the convulsant drug,

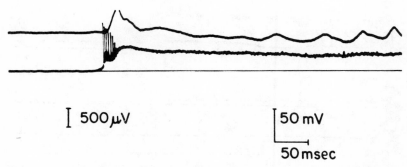

I 500 μV          [50 mV
                  50 msec

**Fig. 5-11** Paroxysmal depolarizing shift occurring in the interictal period follow-ing i.v. Metrazol (cat). Upper trace surface record; lower trace, intracellular. The paroxysmal depolarizing shift occurs concurrently with a convulsive "spike" in the surface trace. (From Goldring, unpublished data.)

Metrazol, which can produce recurring seizure discharges. In the interictal periods, convulsive "spikes" appear in the electroencepha-logram concurrently with large and prolonged membrane depolari-zations, the start of each such depolarization giving rise to a high frequency cell discharge (Fig. 5-11). An electrical stimulus applied to the cortical surface during these interictal periods produces an identical depolarization and cell discharge. Such depolarizations (spontaneous and evoked), called paroxysmal depolarizing shifts, have been studied extensively during seizure activity produced by the topical application of penicillin, and recent data indicate that they are probably giant excitatory post-synaptic potentials. The sig-nificance some workers impute to these findings is that seizure ac-tivity represents an altered state of synaptic transmission rather than a deficiency of the post-synaptic membrane. In other words, the individual neuron is not "epileptic." Instead, the epilepto-genicity stems from an altered state of synaptic interaction, which is reversible.

## Why does a seizure stop?

Seizure activity induced in the hippocampus by repetitive stimu-lation of the fornix also begins with sustained membrane depolari-zation. Of particular importance to our discussion is the fact that seizure termination is associated with a large, enduring membrane hyperpolarization. The hyperpolarization lasts many seconds; dur-

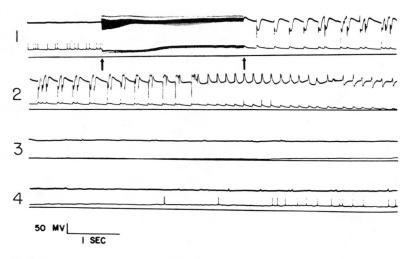

**Fig. 5-12** Seizure in an intact fornix preparation (cat). Top record in each numbered row, the surface electrode; bottom record, intracellular microelectrode. The line underneath the microelectrode record is an arbitrary baseline. Arrows indicate the period of stimulation. The voltage calibration refers to both surface (2 mV) and intracellular (50 mV) records. (From Kandel and Spencer, 1961.) At the onset of a stimulation, the membrane first hyperpolarizes, but the depolarizing effect of the electrical stimulus soon overwhelms the cell's protective inhibitory mechanism, producing a sustained membrane depolarization and seizure activity. Termination of the seizure is associated with membrane hyperpolarization (the intracellular trace approaches baseline).

ing this time, the cell stops firing, and surface brain potentials are suppressed (Fig. 5-12). Seizures induced by application of penicillin to the surface of cerebral cortex terminate similarly. Ayala and his colleagues have suggested that the hyperpolarization may be generated by an electrogenic sodium pump, and Ransom and Goldring have come to a similar conclusion because they found that membrane resistance does not change during such hyperpolarization. This would not be the case if the hyperpolarization were a result of synaptic inhibition because the latter is a function of increased $Cl^-$ permeability, which changes membrane resistance.

## What keeps a seizure from spreading?

In penicillin-induced epileptogenic foci, the paroxysmal depolarizing shifts are usually followed by an equally long, or longer hyper-

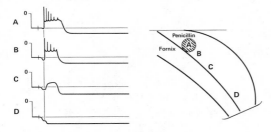

**Fig. 5-13.** Schematic diagram of surface and intracellular recordings from cells in and around a penicillin focus. *Right:* Diagram of the exposed dorsal hippo campus and fornix with the recording sites indicated by letter. (A) A typical response from the pyramidal cells within the penicillin focus illustrates the early depolarizing potential, with action potentials arising from a flat background followed by a long-lasting hyperpolarization. Successive action potentials of a burst would be smaller due to the inactivation of the soma spike-generating mechanism; (B) intermediate form consisting of early hyperpolarization, the depolarizing potential with action potentials, and finally a late hyperpolarization; (C) another intermediate form consisting of a more delayed and somewhat reduced depolarizing potential arising out of hyperpolarization; (D) pure hyperpolarizing response characteristic of cells at the periphery of the focus. Often the inhibitory post-synaptic potential appeared to be double—one due to fornix triggering and one to the peripheral inhibition generated by the cells in the center of the focus during the paroxysmal discharge. (From Dichter and Spencer, 1969.)

polarization. Depending upon the site of electrical recording in relation to the penicillin focus, these convulsive potentials will show greater or lesser degrees of hyperpolarization. For example, within the penicillin focus itself, the depolarization is followed by hyperpolarization with the former predominating. As one moves farther and farther away from the penicillin focus, however, cells will eventually show only hyperpolarization. That is, there is an inhibitory surround (Fig. 5-13), which could function to prevent spread of seizure activity to distant sites.

### Are glia also involved?

Recently, glia in leech, amphibia, and mammalian cerebral cortex have been shown to be exquisitely sensitive to $K^+$. In fact, in leech and amphibia (and probably also in mammalian cortex), the glial membrane is almost exclusively permeable to potassium, and the membrane potential equals the equilibrium potential for $K^+$ (—90

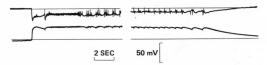

**Fig. 5-14** Glial depolarization associated with seizure discharge in the cerebral cortex (cat). Upper trace, surface record; lower trace, intracellular record. The break in the middle of the traces is an omission of many seconds of record during which time there was no significant change from that shown before and after the break. The glial cell is massively depolarized (45 mV) during seizure activity. Observe the much closer correspondence between the glial depolarization and the surface-negative dc shift (this figure) than between the neuronal depolarization and surface dc shift (Fig. 5-10); this indicates that surface dc changes associated with seizure discharge reflect predominantly glial membrane changes. (From Ransom and Goldring, unpublished.)

mV). It has also been demonstrated that there is electrical continuity between glia. Thus, a focal gial depolarization resulting from an increase in extracellular $K^+$ (i.e., by excessive neuronal activity) (Fig. 5-14) will draw current from neighboring unaffected glia, and $K^+$ will move into cells in the region of high $K^+$ concentration and outwardly from unaffected, but electrically coupled glia. That is, glia passively transfer excess $K^+$ away from a region of excitation and help maintain extracellular homeostasis. Such spatial buffering of extracellular $K^+$ could play a role in preventing the onset of seizure activity, since an increase in extracellular $K^+$ also depolarizes the neuronal membrane, and excessive neuronal depolarization is epileptogenic.

## General references

Ajmone-Marsan, C. 1969. Acute effects of topical epileptogenic agents. Pages 299-319 *in* H. H. Jasper, A. A. Ward, Jr., and A. Pope, eds. Basic mechanisms of the epilepsies. Little, Brown, Boston.

Ayala, G. F., H. Matsumoto, and R. J. Gumnit. 1970. Excitability changes and inhibitory mechanisms in neocortical neurons during seizures. J. Neurophysiol. 33:73-85.

Castelluci, V. F. and S. Goldring. 1970. Contribution to steady potential shifts of slow depolarization in cells presumed to be glia. Electro-enceph. clin. Neurophysiol. 28:109-118.

Dichter, M. and W. A. Spencer. 1969. Penicillin-induced interictal discharges from the cat hippocampus. 1. Characteristics and topographical features. J. Neurophysiol. 32:649-662.

Eccles, J. C. 1969. Excitatory and inhibitory mechanisms in brain. Pages 229-252 *in* H. H. Jasper, A. A. Ward, Jr., and A. Pope, eds. 1969. Basic mechanisms of the epilepsies. Little, Brown, Boston.

Kandel, E. R. and W. A. Spencer. 1961. Excitation and inhibition of single pyramidal cells during hippocampal seizure. Exp. Neurol. 4:162-179.

Katz, B. 1966. Nerve, muscle and synapse. McGraw-Hill, New York.

Kuffler, S. W. and J. G. Nicholls. 1966. The physiology of neuroglial cells. *In* Reviews of physiology biochemistry and experimental pharmacology. Springer-Verlag, Berlin/New York.

Matsumoto, H. and C. Ajmone-Marsan. 1964. Cortical cellular phenomena in experimental epilepsy: Interictal manifestations. Exp. Neurol. 9:286-304.

Pape, L. and R. Katzman. 1972. Response of glia in cat sensorimotor cortex to increased extracellular potassium. Brain Res. 38:71-92.

Prince, D. A. and B. J. Wilder. 1967. Control mechanisms in cortical epileptogenic foci. Arch. Neurol. 16:194-202.

Ransom, B. R. and S. Goldring. 1900. Ionic determinants of the membrane potential of cells presumed to be glia in cerebral cortex of cat. J. Neurophysiol.

Ransom, B. R. and S. Goldring. 1900. Slow hyperpolarization in cells presumed to be glia in cerebral cortex of cat. J. Neurophysiol.

Spencer, W. A. and E. R. Kandel. 1969. Synaptic inhibition in seizures. Pages 575-603 *in* H. H. Jasper, A. A. Ward, Jr., and A. Pope, eds. 1969. Basic mechanisms of the epilepsies. Little, Brown, Boston.

Sugaya, E., S. Goldring, and J. L. O'Leary. 1964. Intracellular potentials associated with direct cortical response and seizure discharge in cat. Electroenceph. clin. Neurophysiol. 17:661-669.

Thomas, R. C. 1972. Electrogenic sodium pump in nerve and muscle cells. Physiol. Rev. 52:563-594.

Ward, A. A., Jr. 1969. The epileptic neuron: Chronic foci in animals and man. Pages 263-298 *in* H. H. Jasper, A. A. Ward, Jr., and A. Pope. eds. 1969. Basic mechanisms of the epilepsies. Little, Brown, Boston.

## NEUROCHEMISTRY OF EPILEPTIC DISCHARGE

JAMES A. FERRENDELLI

Seizures result from the rapid and repetitive depolarization of neurons. As has been discussed, depolarization is accompanied by an accumulation of sodium ions within the cell and a decrease of intracellular potassium. During repolarization, as the membrane returns to its normal resting potential, $Na^+$ ions are "pumped out," and $K^+$ ions enter neurons. This is an energy-consuming process and is preceded by an increase in $Na^+$-$K^+$ adenosine triphosphatase activity.

During an epileptic seizure, involved neurons are more easily depolarized and less apt to return to a normal resting membrane potential between discharges. Despite intensive investigation and numerous thories, the basic chemical mechanisms that initiate and sustain seizure discharge remain unknown. Epileptic discharges can be initiated experimentally by a number of techniques, which either enhance excitatory impulses impinging upon the neuron or decrease the influence of inhibitory synapses. Convulsants may act presynaptically to influence the amount of transmitter generated or, like strychnine, post-synaptically to reduce the inhibitory postsynaptic potential. Topical application to the cortical surface of acetylcholine, which normally may serve as an excitatory transmitter in the cerebral cortex, produces focal seizure activity. A variety of chemicals that deplete the brain of $\gamma$-aminobutyric acid, a putative inhibitory transmitter, also initiate seizure activity when applied topically or given systemically. Substances that interfere with neuronal energy metabolism result in a greater propensity for epileptic discharge, as do such drugs as ouabain, which directly interfere with membrane transport of $Na^+$ and $K^+$. Nevertheless, it has not been shown that exquisite sensitivity to possible excitatory transmitters or a decrease in putative inhibitory transmitters precedes naturally occurring or electrically induced seizures in man or experimental animals. Nor is it clear that epileptic activity is preceded by a change in conductance of either $Na^+$ or $K^+$, or by a decrease in the formation of high energy phosphate bonds as a result of a block in the oxidative metabolism of glucose.

Neurons involved in an epileptic seizure utilize considerably more energy than they would if the cerebrum were functioning at its normal resting level. In addition to increased ionic transport, other cellular metabolic processes are accelerated during seizure activity. These include the synthesis of neuro-transmitters, the turnover of lipids and proteins, and axoplasmic transport. These processes, directly or indirectly, require the use of chemically generated energy.

During the seizure, there is an increase in energy production. As in other tissues, the major direct source of energy in brain is adenosine triphosphate (ATP). Unlike most other tissues, however, the brain depends almost entirely upon the metabolism of glucose for the production of high energy phosphate bonds. Increased amounts of glucose are utilized by the central nervous system during seizure activity. As long as energy utilization does not exceed the capacity of energy-producing systems in brain, no energy debt occurs. During major motor seizures induced in mice by electric shock, however, there is a rapid decrease in brain levels of ATP, phosphocreatine, and glucose, and a concomitant accumulation of lactate. This indicates that the rate of utilization of high energy phosphate during seizure activity is greater than its rate of production. This occurs in all subcortical areas examined, as well as in the cerebral cortex. In contrast, the generalized motor seizures elicited in susceptible mice by a loud sound, although clinically identical to the seizures produced by electric shock, differ chemically in that there is a decrease in ATP, phosphocreatine, and glucose only in the subcortical regions of the brain. The concentration of the substrates in the cerebral cortex remains unchanged. Little is known of the regional metabolism of the brain during generalized tonic-clonic seizures induced by other mechanisms or of the metabolic changes associated with other types of seizure activity (focal, psychomotor, petit mal).

Recent studies have indicated that the central nervous system energy debt occurring during generalized motor seizures may be accentuated by systemic factors. Grand mal seizures in unanesthetized, nonparalyzed animals or man are accompanied by vigorous muscle activity and, during the tonic phase of the seizure, a period of apnea that results in transient hypoxemia. Apparently, increased metabolic activity in skeletal muscle, in association with hypoxemia, results in the central nervous system receiving insufficient oxygen to maintain the rate of oxidative phosphorylation needed to keep up with the increase in energy used. Anaerobic glycolysis alone does not produce enough high energy phosphate bonds to maintain normal levels of ATP.

It has been observed that seizures produced in paralyzed, anesthetized animals with an adequate oxygen supply are not accompanied by a fall in high energy phosphates and glucose or a rise in lactate in brain, although cerebral blood flow and cerebral oxygen and glucose consumption do increase. These experiments are also interesting in a negative sense with respect to the cessation of seizure activity and the decrease in neuronal function that is often observed after an epileptic discharge. It has sometimes been assumed that, at the conclusion of a seizure, the neuron does not function

normally because it has incurred a severe oxygen debt, or there is
an accumulation of acid metabolites, which interfere with the normal metabolic processes of the cell. Since seizures conclude spontaneously, and subsequently decreased neuronal activity occurs in
anesthetized, well-ventilated animals, who do not accumulate excessive lactate or incur an oxygen debt, these theories concerning
the termination of seizures and post-epileptic paralysis no longer
appear tenable.

## General references

Alpers, R. W., G. J. Siegel, R. Katzman, and B. W. Agranoff, eds. 1972.
    Basic neurochemistry. Little, Brown, Boston.
Jasper, H. H., A. A. Ward, Jr., and A. Pope, eds. 1969. Basic mechanisms of
    the epilepsies. Little, Brown, Boston.
McIlwain, H. and H. S. Bachelard. 1971. Biochemistry of the central nerv-
    ous system. Williams & Wilkins, Baltimore.
Schmidt, R. P. and B. J. Wilder. 1968. Epilepsy. Contemporary neurology
    series Vol. 2. F. A. Davis, Philadelphia.
Tower, D. B. 1960. Neurochemistry of epilepsy. Charles C. Thomas, Spring-
    field, Ill.

## THE HIGHER-ORDER DYSFUNCTIONS: APRAXIA, AGNOSIA, AND APHASIA

WILLIAM B. HARDIN, JR., AND RICHARD M. MERSON

### Introduction

The neural mechanisms that underlie movement, perception, and
such higher-order activities as language and cognition have tradi-
tionally been the province of philosophers and psychologists. Only
recently have experimental physiologists begun to explore these
mechanisms, and, thus far, we have no firmly based neurophysiological explanations for such disorders of higher-order functions as
the apraxias, agnosias, and aphasias.

Clinical neurologists customarily think of the central nervous
system in terms of its structural and functional interrelationships.
There are basically two opposing viewpoints in this regard. According to one, the brain is a composite organ made up of modular
parts, each serving a distinct function according to its internal
structure and location. Thus, there is an area (modular part) that

functions to make judgments regarding the color of objects, another to discern the meaning of spoken language, still another to guide the movements of the arm and hand during writing, and so on through the infinite variety of perceptions, cognitive decisions, and skilled movements the adult brain controls.

According to the second view, the brain is, for all intent and purposes, a single large integrative unit, no part of which operates as a distinct "center" for integration or association. That some regions of the cortico-thalamic feedback systems appear to function more in the visual mode or the tactual mode or the auditory mode is merely an artifact of our testing methods. In reality, every thought, every perceptual experience, is, in fact, a total neurophysiological experience evoking memory traces from innumerable memory banks scattered throughout the brain. Destruction of the primary visual cortex, for example, prevents or impedes appropriate visual input, thereby causing a hiatus within the total experience we call "visual." Yet we can still "revisualize," we can still dream "pictorial events," and we can still speak and think in primarily "visual" terms because the memories of prior visual experiences still await recall among the many recesses of our brains.

The former viewpoint (specific localization of functions to centers of integration) is the more comfortable one for the clinical neurologist, who must, out of practical necessity, evaluate his patient's central nervous system function by means of a highly restricted, stereotyped examination. The neurologist, finding in his patient a disorganization in the smooth performance of one or more neurological tests, infers the "dysfunction of a center" (a locus of neurons with a particular job to do) at a specific place(s) within the nervous system.

The experimental physiologist, working with a whole brain, is impressed by the variability of the central nervous system's responses to apparently identical stimuli. For example, the larger positive electrical potential elicited from the cochlear nucleus (in the brain stem) of a cat, alone and disturbed only by a click sound, is virtually eliminated when the cat's attention is directed to a live mouse placed in a glass jar in front of him. The first electrical potential recorded from the surface of the cerebral cortex in response to a click, a light flash, or a peripheral nerve shock is followed by a series of "afterpotentials." After a succession of 60 or more stimuli, however, the afterpotentials disappear. Clearly, the animal's brain somehow adapts to the repeating stimulus input in a way that changes its measured electrical output over a short period of time. Thus, the physiologist interprets the brain's functions in terms of their variability (plasticity), the input from one sensory modality modifying the results of an input from another. From this viewpoint, the idea of "centers" with specific, fixed jobs to perform becomes tenuous at best. Upon taking a critical look, one can see that a "center" is really defined (inferred) by all the functions remaining after the presumed anatomical location for that center is destroyed.

In this section, we will discuss first a disorder of movement characterized by inability to perform previously learned, skilled, voluntary acts (in the absence of paresis) due to a central nervous system dysfunction known as apraxia. Later, we will describe several disorders of perception called agnosias, which are characterized by the inability to comprehend the significance of a previously experienced sensation, again due to a central nervous system lesion. Finally, we will delve briefly into various disorders of language capability, the aphasias, that result primarily from destructive lesions of the left cerebral hemisphere.

### Apraxia

The complex act of performing a skilled, learned, voluntary movement is basically cognitive, even though it may be performed effortlessly and automatically. The term apraxia derives from the Greek *prassein* meaning "to do," *a*praxia carrying the negative connotation "without doing" or "being unable to do." Clinically, the concept of apraxia in its purest hypothetical form refers to a curious lack of ability to perform familiar (previously learned) tasks or exercise skills as a result of an acquired brain disorder, even though there is no intellectual impairment, psychotic disorder, paralysis, cerebellar incoordination, peripheral sensory loss, disordered muscular tone, or interference by involuntary movements (i.e., tremor, choreoathetosis). As with the agnosias, brain lesions resulting in apraxias may be focal or generalized or structural or pathophysiological (i.e., there is no demonstrable destructive lesion at postmortem examination). Although any voluntary function or movable

body part can theoretically be apraxic, only a few have been identified clinically.

There is no satisfactory experimental animal model of apraxia.
Destructive brain lesions large enough or located precisely enough
to cause loss of a previously learned skill produce either dementia
or significant paresis of motor functions. Furthermore, animals have
no way of describing verbally how they would go about completing
a task even if they were not so incapacitated. Apraxia, therefore, is
presently a clinical rather than a physiological concept. In theory,
it occurs when the brain's memory banks, which presumably store
images and patterns of skilled movements, are made unavailable to
language-integrating centers.

## LIMB KINETIC APRAXIA

Uncomplicated motor or limb kinetic apraxia involves one or
both limbs on one side of the body only, the contralateral limb(s)
remaining unaffected. The involved limb(s) cannot perform previously learned, usually skilled acts [which can often be accomplished
by the opposite limb(s) quite easily]. The involved limb is usually
clumsy and interferes with the smooth performance of attempted
bimanual activities. Gestures and some automatic actions can be
performed with ease, especially if they are done without the individual first "thinking" about them. The responsible lesion is generally in the cerebral hemisphere contralateral to the apraxic
limb(s). Small lesions causing Broca's aphasia (see below) may also
cause ipsilateral (as well as contralateral) upper extremity motor
apraxia. Occasionally, a few abnormal motor or sensory neurological signs may be found in the apraxic extremity. A characteristic
of this form of apraxia is that the impaired acts or skills can be
verbally described by the person if he is not aphasic) in precise
step-by-step detail.

## IDEOKINETIC APRAXIA

In contrast to limb kinetic apraxia, ideokinetic apraxia refers to
the loss of previously learned, bilaterally, as well as unilaterally,
performed motor skills. The ideokinetic apraxic individual seems
to know what he has been commanded to do (or voluntarily wishes
to do); he can formulate and even describe it (if not aphasic) but is
unable to carry out the plan of action. Often, the harder he tries

the more apraxic he becomes. On the other hand, he might un-
thinkingly perform the task perfectly well a moment or two later.
This peculiar variability in performance may give the physician
the mistaken impression that the patient is deliberately misleading
him by playing games. In the majority of such cases, the lesion is
in or near the juncture of the temporal, parietal, and occipital
lobes of the dominant hemisphere; hence, the patient may be aphasic or even have a mild degree of hemiparesis. It is not uncommonly
seen with diffuse, unlocalized, cerebral hemisphere disease (usually
in the absence of hemiparesis).

*Constructional apraxia.* This is a specific variant of ideokinetic
apraxia, diagnosed when patients are unable to copy two-dimensional geometric figures drawn on paper by the examiner or to construct copies of three-dimensional figures or designs with small
(children's) building blocks. Most of these patients find it difficult
to dress themselves (especially if one sleeve of their coat is pulled
inside out). There is now weakness or apraxia for individual movements (pencils, blocks, and clothes are handled normally), but the
spatial part of the task is missed. This differs from agnosia i.e., loss
of spatial perception) because the patients usually realize they are
making mistakes they cannot correct, try as they may. Constructional apraxia is seen primarily with lesions involving the right
parietal lobe.

IDEATIONAL APRAXIA

Ideational apraxia is thought to result from a loss of the ability
to formulate, even subconsciously, a plan for action. Persons with
ideational apraxia may differ very little from those with ideokinetic
apraxia as far as their performance of a task upon command is concerned. Unlike the ideokinetic apraxic, however, the ideational
apraxic cannot describe the task (language difficulty or no) because
he never really comprehends the entire idea of it. He is confused,
remains so, and rarely carries out the task automatically at some
later time. It is difficult to differentiate this condition from a cognitive disorder (i.e., dementia), since the patient behaves as if he were
extremely absent-minded, and his judgment, memory, and speech
may also be impaired. The lesion(s) is frequently diffuse, but a large
focal destructive process of one inferior parietal lobe can produce
the syndrome.

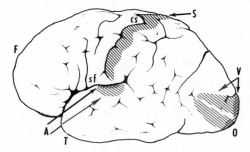

**Fig. 5-15** View of left cerebral hemisphere showing the frontal (F), temporal (T), and occipital (O) poles; the central sulcus (cs) and the Sylvian fissure (sf); and the three primary sensory projection areas, somatosensory (S), visual (V), and auditory (A). Note that the visual area lies mainly on the medial aspect of the cerebral hemisphere, and the auditory area lies mainly within the depths of the Sylvian fissure. Most of the unshaded areas, with the exception of a small region immediately rostral to the central sulcus, are association areas.

## Agnosia

The concept of agnosia is based upon the hypothesis that perception occurs when sense data coming to the brain from the sensory receptors and their peripheral and spinal pathways are brought to primary sensory receiving cortex (for analysis and assortment) and thence to association areas (containing memory banks) for higher-order interpretation, including translation into the codes and symbols of language (see Fig. 5-15). Freud's definition of agnosia implies that one or more of the primary sensory receiving areas or their related association areas (as well as the anatomical or functional connections of either with the thalamus) must be nonfunctioning. The definition categorically excludes dysfunction of the sensory receptors, peripheral and cranial nerves, and their centripetal.pathways to the thalamus via the spinal cord and brain stem. Lissauer (1889) proposed that a clinical distinction be made between two hypothetical mechanisms for agnosia, on the belief that primary receiving and association areas, being anatomically distinguishable, probably had different functions as well. He called the loss of ability to recognize the meanings of specific sensory data, due to malfunction of the primary receiving cortex (or its projecting circuitry to association cortex) apperceptive agnosia. Loss of the capacity to make sense out of internal sensory data because of malfunction of the association areas was named associative agnosia.

Initially, these two groupings gained support because two groups of patients seemed to be distinguishable. For example, patients with apperceptive agnosia were more likely to have clinically demonstrable sensory deficits in addition to their agnosia, whereas those patients with the so-called associative agnosia appeared to have few, if any, such deficits. Today, Lissauer's division of agnosia into two types has little empirical basis of support. With newer and more sophisticated sensory testing methods, sensory defects of some degree can be demonstrated in virtually all persons with agnosias. Furthermore, it is difficult, if not impossible, in many cases, to be certain that persons with associative agnosia do not have a significant cognitive defect (i.e., dementia) as well.

At this point, we might pause to ask whether agnosias exist at all. Yes, they do, but their pathophysiological basis is obscure. They represent a clinical concept that had its origin in observations that some patients with destructive focal brain lesions (i.e., infarctions, tumors, gunshot wounds) were unable to appreciate a sensory concept via one sensory modality (i.e., vision or hearing) that they could easily understand by way of another modality (i.e., touch or smell).

### VISUAL AGNOSIA

The classical prototype of all agnosias is visual agnosia. In its purest form, it is characterized by an inability to recognize any object or shape by sight alone, although they can be recognized at once (i.e., named, and their uses described or demonstrated) through other than visual modalities. Of course, this presupposes the absence of blindness or of "significant" visual impairments.

### TACTUAL AGNOSIA

Tactual agnosia (astereognosia) is the loss of the ability to identify objects by touch and manipulation alone. Notice the familiar phrase, "loss of ability." Agnosia implies the loss of some previously acquired visual, tactual, gustatory, olfactory, etc. information from the brain's memory stores. Thus, new sensory data reaching the brain via a particular sensory system that has been programmed (through prior learning and experience) to make use of a specific memory bank will have no meaning if that memory bank is not available to it (i.e., destroyed by a structural lesion or already being put to use by some other neural system).

## PARTIAL OR MIXED AGNOSIAS

Among the vast array of agnosias described in detail in the neurological literature of the twentieth century, many partial and mixed forms derived their names from the patient's most outstanding (or most interesting) perceptual problem. Pallis (1955) reported a curious type of visual agnosia in an engineer who had had a cerebral embolism from mitral stenosis. His only complaint was his inability to recognize human (and even animal) faces. All other visual functions, including reading, appeared to be intact. In the patient's words, he saw "the eyes, nose, mouth and all, but they just don't add up, and they seem chalked in, like on a blackboard." He could revisualize the faces of people he knew but could not recognize them in photographs, nor could he recognize himself in a mirror or in photographs. Pallis called this prosopagnosia (agnosia for faces). Another visual agnosia, called simultanagnosia by Wolpert, is presumably a loss of ability to comprehend the total meaning of a composite picture (or scene) or the theme of a sequence of photographs as in a silent movie. The patient with simultanagnosia can recognize, and even name, the individual elements, but he cannot synthesize them into a whole and extract the meanings from their interrelationships. Anosognosia is the name given to a condition in which the patient with a brain lesion, which results in paresis of one or more parts of his body, fails to realize that he is paralyzed and often vigorously denies any illness or disability whatsoever. Anosognosia is more clearly evident with lesions of the nondominant (right) cerebral hemisphere, because language areas are unaffected, and the patient can verbally express his denial (or ignorance) of illness.

Agnosias derive their terminology from almost any conceivable perceptual experience subject to psychophysiological testing. They include barognosia (inability to discriminate among different weights), achromatopsia (agnosia for colors in the absence of congenital color blindness), and somatotopagnosia inability to identify or recognize the parts of the body). It is evident that what we call "agnosia" can accompany localized as well as diffuse lesions of the cerebral hemispheres. The trouble with the entire concept of agnosia is simply that the descriptive names given to agnosias have misled us in thinking about them: the concept of specifically functioning centers has been the implication behind descriptions and discussions of agnosias in neurological and psychological literature from the beginning.

## Aphasia

Language is a highly ordered and rule-bound system of symbols conveyed by two expressive codes, the written and the spoken, and interpreted in two receptive modes, reading and listening. Besides the system of language, other channels of communication used to convey meaning include facial expression, emotional declarations (e.g., laughter, crying, moaning, sighing), gestures, and sign "language." Brain-damaged patients often retain a considerable ability to communicate meaning through gesture or other emotive expression, while formal language is markedly reduced. Similarly, a patient's problem-solving ability, orientation in time and place, interpersonal relationships, and capacity to appreciate humor are not necessarily affected by language disabilities. The aphasic patient is impaired in his ability to communicate (receive and express) by means of language.

Aphasia may be characterized as a varying degree of loss of the ability to comprehend and integrate receptive language and to formulate and use expressive language. The receptive language modalities include reading (visual integration and comprehension of printed symbols) and listening (auditory integration and comprehension of verbal symbols); the expressive language modalities include writing (visual-motor formulation and use of printed symbols) and speaking (oral-motor formulation and use of verbal symbols). All four of the language modalities are affected, frequently unequally, in patients with aphasia. Aphasia is not a specific language disability involving an isolated impairment in reading (dyslexia) or writing (dysgraphia), nor does it apply to patients suffering specific sensory loss (auditory agnosia, astereognosis, visual agnosia, etc.) or specific motor speech disorders (dysarthrias, as seen in patients with parkinsonism, cerebellar disorders, myasthenia gravis, and hypokinetic or flaccid dysarthria). Furthermore, the term aphasia is not applicable to patients with irrelevant confabulated speech, as in dementia, or memory loss for premorbid events and names, as in amnesia. Likewise, patients who exhibit a generalized intellectual impairment characterized by pronounced reading difficulties, faulty calculation, disorientation, and confusion when attempting to perform abstract reasoning and problem-solving tasks should not be considered aphasic. These disorders (dementia, intellectual impairment, dysarthria, amnesia for events and names) often coexist with aphasic syndromes but are not themselves considered symbolic language disorders.

## LOCALIZATION OF LESIONS IN APHASIA

Since the reports of Broca and Wernicke in the late 1800's, there has been general agreement among neurologists that the left cerebral hemisphere is dominant (or at least more important than the right) in the reception and expression of language. Several investigations in the last 20 years have demonstrated this point quite clearly. Brown and Simonson (1957) collected neurological diagnostic data (X-ray's, electroencephalograms, operative reports, neurological examinations, and scores on language examinations) on 100 patients with aphasia at the Mayo Clinic. Patients in whom lateralization of the lesion was undetermined or in whom cortical damage was bilateral were excluded. In these 100 aphasic patients, lesions were found in the left hemisphere in 96% of the right-handed patients and in 73% of the left-handed or ambidexterous patients. Brown and Simonson concluded, as is generally accepted, that regardless of handedness the great probability is that the causative lesion in aphasia will be located in the left cerebral hemisphere. They correlated three clinical syndromes of aphasia with lesions and other neurological deficits in the following manner:

> Aphasia manifested mainly by defects in reading was often associated with homonymous hemianopsia, and most often was caused by relatively small lesions. In 84% of these cases the lesions involved the posterior temporo-parietal or anterior occipital region. . . .
>
> Patients with predominant defects in speaking or writing or both often had associated milder neurologic deficits including hemiparesis, hypesthesia for discriminative sensation . . . and were associated with a lesion implicating but not necessarily limited to the mid-temporal anterior parietal region in 95% of the patients. . . .

> Global aphasia (severe defect in reading, writing, speaking and listening) was associated with severe neurologic signs, including hemiplegia, hemianesthesia, and at times hemianopsia. The lesions in 74% of the patients with global aphasia were large . . . involved the mid-temporal anterior parietal region in 87% of the cases.

Russell and Espir (1961) reviewed 693 case records of patients with penetrating head wounds. Aphasia occurred in 60% of patients with entry wounds and fragment lesions in the left cerebral hemisphere.

Wilder Penfield and Lamar Roberts made a significant contribution to our understanding of cerebral localization and language function by meticulously recording verbal responses and mapping cortical sites of stimulation (electrical current) during craniotomy procedures in conscious patients and by followup testing of residual aphasic symptoms after circumscribed cortical excisions. In *Speech and Brain Mechanism* (1959), Penfield and Roberts reported on 569 patients exhibiting aphasic symptoms after or during operations in both the dominant and minor hemispheres. Aphasia occurred after surgery in the left hemisphere in 73% of the right-handed and 72% of the left-handed patients. Aphasia occurred after surgery in the right hemisphere in 0.5% of the right-handed patients and 6.7% of the left-handed patients. These data support previous research that the left hemisphere is usually dominant for speech, regardless of handedness. The authors observed that inability to name (with the ability to speak being otherwise intact), confusion in counting out loud, and perseveration and misnaming (paraphasia) were produced by the application of electrical current to three areas of the left hemisphere—Broca's area, the supplementary motor area, and the inferior parietal-posterior temporal area (see Fig. 5-16).

Subcortical structures contributory to language functions have been inferred by Schuell (1967), Samra (1969), and others, based on clinical pathological data on patients with lesions primarily involving the thalamus and white matter, but the physiological mechanisms and relationships of these structures to the cortical language areas are not as yet defined. It makes sense, hypothetically, to postulate physiological interdependence of cortical language areas and subcortical (thalamic) nuclei in the production of language, since two-way anatomical connections exist between them. It is more correct to speak of hemispheral control of language, keeping in mind

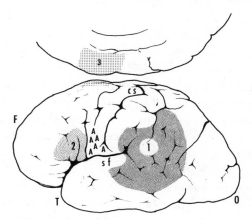

**Fig. 5-16** Medial (above) and lateral convexity views of hemisphere usually dominant for language functions as interpreted by Penfield and Roberts from electrical stimulation of the cerebral cortex: 1. Wernicke's and its surrounding areas, 2. Broca's area, and 3. supplementary motor area. Articulation distortions or repetitions of words and syllables occur at stimulation points (A). F, frontal, T, temporal, and O, occipital poles; cs and sf indicate the central sulcus and sylvian fissure, respectively.

that the cerebral cortex, together with its U-fiber interconnections, is far more important than subcortical structures. Although the studies of Brown and his colleagues, Russell, and Penfield documented rather well the fact that the left cerebral hemisphere was dominant for speech and language functions, the question of complete unilateral control of language by only one cerebral hemisphere remains debatable. Commissurotomized patients (those with complete transection of the corpus callosum) are still able to perceive, learn, and recall visual and auditory sense data, and they act appropriately upon these memories even though they may be unable, in some instances, to write or speak about them. Furthermore, clinical experience has shown that left-handed persons who become aphasic as a result of left hemisphere lesions tend (as a group) to recover more language function than right-handed persons rendered aphasic by similarly placed lesions.

## DIAGNOSIS OF SPEECH AND LANGUAGE

The neurologist's primary concern is that of differentially diagnosing discrete, well-localized lesions from those that are diffuse or disseminated (multiple focal). Consider four categories of speech and language manifestations of neurological disease: dysarthria, apraxia of speech, general intellectual impairment, and confused language of the demented person. Dysarthria is a motor speech disorder resulting in articulation, resonance (nasality), or voice dysfunction due to upper or lower motor neuron disease. Dysarthrias are the direct result of paralysis, paresis, or incoordination of the articulatory (oral-facial), resonatory (palatopharyngeal), or phonatory (laryngeal) muscles. They can occur as a result of lesions at any level of the neuraxis from bulbar musculature to cerebral cortex. Spastic dysarthria, as found in the pseudobulbar palsies (bilateral upper motor neuron disorders), is typically characterized by slowed and imprecise articulation and harsh, strained phonation and is often accompanied by hypernasality. Flaccid dysarthria, as manifested in diseases like myasthenia gravis or the bulbar palsies, is characterized by hypernasality, weak consonant production due to nasal escape of air, and a breathy dysphonia that deteriorates over time. Cerebellar and extrapyramidal disease can also produce characteristic dysarthria. Keep in mind that dysarthria, by definition, is only a motor expressive (articulatory) disorder, but dysarthrias may (and often do) accompany aphasia and, when severe, can make the diagnosis of aphasia difficult. The unintelligible speech of the "dysarthric-aphasic" must be separated if possible into paraphasic symptoms (e.g., language disorder) and purely motor symptoms (e.g., articulatory disorder). The signs of a language disorder (aphasia) in these difficult cases may be clearly distinguished from those of dysarthria by the demonstration of a problem with writing or reading or even with auditory comprehension.

Apraxia of speech is a symptomatic articulatory disorder distinct from dysarthria but often seen with expressive aphasia. According to Derenzi (1967) and Johns and Darley (1969), speech apraxia is a phoneme sequence programming disorder caused by lesions of one or both cerebral hemispheres. Unlike dysarthria, it cannot be accounted for by simple paresis or cerebellar incoordination of the muscles of speech articulation. To use an analogy, patients with speech apraxia "handle" the sounds of language (phonemes) with much the same misdirection (trial and error) as patients with constructional apraxia handle sticks in an attempt to form two-dimensional figures. In contrast to the expressive aphasic, the speech apraxic has little trouble recalling a particular word from memory, using it correctly in a sentence, or producing a normal flow of phonemes. He does have trouble making himself understood because he cannot decode (express in brain language) and then verbalize the phonemes that make up the word. The locations of lesions solely responsible for speech apraxia (without aphasia) are not known with certainty. Wertz and his associates (1970) found indirect evidence from X-ray and electroencephalogram records that lesions occurring in the parietal, frontal, and temporal lobes coincided with symptoms of apraxia of speech. Usually it is so difficult to make a clinical distinction between phoneme retrieval and sequencing, on the one hand, and word recall and verbalization, on the other, that many investigators still believe apraxia of speech to be a misnomer. They contend that the patient who must grope in order to articulate sequential consonant sounds is merely manifesting Broca's aphasia. The issue remains unresolved, and few neuropathological studies comparing the two clinical syndromes are available to resolve the issue.

On the basis of clinical evidence, Halpern (1972) has described two communication disorders that are distinct from classical aphasia: confused language in patients with brain syndromes and intellectual impairment in patients with generalized dementias. Patients with generalized intellectual impairment, unlike those with aphasia, exhibit pronounced difficulty with reading comprehension and arithmetic calculations but only moderate impairment of auditory comprehension, intact writing ability, and relevant speech utterances, and no naming difficulties. Halpern reported that the majority of these patients exhibited diffuse, degenerative lesions. In contrast, patients with confused language, who had a variety of brain syndromes including dementia, were distinguished from aphasics by the preponderance of bizarre, confabulated, and irrelevant spoken language in the absence of any significant syntactical breakdown or work-finding errors. In this latter type of communication disorder, Halpern found that the neurologist's report indicated primarily disseminated lesions of traumatic origin characterized by hemorrhage and hematoma.

CENTRAL NERVOUS SYSTEM DISORDERS

Since so many combinations of etiologies (neoplastic, vascular, traumatic) and locations of lesions (discrete, diffuse, disseminated, superficial, etc.) can take place, it is easy to appreciate that a large variety of disordered language patterns may occur in aphasic patients. Since the late nineteenth century, neurologists (and, more recently, speech pathologists) have proposed a number of descriptive categories for aphasia. For the most part these classification systems have been intended to serve at least one of three basic clinical needs: (1) to define the syndrome's most prominent characteristics; (2) to provide a clinical method of localizing the position and size of the cerebral lesion; and (3) to describe the language deficit pattern in order to prescribe therapy and predict language recovery.

Trousseau (1864) coined the term aphasia to refer to the loss of spoken language as the patient's prominent symptom, instead of what Broca (1861) had called aphemia. Broca, however, had used the term aphemia to mean a specific impairment of "the faculty of articulated language," which is quite distinct from our definition of aphasia as an impairment in language in general. Today many neurologists use the term Broca's aphasia (Geschwind, 1972; Goodglass et. al., 1972) to mean primarily an expressive disorder of language, whereas other neurologists use "apraxia of speech" (Johns and Darley, 1970; Denny-Brown, 1965) to denote the type of articulation programming difficulty Broca described.

Later in the nineteenth century, Wernicke described another aphasic disorder characterized by impairment of language comprehension and frequent use of jargon-like utterances (unintelligible or neologistic utterances). This led to the acceptance of the term Wernicke's aphasia to characterize patients with predominantly receptive language deficits. In 1935, Weisenberg and McBride developed an aphasia test battery and introduced what is now perhaps the most popular classification of aphasia: predominantly expressive aphasia and predominantly receptive aphasia, which are comparable to the Broca and Wernicke dichotomy. Weisenberg and McBride also included a category of amnesic (loss of memory) aphasia for patients with particular problems recalling names (anomia: loss of the ability to evoke the appropriate word in naming pictures, objects, using adjectives, and defining relationships) and another category for the most severely affected patient, the expressive-receptive aphasic.

Goodglass and Kaplan (1972) have recently suggested that two

TABLE 5-1 *Aphasia Classification System, Locus of Lesion, and Aphasic Symptomatology as Used on the Boston Diagnostic Test of Aphasia*[a]

| TYPE OF APHASIA | SYMPTOMS | LOCUS OF LESION |
|---|---|---|
| Broca's | Nonfluent spontaneous speech, intact comprehension, repetition limited, naming limited | Posterior inferior frontal area |
| Wernicke's | Fluent spontaneous speech, comprehension impaired, repetition and naming impaired | Posterior superior temporal area |
| Conduction | Fluent spontaneous speech, comprehension intact, repetition and naming impaired | Arcuate fasciculus |
| Isolation | Fluent spontaneous speech (but echolalic), comprehension impaired, repetition intact, naming impaired | Association cortex |
| Anomic | Fluent spontaneous speech, comprehension intact, repetition intact, naming impaired | Angular gyrus |

[a] After Goodglass and Kaplan, 1972.

broad categories of aphasia (specifically, nonfluent aphasia and fluent aphasia) be used to indicate anterior and posterior lesions, respectively. The use of their scheme is a simple way of classifying many aphasic disorders according to their most prominent symptom, but the scheme neglects a large percentage of aphasic syndromes that cannot be so easily categorized. Benson (1967) found that this dichotomous system encompasses approximately 64% of those lesions confirmed on radioisotope brain scan. Thus, it appears that in about one-third of these patients we will be unable to localize the lesion or categorize the aphasia. Of increasing importance is the neurologist's attempt to correlate specific aphasic syndromes with specific localization of the lesion within the dominant cerebral hemisphere for language. Goodglass, Kaplan, and Geschwind (1972) are proponents of such a classification system, which is outlined according to the language syndrome and the focus of lesion in Table 5-1.

## General references

Bender, M. B. and M. Feldman. 1972. The so-called "visual agnosias." Brain 95:173-186.

Benson, D. F. and J. P. Greenberg. 1969. Visual form agnosia. Arch. Neurol. 20:82-89.

Brown, J. R. and J. Simonson. 1957. A clinical study of 100 aphasic patients: Observations on lateralization and localization of lesion. Neurology 7:777-783.

Darley, F. L., A. E. Aronson, and J. R. Brown. 1969. Differential diagnostic patterns of dysarthria. J. Speech and Hearing Resch. 12:264-269.

Denny-Brown, D. 1958. The nature of apraxia. J. Nerv. Ment. Dis. 126: 9-32.

Halpern, H. 1972. Adult aphasia. Bobbs-Merrill, Indianapolis.

McFie, J. and M. F. Piercy. 1952. Intellectual impairment with localized cerebral lesions. Brain 75:292-317.

Nielsen, J. M. 1962. Agnosia, apraxia, aphasia, 2nd ed. Hafner, New York.

Penfield, W. and L. Roberts. 1959. Speech and brain mechanisms. Princeton University Press, Princeton.

Vinken, P. J. and G. W. Bruyn, eds. 1969. Disorders of speech, perception, and symbolic behavior. In Handbook of clinical neurology. Vol. 4. Wiley, New York, 481 pp.

# 6

# The Special Senses

## THE AFFERENT VISUAL SYSTEM

CARL ELLENBERGER, JR.

### Clinical anatomy

The neural visual pathway begins at the retina, a delicate, transparent tissue that covers the inner surface of the posterior wall of the globe. Although very thin (0.1–0.5 mm), the retina contains five types of neurons in three well-defined nuclear layers separated by two plexiform layers of cell processes and synapses. These neural elements are bounded by limiting membranes; the inner membrane (toward the center of the globe) and the outer limiting membrane are connected by glia (Müller cells) extending vertically through the retinal layers. The presence of neurons and glia remind us that the retina is actually part of the brain, derived from the optic vesicles that evaginate from the forebrain before the fourth week of embryonic life. (This embryogenetic relationship explains, in part, why the eyes are affected by such a wide range of neurological diseases.) A tract of white matter, the optic nerve, transmits visual impulses from the eye to the brain.

RODS AND CONES

The outermost nuclear layer of the retina is comprised of rods and cones, the receptor cells (Fig. 6-1). Their outer segments con-

187

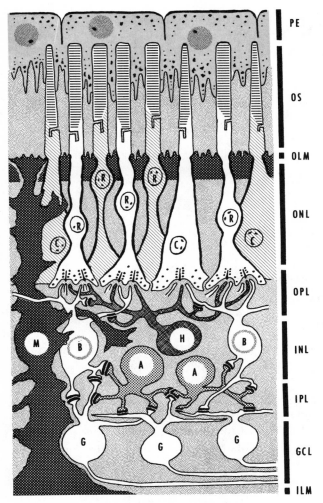

**Fig. 6-1** Diagrammatic cross section of the primate retina. PE, pigment epithelium; OS, outer segments of the rods and cones; OLM, outer limiting membrane; ONL, outer nuclear layer; OPL, outer plexiform layer; INL, inner nuclear layer; IPL, inner plexiform layer; GCL, ganglion cell layer; ILM, inner limiting membrane M, Müller cell; G, ganglion cell; A, amacrine cell; H, horizontal cell; B, bipolar cell; R, rod; C, cone. Light travels from the bottom to the top of the figure.

taining the photoreceptive pigments project outward from the outer limiting membrane to the pigment epithelium. The pigment epithelium has an extremely high rate of metabolism and many functions; for example, it supplies nutrients to the receptors and phagocytizes and digests their continually growing outer segments. Disease of the pigment epithelium that may seriously reduce vision can be detected by fluorescein angiography because the absence of the normal uniform distribution of pigment allows fluorescence in the vessels of the choroid (the layer behind the retina) to show through affected areas after intravenous injection of fluorescein hydrochloride. These defects may be caused by several of the hereditary retinal degenerations, some inflammatory diseases (e.g., rubella), and a wide range of drugs (including the phenothiazines).

## BIPOLAR CELLS

These cells in the middle retinal layer transmit impulses from the receptors to the ganglion cells, the axons of which carry impulses through the optic nerves to the brain. The bipolar cells do not merely pass along information in "bucket brigade" fashion from receptors to transmitters, but they, along with the amacrine and horizontal cells in the middle layer, are part of a highly organized complex circuitry that begins processing visual information before it leaves the eye. Impulses from 130,000,000 receptor cells in each retina converge through the retinal circuitry onto about 1,000,000 ganglion cells. In lower animals, not endowed with as complex a cerebrum as man, the responsibility of the retina is greater. In the laboratory, their retinas respond best to stimuli with properties that resemble those that would, under natural conditions, elicit the snapping response for catching food. Retinas of fish and amphibians are especially sensitive to movement; the retina of the frog, for example, is essentially a "bug detector." When examining Fig. 6-1, remember that a synapse may be excitatory or inhibitory, that many nerve terminals synapse with a single cell body or dendrite, and that the postsynaptic cell depolarizes in response to the sum of all excitatory and inhibitory influences.

## THE MACULA LUTEA

This yellow spot (2.0 by 1.0 mm), which usually appears gray through the ophthalmoscope, lies in the center of the retina at the posterior pole of the globe. In the center of the macula, the fovea centralis, a small pit, contains a high concentration of small cone receptors without rods or overlying blood vessels and cell nuclei.

Images on the fovea separated by as little as one minute of arc, approximately the diameter of one cone, can be resolved by the visual system. The oculomotor system moves the globe so that the point of interest is projected onto the fovea; the imaginary line connecting this point and the fovea is the visual axis. The power of resolution is proportional to the concentration of cones, which decreases sharply in all directions from the fovea. Thus, patients with small lesions in the macula, solar burns, for example, are usually disabled by poor acuity despite the fact that the lesion is often less than 1.0 mm in diameter. Many of a wide spectrum of hereditary degenerative retinal diseases have an unexplained localization to the macula.

The 7,000,000 cones in each macula are receptors of photopic or light-adapted vision, which is characterized by high resolution, color perception, and relatively low sensitivity. Rods, which predominate in the peripheral portion of the retina, are receptors for scotopic or dark-adapted vision. Rods are more sensitive to a low intensity of light, but their ability to resolve images is poor when compared to cones. If the visual system is dark adapted (this requires 20 to 30 minutes of darkness), stars appear brighter when perceived peripherally by the scotopic system. Scotopic vision is selectively affected in patients with early stages of the various forms of hereditary retinal pigmentary degeneration (retinitis pigmentosa), which, when progressive, usually begin in the outer layers of the retina in the periphery. These patients eventually become blind in darkness and have reduced peripheral vision. Pigment, usually uniformly distributed in the pigment epithelium, is clumped into a "bone spicule" or "salt and pepper" pattern. In childhood, diseases of cerebral gray matter may be associated with a similar pigmentary retinal degeneration, whereas diseases of white matter more often affect ganglion cells and thus cause pallor of the optic disc (see below).

Axons of the retinal ganglion cells comprise about 38% of all fibers, motor and sensory, that enter and leave the central nervous system. Most of the ganglion cell fibers (about 90%) are of relatively small caliber and originate from "midget" ganglion cells closely packed in the macula. These axons arch from their site of origin across the surface of the retina to the optic disc (also called the papilla), which marks the 1.5-mm hole in the wall of the globe where these fibers leave to join the optic nerve [Fig. 6-2(A)]. Arcuate defects radiating from the blind spot in the visual field indicate inter-

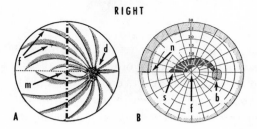

**Fig. 6-2** (A) Diagram showing radiation of arcuate ganglion cell fibers (f) on the surface of the retina to the right optic disc (d). Fibers originating to the right of the dashed vertical line cross in the optic chiasm. The "papillomacular bundle" contains the fibers between the disc and the macula (m). (B) A right visual field with an arcuate scotoma (s) that would result from interruption of a small segment of ganglion cell fibers (sometimes called "fiber bundle") in the inferior half of the optic nerve. The nasal step (n) provides another clue to the presence of lesions in the optic nerve; f is the point of fixation; b is the normal blind spot.

ruption of these arching ganglion cell fibers and identify the retina or optic nerve as the site of the lesion [Fig. 6-2(B)].

### THE OPTIC DISC

The optic disc is one of the single most important structures in neurological and ophthalmic diagnosis. Normally yellow-gray, and flat, it becomes pink, enlarged, and elevated when intracranial pressure is abnormally high. This hemorrhagic swelling of the optic disc called papilledema, when not long-standing or unusually severe, does not interfere with visual function as evidenced by normal visual acuity and visual fields. Papillitis, in contrast, occurs with acute lesions, usually inflammatory (optic neuritis) or ischemic (ischemic optic neuropathy), in the anterior part of the optic nerve, and, although ophthalmoscopically indistinguishable from papilledema, it is associated with severe visual impairment. Chronic processes as, for example, progressive compression or repeated inflammation of the optic nerve, cause pallor of the disc and eventually optic atrophy, with dropout of nerve fibers and small vessels and proliferation of glia causing the optic disc to appear white. Chronic glaucoma causes progressive enlargement of the normal optic cup, a circular depression in the center of the optic disc out of which the retinal vessels emerge as they enter the globe. Normally the cup is no larger than 30% of the diameter of the disc itself.

THE OPTIC NERVE

Immediately after entering the optic nerve, retinal ganglion cell fibers acquire a myelin sheath and, thus, are vulnerable to all diseases, for example, multiple sclerosis, that affect cerebral white matter. Because macular fibers, though concentrated in the center of the optic nerve, are distributed throughout its cross section, such intrinsic compressing lesions as tumors or aneurysms, as well as lesions within the nerve, cause early impairment of central vision. If a central defect in the visual field does not extend out to the periphery, it is called a scotoma (blind spot). Scotomas almost always indicate lesions in the retina or the optic nerve, although occasionally the optic chiasm may be involved. Impairment of central vision by optic nerve lesions is detectable not only by defects in the visual fields, but also by impairment of visual acuity, perception of brightness, and discrimination of colors.

Fibers from the retina maintain the same relative positions in the optic nerves and, with minor exceptions, all the way to the occipital lobes. For example, fibers from the superior half of each retina are superior in the optic nerve and synapse in the lateral geniculate nucleus with fibers that terminate in the superior half of the visual cortex. The posterior portion of the optic nerve passes from the orbit into the cranium through the optic canal in the sphenoid bone, an important landmark that may show early radiographic abnormalities in the presence of expanding lesions in and around the optic nerves, particularly tumors and aneurysms.

In man, whose visual fields almost completely overlap, about 50% of optic nerve fibers cross the midline in the optic chiasm [Fig. 6-3(A)]; the remainder travel to the ipsilateral half of the cerebrum. As a result of this partial decussation, the right hemisphere receives input only from the left visual field of both eyes and vice versa. The partial decussation is important for stereopsis because each hemisphere receives visual information from each eye and therefore from two slightly different points of view. The normal brain translates this disparity, combined with other clues, into perception of depth. In lower animals without overlapping visual fields (animals whose vision is adapted for detection rather than stereopsis and high acuity), most or all optic nerve fibers cross to the opposite side.

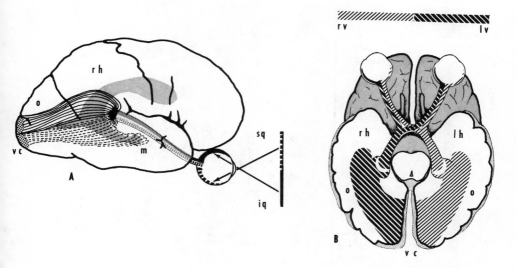

**Fig. 6-3** (A) Horizontal section of the brain from below showing the visual pathways. (B) Camera lucida drawing of the right cerebral hemisphere to show the location of the optic radiations; rv and lv, right and left visual fields; sq and iq, superior and inferior visual fields; rh and lh, right and left hemispheres; vc, visual cortex, m, Meyer's loop; o, occipital lobe.

### THE OPTIC CHIASM

This is another important structure in neuro-ophthalmic diagnosis. It lies in a variable position on a plane sloping almost 45° upward about 1 cm above the sella turcica and forms part of the anterior, inferior wall of the third ventricle. Because its superior and inferior surfaces are in contact with the cerebrospinal fluid, its position can be accurately determined by replacing the fluid with air and taking radiographs of the region (pneumoencephalography) (Fig. 6-4). The optic chiasm can be compressed and displaced by lesions expanding upwards out of the sella turcica (suprasellar lesions), usually tumors of the pituitary gland, and by lesions originating beside the sella (parasellar lesions), aneurysms or meningiomas, for example. When these lesions interrupt only the fibers crossing in the chiasm, bitemporal hemianopsia, loss of vision in both temporal fields, is the result. Although such visual field defects may be the first sign of intrasellar tumors, these masses must reach considerable

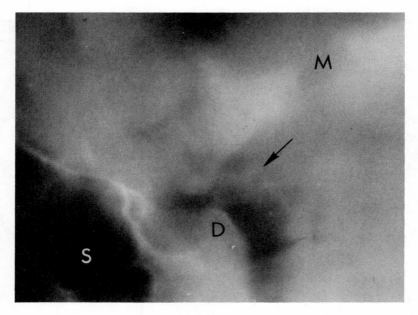

**Fig. 6-4** Pneumoencephalogram of a normal suprasellar region. Air fills the ventricles and subarachnoid cisterns making them appear darker than the surrounding brain, and structures lateral to the midline are blurred out by movement. The arrow, overlying the third ventricle, points to the posterior aspect of the optic chiasm, which lies above and slightly behind the cup-shaped sella turcica; S, sphenoid sinus; M, foramen of Monro; D, dorsum sellae.

size before interfering with visual function. Lesions anterior to the sella, however, may impair the function of one optic nerve when still small. Tumors in the region of the chiasm are common causes of progressive loss of vision but often are not discovered until visual loss is extensive and irreversible. They should be suspected in all cases of unexplained visual impairment.

### THE OPTIC TRACTS

These diverge posteriorly from the chiasm and encircle the peduncles of the midbrain on their way to the lateral geniculate nuclei on each side of the thalamus [Fig. 6-3(A)]. Before each tract reaches the lateral geniculate, fibers of the afferent limb of the pupillary reflex, which are probably collateral branches of ganglion cell neurons, leave and travel to the pretectal region of the midbrain. Through one intercalated neuron, this afferent pupillary pathway projects to ipsilateral and contralateral Edinger-Westphal nuclei, the paramedian, parasympathetic motor nuclei in the tectum of the midbrain that innervate pupillary constriction. Because of this bilateral projection, lesions in one retina or optic nerve reduce the response of both pupils to light shown in the affected eye. This is the Marcus Gunn pupillary sign, an important indication of lesions in the optic nerve (see below).

Other fibers leave the optic tract and travel to the superior colliculi in the tectum of the midbrain, where their termination is precisely organized. This retinal-tectal pathway is dominant in many lower animals with a large tectum and a relatively small cerebral cortex. In primates, axons from the superior colliculi project to the visual cortex of the occipital lobes. Each part of Brodmann's area 17 of the visual cortex, in turn, projects back to a topographically corresponding part of the superior colliculus. These reciprocal connections between cortex and midbrain allow an interaction between visual stimulation and eye movement that is important in the act of turning the eyes to look at a visual stimulus of potential interest.

The majority of fibers in the optic tracts continue to the two lateral geniculate nuclei. The evolution of the retinal-geniculate pathway has paralleled the evolution of such complex abilities of primates as stereoscopic vision and increased discrimination. Each lateral geniculate nucleus resembles a cupola comprised of six layers of cells in a stack. Ganglion cell fibers from each eye synapse with cells in three of these layers; the fibers from the ipsilateral eye are segregated from those from the contralateral eye.

OPTIC RADIATIONS

Axons of neurons with cell bodies in the lateral geniculate nuclei project to the occipital cortex as optic radiations [Fig. 6-3(B)]. The lower half of each optic radiation first extends forward from each lateral geniculate nucleus in Meyer's loop into the tip of the temporal lobe. When the fibers of Meyer's loop are interrupted by tumors at the tip of the temporal lobe or by resection of part of the temporal lobe to alleviate intractible seizures, a defect may appear in the superior part of the contralateral half of the visual field of both eyes (homonymous quadrantanopsia). From the temporal lobe, fibers pass through the junction of the temporal, parietal, and occipital lobes and continue to area 17 of the visual cortex, an area that abuts the calcarine fissure on the medial surface of the occipital lobe. This area is also called the calcarine or striate cortex, the latter term derived from the white line of Gennari seen only in this area on gross specimens. In accordance with the greater discriminative capability of the macula, fibers from the maculas project to an area of the cerebral cortex equal in size to the area of the cortex that receives fibers from all other retinal areas combined. The fibers in the optic radiations and their termination in the visual cortex are so well organized that examination of the visual fields is an accurate method of localizing lesions in the posterior part of the cerebrum. Complete interruption of one optic radiation between the chiasm and the visual cortex results in homonymous hemianopsia, the total loss of vision in the contralateral half of the visual field of both eyes. In contrast to lesions in the optic nerves or chiasm, unilateral cerebral lesions do not reduce acuity or color perception because macular fibers to the opposite hemisphere remain intact.

Upon arriving at area 17, the primary receiving area of the visual cortex, visual information continues anteriorly into areas 18 and 19 for further processing. These regions are called "association" areas because they help integrate vision with other functions of the cerebral cortex.

## Clinical neurophysiology

Light passes through the ocular media and inner layers of the retina and excites a photochemical reaction of four visual pigments contained in the outer segments of the rods and cones. The first clue to the nature of these pigments was the discovery that dietary night blindness occurring during World War I resulted from a deficiency of vitamin A. Then vitamin A was identified in the retinal pigment epithelium where it is converted into a form that can be utilized by the photoreceptors for synthesis of visual pigment. The aldehyde of vitamin A, now called retinal, is a chromophore (a functional group that gives color to the compound) bound to lipoprotein, an opsin; this complex of chromophore and opsin is the common plan of all known visual pigments. Opsin is species specific and is different for each pigment within a species; rhodopsin is found in human rods, and three other pigments most sensitive to red, green, or blue are contained in the cones. Inherited human color blindness is probably related to the absence or deficiency of one or more pigments resulting from faulty genetic specification of the amino acid sequence of one or more opsins because of an autosomal recessive mutation. Interestingly, segments of the normal human retina are "color blind"; cones in the very center of the fovea, for example, cannot perceive blue.

The only action of light is to cause stereoisomerization of the chromophore from 11-cis retinal in the dark to an 11-trans retinal, a change in the configuration of the molecule but not in its chemical composition (Wald, 1968). How does this change in the shape of the chromophore produce a flow of current? This problem is under investigation; some workers have preliminary evidence that cyclic AMP may play an intermediate role in altering the conductance of the membrane or receptor cell.

As we follow a visual impulse that has been translated from light energy to electrical energy by a photochemical reaction, we come again to the complex neural network of the retina. Some indication of the function of this network has come from a study of single ganglion cells in animals (Hubel and Wiesel, 1963). The normal resting firing rate of a ganglion cell (20-30/second) does not change when the entire retina is illuminated uniformly, but each ganglion cell responds to a spot of light precisely focused on a particular area of retina; the area is that cell's receptive field. Receptive fields of ganglion cells are subdivided into two concentric regions: an "on" region within which light increases the firing rate of the cell and an "off" region within which light decreases the rate [Fig. 6-5(A)]. Ganglion cells in the cat and monkey can be grouped into two classes, those with fields having a central circular on region and surrounding off region and those with a central off region surrounded by an on region. Diffuse light that illuminates the entire receptive field, excitatory and inhibitory areas together, does not elicit nearly as great a response as does a point of light focused precisely on an on center. The response of the cell varies according to the number of off and on sections illuminated at one time.

Some ganglion cells respond by increasing their firing rate when their receptive field is stimulated by light of a certain color. Illumination of the same receptive field by light of another color will usually decrease the firing rate; accordingly, these cells are called opponent color cells. Double-opponent color cells have a more complex response to pairs of colored stimuli.

Psychological experiments indicate that a similar receptive field organization exists in the human retina. The mean diameter of human fields increases linearly toward the periphery from 10 to 20 minutes of arc in the fovea. The center of a receptive field in the fovea of a monkey approaches the diameter of one cone. One obvious consequence of the retinal receptive field organization is the detection and enhancement of contrast. Larger receptive fields in the periphery imply increased spatial summation; a single ganglion cell gathers impulses from a greater number of receptors and, therefore, responds to lower levels of illumination of each individual receptor. This anatomical arrangement tends to increase sensitivity at the expense of resolution in the peripheral retina.

If the recording electrode is moved from the optic nerve to a neuron in the lateral geniculate body, a similar receptive field is found, but stronger illumination of the periphery of the cell's receptive field cancels the effects of illuminating the center. That is, the lateral geniculate body further enhances the contrast between on and off regions.

Recording from the calcarine cortex of the occipital lobe, we find different receptive fields [Fig. 6-5(B)]. Two main groups of cells have been identified. "Simple" cortical cells respond to linear stimuli (slits, dark bars, or edges). Each simple cell requires that these stimuli be exactly oriented (e.g., vertical, oblique, horizontal) and in one specific location on the retina. The receptive fields of simple cortical cells consist of a long on area bordered by larger off areas. "Complex" cells in the cortex also respond to line stimuli at only one orientation but do not discriminate as to the position of the stimulus. Unlike the simple cells, they respond with sustained firing to moving lines. Impulses pass forward and farther up the hierarchy of cortical cells into area 18. "Hypercomplex" cells found here are more specific in their required orientation and length of stimuli but even less specific for the position of the stimulus on the retina.

The operation of the visual cortex (areas 17, 18, and 19) depends upon the coordinated action of very large numbers of precisely organized neurons because a separate pathway or combination of neurons probably exists for each possible visual pattern. For example, a simple cortical cell, responding to a dark vertical bar at 90°

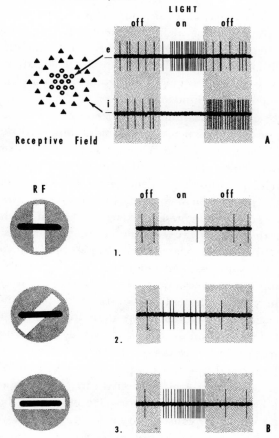

**Fig. 6-5** (A) Diagram (Ellenberger) of the receptive field of a primate "on" center type of retinal ganglion cell. When a spot of light strikes the center of the receptive field (e) firing rate increases; when light strikes the concentric surrounding area (i) firing is suppressed until the light goes off. (B) Receptive field (Ellenberger) of a "simple" cortical cell that responds best when illuminated by a white bar of light oriented horizontally (3).

at one point in space, probably receives input from off-center ganglion cells with receptive fields along a vertical line on the retina. Similarly, a set of simple cells in the calcarine cortex responding to a dark bar at one orientation on just one point on the retina may converge onto a complex cell that responds to a dark bar anywhere on the retina. Good evidence suggests that this hypothesis is correct: Hubel and Wiesel (1963) found that all cells detected by an electrode passed perpendicularly through the cortex at any given point responded to a stimulus of identical orientation, an ideal arrangement if they are to be closely interconnected. The principles of operation of the visual system have been compared with pattern analysis by computers; both systems magnify singularities, contrasts, and discontinuities and reduce redundancies.

Although receptive field organization and directional preferences are found in the cortical cells of newborn animals, continued development of the full potential of the visual system depends on early visual experience. Amblyopia, reduced visual acuity without apparent morphological abnormalities in the ocular fundus, develops in 2 to 3% of the population before the age of 5 years. Strabismic amblyopia may occur in the presence of tropia, lack of fusion of the images from both eyes; one eye fixes on the object of interest, but the visual axis of the other deviates in (esotropia) or out (exotropia), and its vision is suppressed to eliminate diplopia (double images). Constant suppression of vision of one eye during a critical period in early life may lead eventually to permanent impairment. If a child learns to use one eye or the other, alternately, however, amblyopia does not develop. Amblyopia may also develop from anisometropia, a difference in the refractive power of the two eyes causing the image on one retina to be sharper than the image on the other retina. If this difference is not corrected early with proper lenses, vision in the eye with the larger refractive error may become permanently impaired after constant suppression. Deprivation of form vision early in life may also cause amblyopia. Congenital cataract, ptosis (drooping eyelid), and, perhaps occasionally, an eye patch prescribed by an ophthalmologist may be responsible for such deprivation.

When stabismus, anisometropia, or deprivation of form vision are present before the age of 5 years, and especially before age 1, amblyopia may result. Temporary patching of the better eye during this critical period eliminates suppression, and may prevent amblyopia, if it is done soon enough. A similar critical period in the development of normal vision has been found in experimental animals. In the normal cat and monkey, 80% of cells in the striate cortex respond to light in either eye. If, however, one eye is sewn shut during the newborn period, even for just a few days, only a fraction of cells in the visual cortex respond to light in either eye, and few cells respond to light from the occluded eye. If development of fusion is prevented by the cutting of one of the extraocular muscles during the newborn period, only about 20% of cortical cells respond binocularly. None of these experiments performed after the critical period in early life will cause reduction of visual acuity; similarly, patching the eye of a child older than 5 years will not damage acuity.

Even in the absence of amblyopia, if stereoscopic vision is not present in children at an early age because the visual axes of the two eyes are not parallel, it will not develop later even if the eyes are perfectly straightened. Presumably, in such cases, one would find a lack of cortical cells that respond binocularly and also a lack of cells that respond best to the slight disparity in the two images from each eye necessary for stereopsis (Pettigrew, 1972). Testing for stereopsis in the clinic is a reliable way of determining whether a patient has ever been able, even intermittently, to align his visual axes, that is, to fuse the image from each eye into one.

Another example of the influence of early visual experiences is Blakemore and Cooper's experiment (1970) in which kittens were maintained from birth in an environment of only vertical lines. After several months, the kittens were totally blind to all horizontal stimuli (edges of tables, shelves, etc.), and no cells responding to horizontal stimuli were found in their visual cortex. The effects of variation in early visual experience in humans need more study; they could be considerable.

The term "amblyopia" should be reserved for the conditions mentioned above that originate in early life. Impaired vision with a normal ocular fundus acquired later in life should be described according to the pattern of defect in the visual field, for example, homonymous hemianopsia. Bilateral lesions completely interrupting the function of both optic radiations cause a so-called cortical blindness, defined as absence of light perception in either eye when pupillary reactions to light are normal. Anoxia and thromboembolic occlusion of both posterior cerebral arteries are common causes of cortical blindness. Occasionally these cortically blind patients deny their inability to see; they have "Anton's syndrome."

In certain vertebrates, the hamster, for example, ablation of the striate cortex does not cause complete blindness. The retinotectal projection to superior colliculi, described above, continues to

mediate the ability to orient toward an object, even though the
cortical lesion destroys the ability to discriminate patterns (Gordon,
1972). Other neurophysiological studies have indicated that the
retinogeniculate pathways transmit information to answer "What
is this visual image?" Information carried by the retinotectal projection answers "Where is it and in what direction is it moving?"
In most lower animals, bilateral destruction of the superior colliculi
results in reduced responsiveness to all visual stimuli with relative
preservation, greater as the phylogenetic scale is ascended, of discriminative abilities. Isolated collicular lesions in man, however,
have not yet been associated with clinical signs. Single unit studies
in monkeys have revealed that collicular neurons have receptive
fields similar to those of ganglion cells. Stimulation of a cell in the
colliculus causes the eyes to move in the direction of that cell's receptive field. Certain collicular cells fire before a voluntary shift
of the visual axes in the direction of their receptive fields, suggesting
that mediation of the shift of visual attention toward the intended
point of refixation by the superior colliculi must precede the actual
displacement of the eyes in a visually guided movement.

## Assessment of visual impairment

Visual function should be assessed before a search is made for other
evidence of structural lesions in the visual pathways. A busy intern
usually reaches for his ophthalmoscope without remembering to
test visual acuity. His usual examination of the eyes is then analogous to performing cystoscopy before testing the urine. It is true
that the eye can be more closely examined by direct inspection than
any other organ, but, nevertheless, impairment of visual function
is the most sensitive indicator of disease in the visual pathway.

The technique of obtaining a complete history of any kind of
visual impairment does not differ from the approach to neurological
diagnosis of defects in other systems. Remember, however, that most
patients can reveal the site of their lesion by describing the nature
of their symptoms. Metamorphopsia (distortion of vision, particularly of straight lines) and positive central scotomas (bright blind
spots) often result from lesions of the macula. Many patients with
central scotomas due to optic nerve lesions recognize that their
peripheral vision is intact and also that colors appear less bright. A

sudden reduction of brightness, "like a shade in front of one eye," is a symptom of acute optic nerve lesions or retinal vascular occlusion. Unilateral progressive loss of vision caused by slowly expanding tumors or aneurysms compressing the optic nerve is sometimes unrecognized until the patient covers one eye, as when sighting a rifle or focusing a camera; onset of the deficit in such cases may then mistakenly be considered sudden. Transient obscurations of vision are reported by at least 25% of patients with papilledema caused by increased intracranial pressure. These 5- to 10-second bilateral or unilateral episodes of blurring or blindness, often after change in position, are a very specific sign of papilledema. In contrast, amaurosis fugax (fleeting blindness), a monocular reduction of vision, usually lasts for 10 or 20 minutes and is highly suggestive of emboli in the retinal circulation that usually originate from an ulcerated atherosclerotic plaque at the bifurcation of the common carotid artery. The emboli can sometimes be seen as bright particles in retinal arterioles. Slowly progressive bitemporal hemianopsia due to chiasmal lesions is often not recognized by patients, but many patients with homonymous hemianopsia associated with a lesion in the optic tract or radiation can describe their defect and may have difficulty reading.

Nonspecific blurring or discomfort when reading may be due to inadequate corrective lenses or advancing presbyopia, a decreasing ability to accommodate for near vision that is universal after the age of 45 to 50 years. Diseases of the anterior segment of the eye that cause impairment of vision are usually easily distinguished because of ocular pain or other obvious signs of local disease.

The first step in the examination of vision is to determine the best corrected visual acuity. Reduction of acuity cannot be attributed to disease unless all refractive error is eliminated. Any letter or number chart is adequate for clinical purposes. Physicians examining vision at the bedside often ask older patients with presbyopia to read a card without proper refractive correction. A $+2.00$ or a $+3.00$ diopter lens should compensate for this lost power of accommodation in most cases if bifocals or reading glasses are not available. If vision is not 20/20 despite the use of the patient's glasses, improvement when looking through a pinhole, which eliminates spherical and chromatic aberration, indicates that at least part of the defect is refractive.

A moving stimulus, especially if it occupies a large portion of the visual field, evokes optokinetic nystagmus; the eyes fixate on a part of the stimulus and follow it until it reaches the limits of excursion of the ocular movements. Then the eyes make a corrective rapid movement (saccade) in the opposite direction to fix on another portion of the moving stimulus. If the stimulus is large enough, optokinetic nystagmus is difficult to voluntarily suppress (try it when looking out of the side window of a moving auto). Therefore, by using moving targets of various sizes (e.g., a striped tape or newspaper) an estimation of visual acuity can be made, even if the patient does not or cannot respond. Vision can usually be demonstrated by this method in hysterical or malingering patients who claim blindness.

Visual fields can be estimated in each eye separately by introducing an object or a finger from the periphery at a distance halfway between patient and examiner and comparing a patient's fields to one's own. A small white or colored object (like a match) can be used to identify the normal blind spot (try it on yourself with one eye closed) and any other scotomas near the center of vision. Incomplete field defects can often be detected by asking the patient to compare the brightness of a colored object in the region of the suspected defect against that of an identical object held in a normal part of the field. If the fields are normal, double simultaneous stimuli may indicate extinction of the right or left homonymous fields when a lesion of the opposite parietal lobe does not completely interrupt the optic radiation.

In the presence of lesions in the visual pathways from the retina to the occipital cortex, pupils are always equal. (A small per cent of normal individuals have slight "physiological" anisocoria, i.e., difference in pupillary size. Acquired anisocoria always indicates a disturbance in the efferent limb of the pupillary reflex, that is, the brain stem, oculomotor nerve, or ciliary body.) Most lesions in the optic nerves and some lesions in the retina, however, will reduce the response of the pupil to light in the affected eye (Marcus Gunn sign). This sign should be sought by the "swinging flashlight test." In a dark room, a bright light is directed alternately in each eye for at least 5 seconds, moving quickly from one eye to the other. In the presence of a lesion in the afferent limb of the pupillary reflex arc, both pupils will constrict when the light is shined into the intact eye, and both pupils will dilate when the light is quickly moved to the affected eye. The Marcus Gunn pupillary sign is often helpful in distinguishing organic from functional or refractive visual impairment, especially when the ocular fundus is normal.

The ocular fundus can often be visualized through an undilated pupil, but for a clear view of the macula and the periphery of the retina, mydriasis (dilation of the pupil) and cycloplegia (paralysis of accommodation) is helpful. A wide range of diseases affecting the ocular fundus can be found in one of the many atlases of fundus pathology. The eye is a "window to the brain" in many respects. A representative sample of cerebral vasculature is visible in the ocular fundus, and close inspection with an ophthalmoscope may reveal evidence of hypertension, diabetes, or embolic disease. Several neurological diseases have specific manifestations in the retina; retinal phakomas (glial tumors) may be seen in tuberous sclerosis, for example, and retinal angiomas are associated with cerebellar hemangioblastomas in the von Hippel-Lindau syndrome. As when reading an X-ray, systematic examination of the fundus is necessary to avoid overlooking important lesions.

## References

Blakemore, C. and G. F. Cooper. 1970. The development of the brain depends on the visual environment. Nature 228:477-478.

Gordon, B. 1972. The superior colliculus of the brain. Scient. American 227:72-82.

Hubel, D. H. and T. N. Wiesel. 1963. The visual cortex of the brain. Scient. American 209:54-62.

Pettigrew, J. D. 1972. The neurophysiology of binocular vision. Scient. American 227:84-95.

Wald, G. 1968. Molecular basis of visual excitation. Science 162:230-239.

## General references

Gregory, R. L. 1966. Eye and brain. McGraw-Hill, New York.

Moses, R. A. 1970. Adler's physiology of the eye, 5th ed. Mosby, St. Louis, Mo.

Walsh, F. B. and W. F. Hoyt. 1969. Clinical neuro-ophthalmology, 3rd ed. Williams & Wilkins, Baltimore.

## EYE MOVEMENTS

RONALD M. BURDE

## Introduction

The oculomotor system in man has but one fundamental purpose and that is to place the image of regard upon the foveas of both eyes simultaneously and to maintain this physiological position under all circumstances.

## Nuclear and infranuclear mechanisms

The final common pathway for eye movements involves the nuclei of the oculomotor, trochlear, and abducent nerves (cranial nerves III, IV, and VI) in the brain stem and the extraocular muscles subservient to these nuclei.

### EXTRAOCULAR MUSCLES

The extraocular muscles controlling eye movement may be grouped into three pairs: (1) the superior and inferior rectus muscles, (2) the lateral and medial rectus muscles, and (3) the superior and inferior oblique muscles. Each muscle is innervated in all extraocular movements, but the action of each muscle may be isolated in one particular field of gaze in order to determine the integrity of its function (Fig. 6-6). The medial and lateral rectus muscles primarily act in horizontal gaze movements; the medial rectus muscle moves the eye toward the nose (adduction), and the lateral rectus muscle moves the eye temporally (abduction). In either eye, the

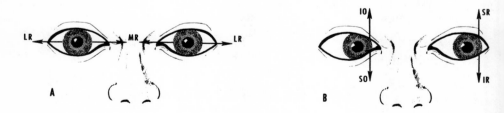

**Fig. 6-6** (A) Horizontal rectus muscles—MR, medial rectus muscle; LR, lateral rectus muscle. (B) Vertical muscles—SR, superior rectus muscle; IR, inferior rectus muscle; SO, superior oblique muscle; IO, inferior oblique muscle.

TABLE 6-1   *Actions of Extraocular Motion*

|  | MEDIAL RECTUS | LATERAL RECTUS | SUPERIOR RECTUS | INFERIOR RECTUS |
|---|---|---|---|---|
| Primary | Adduction | Abduction | Elevation | Depression |
| Secondary |  |  | Adduction | Adduction |
|  |  |  | Intorsion | Extorsion |

|  | SUPERIOR OBLIQUE | INFERIOR OBLIQUE |
|---|---|---|
| Primary | Intorsion | Extorsion |
| Secondary | Depression | Elevation |
|  | Abduction | Abduction |

medial and lateral muscles function as an agonist and antagonist pair according to Sherrington's Law of Reciprocal Innervation, that is activation of the agonist is accompanied by inhibition of the antagonist. Similarly, the superior and inferior muscles act primarily in up and down gaze or in torsional movements but have other secondary actions (Table 6-1). From the table one can make certain generalizations. The superior muscles, rectus and oblique, act as intorters, and the inferior muscle groups act as extorters (i.e., turn the vertical axis of the globe at 12 o'clock laterally). The vertical recti act as secondary adductors, whereas the oblique muscles act as abductors. The function of the individual muscles may be isolated in particular fields of gaze, according to the diagram shown in Fig. 6-6.

Movements of both eyes together are called "conjugate movements" and are activated by innervation of pairs of homologous muscles. In left lateral gaze, for instance, the left lateral and right medial rectus muscles are innervated, while the left medial and right lateral rectus muscles are inhibited. These muscle pairs are called "yoke muscles," and their innervation patterns are determined according to Hering's Law with equal innervation and inhibition going to the appropriate yoke pairs. Other yoke muscle pairs are the left superior rectus and the right inferior oblique muscles (similarly, the right superior rectus and left inferior oblique) and the left inferior rectus and right superior oblique muscles (similarly, the right inferior rectus and left superior oblique).

Since these muscle groups function according to Hering's Law, a paresis of one of the extraocular muscles will produce a differential deviation depending upon which eye is used for fixation. That is,

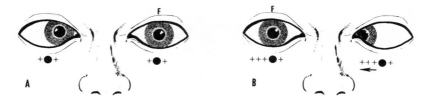

**Fig. 6-7** (A) Paretic lateral rectus muscle, primary deviation. Left eye fixing (F) in straight ahead gaze. Innervation is equal to all four horizontal rectus muscles. Since the right lateral rectus muscle cannot respond normally to the input designated by the "+" signs, the right eye will be deviated medially by a given amount, *X*. (B) Paretic right lateral rectus muscle, secondary deviation. Right eye fixing (F) in straight ahead position. Since it will require a greater input to the right lateral rectus muscle to maintain the right eye in the straight ahead position, a greater innervation will be sent to the yoke or left medial rectus muscle and result in a greater absolute deviation.

there will be a difference in the measured prismatic deviation if the uninvolved eye is used for fixation, "primary deviation," or if the involved eye is used for fixation, "secondary deviation" (Fig. 6-7). The secondary deviation (the deviation measured with the eye with the paretic muscle fixating) will always be greater than the primary deviation. With the passing of time after the acute lesion, this difference in deviation between fixation with the paretic and nonparetic eye fixing becomes blurred. It is beyond the scope of this book to discuss the methods of testing these deviations. For a more complete review see Cogan (1956), Walsh and Hoyt (1969), and Moses (1970). Similarly, primary and secondary deviations can be demonstrated for all of the extraocular muscles and can be emphasized in their fields of relatively isolated action (Fig. 6-6). Patients with concomitant strabismus, for example primary esotropia (cross-eyes) or exotropia (wall-eyes), do not show this differential deviation.

Movements of the eyes in opposite directions are called "disjunctive movements." Horizontal disjunctive movements are typically convergence or bilateral adduction when the image of regard is nearer than 6 m (assumed distance for parallel ocular movements) or divergence or bilateral abduction as an image of regard recedes to 6 m from a near point of fixation. The eyes also have the ability to tort in a clockwise or counterclockwise direction in order to maintain the objective vertical plane straight up and down (Fig. 6-8).

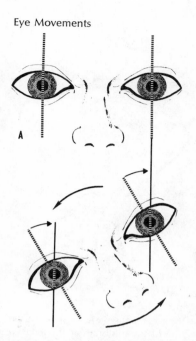

**Fig. 6-8** (A) Dashed line represents the vertical meridian of the retina in primary position. (B) With head tilt to the right shoulder, the right eye must intort or conclinate, while the left eye must extort or disclinate in order to bring the vertical meridian perpendicular to the horizon. These movements are under the control of the vestibular system.

## Cranial nerves III, IV, and VI and their nuclei

As mentioned previously, the nerves supplying the extraocular muscles have their nuclei in the brain stem (Fig. 6-9). The oculomotor nerve (cranial nerve III) supplies the superior, inferior, and medial recti muscles as well as the inferior oblique muscle and levator palpebrae superioris muscle. It also supplies the parasympathetic outflow to the internal muscles of the eye, i.e., the ciliary muscle, which controls accommodation, and the sphincter muscle of the iris, which controls, for the most part, the size of the pupillary aperture. Fibers arise from a paired group of motor neurons in the mesencephalon just below the superior colliculus. The fibers course ventrally, passing through the medial longitudinal fasciculus, the red nucleus, the substantia nigrae, and the pons, to form the oculomotor nerve in the intrapeduncular fossa. This nerve travels anteriorly in the subarach-

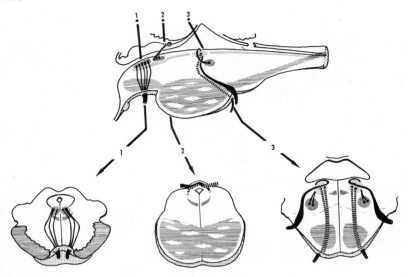

**Fig. 6-9** Location of the oculomotor nuclei and nerves (schematic sagittal section through the midbrain and pons). 1. Cross section of the midbrain at the level of the oculomotor nucleus (cranial nerve III). The fascicles of the nerve travel ventrally through the red nucleus and pyramidal tracts (not shown) to emerge as the oculomotor nerve in the intrapeduncular fossa. The lightly shaded tract is the medial longitudinal fasciculus. 2. Cross section of the caudal midbrain demonstrating the total decussation of the fascicles of the trochlear nerve (cranial nerve IV) in the superior medullary velum. This schematic representation shows part of the trochlear nerve nucleus for orientation, but, in life, it does not extend this far caudally. 3. Cross section of the pons at the level of the nucleus of the abducent nerve (cranial nerve VI) shown leaving the pons at its base close to the midline (dashed line) with respect to facial nerve (cranial nerve VII) (solid line), which is shown enveloping the abducent (cranial nerve VI) nucleus.

noid space, being suspended over and under the superior cerebellar anterior and posterior cerebral artery (early pressure in threatened herniation leads to pupillary signs), to enter the lateral wall of the cavernous sinus. The pupillary fibers are believed to travel superficially in the superior portion of the nerve. The nerve enters the orbit through the superior orbital fissure and divides into a superior branch (superior rectus muscle and levator palpebrae superioris) and an inferior branch carrying the parasympathetic innervation as well as fibers to the medial and inferior recti and the inferior oblique muscle. The parasympathetic fibers travel with the fibers to the inferior oblique muscle from which they exit as the motor root to the ciliary ganglion. Here they synapse and enter the globe by way of the short ciliary nerves.

The trochlear nerve (cranial nerve IV) (Fig. 6-9) arises from a pair of grouped motor cells just beneath the central gray substance under the mid-portion of the inferior colliculus. The cells are almost continuous with those of the oculomotor nerve. The fibers course dorsally and cross completely in the superior medullary velum. The trochlear nerve is the only cranial nerve that exists dorsally and decussates completely as well. It travels anteriorly and ventrally in the subarachnoid space to pierce the dura and enter the cavernous sinus just caudal to the posterior clinoid processes. It lies in the lateral wall of the sinus and enters the orbit through the superior orbital fissure to innervate the superior oblique muscle.

The abducent nerve (cranial nerve VI) arises from a group of paired motor cells situated in the floor of the fourth ventricle (Fig. 6-9). These nuclei are demarcated on the floor of the fourth ventricle by the facial colliculi. The fibers course ventrally through the pons to emerge at its base. They travel anteriorly and laterally over the tip of the petrous portions of the temporal bone. The abducent nerve is bound to the tip by the petrosphenoidal ligament. It pierces the dura at the level of the dorsum sellae to enter the cavernous sinus traveling within the sinus near the carotid artery. It enters the orbit through the superior orbital fissure and supplies the lateral rectus muscle. It has the longest intracranial course and is often subject to embarrassment with raised intracranial pressure.

Disturbances of the efferent input to the extraocular muscles from the nucleus to the periphery will cause diplopia (double vision). This contrasts with supranuclear disorders in which gaze palsies (i.e., inability to move both eyes in one direction) are evident, but diplopia is not. Diplopia, for all practical purposes, is pathognomonic of nuclear or infranuclear lesions.

## Supranuclear mechanisms

The control mechanisms for eye movements fit into five functionally distinct groups. These are (1) the saccadic system, (2) the smooth pursuit system, (3) the vestibular system, (4) the vergence system, and (5) the position maintenance fixation system. These five systems are defined by the functional stimuli that evoke the activation of

TABLE 6-2   *Control Mechanism*

|  | SACCADIC | PURSUIT | VESTIBULAR | VERGENCE | POSITION MAINTENANCE |
|---|---|---|---|---|---|
| Function | Place object of interest on fovea rapidly | Maintain object of regard near fovea; matches eye and target | Maintain eye position with respect to changes in head and body posture | Align visual axes to maintain bifoveal fixation | Maintain eye position vis-à-vis target |
| Stimulus | Object of interest in peripheral field | Moving object near fovea | Stimulation of semicircular canals | Retinal disparity | Visual interest and attention? |
| Latency (from stimulus to onset of eye movement) | 200 msec | 125 msec | Very short | 160 msec | |
| Velocity | To 400°/second | To 100°/second, accurately to 30°/second | To 300°/second[a] | Around 20°/second | Both rapid (flicks, microsaccades) and slow (drifts) |
| Feedback | Sampled data | Continuous | | | |
| Substrate | Frontal lobe | Occipitoparietal junction | Vestibular apparatus muscle receptors in neck, cerebellum? | Unknown | Occipitoparietal junction; superior colliculus |

[a] Slow phase only. The fast phase, although initiated in the pontine reticular formation, is discharged vis-à-vis the saccadic mechanism.

these systems and by the response characteristics of the oculomotor movements initiated (Table 6-2). The control mechanisms are represented in supranuclear centers, which specify the function of coordinated muscle groups rather than individual muscles. Therefore, interruption of these centers or their pathways will result in a loss of gaze function, not in diplopia.

The output of these systems is translated into action in one of two modes—rapid eye movements and slow eye movements. Rapid eye movement is due to a pulsatile output whose amplitude is determined by burst activity. Slow eye movements, on the other hand, are mediated by a continuous graded response.

## Supranuclear connections

### MEDIAL LONGITUDINAL FASCICULUS

This tract runs from the thalamus to the anterior horn cells of the spinal column. It extends on either side of the midline forming, grossly, a "V-shaped" pattern, which is especially well developed between the region of the vestibular and oculomotor nuclei. This tract serves to coordinate the nuclei of the oculomotor, trochlear, and abducent nerves between themselves and other brain-stem nuclei and centers.

## Horizontal gaze

### BRAIN-STEM CENTERS

*Pontine gaze centers.* Lateral gaze movements are coordinated through the pontine centers of horizontal gaze. Good experimental evidence for the existence of such centers is available. They are located in the paramedial zone of the pontine reticular formation, just rostral to the abducent nerve nuclei bilaterally. Each center controls ipsilateral conjugate gaze, sending fibers to the ipsilateral abducent nucleus and to the contralateral oculomotor nucleus (those cells associated with the medial rectus muscle) (Fig. 6-10).

Lesions of the medial longitudinal fasciculus between the abducent nerve nucleus caudally and the oculomotor nerve nucleus rostrally produce a characteristic movement deficit in horizontal gaze called "internuclear ophthalmoplegia." This involves weakness of

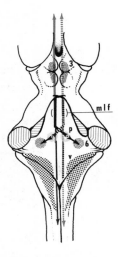

**Fig. 6-10** Fibers from the pontine gaze center (p) run to the ipsilateral abducent nerve (cranial nerve VI) (6) nucleus and, via the medial longitudinal fasciculus (mlf), to the contralateral oculomotor nerve (cranial nerve III) (3) nucleus (motor neurons to the medial rectus muscle); v, vestibular nuclei.

the ipsilateral medial rectus muscle, as demonstrated by a lag in response, and a nystagmus of the abducting eye in conjugate gaze movement. Bilateral lesions of the medial longitudinal fasciculus are almost pathognomonic of demyelinating disease. Unilateral internuclear ophthalmoplegia is usually indicative of small vessel occlusive disease.

*Cerebellum.* The role of the cerebellum in oculomotor function is not yet understood. Most likely, it coordinates input from afferent ocular muscle spindles, from the vestibular apparatus, from tonic neck receptors, and from gaze center outflow, integrates this information, and, through its efferent output, controls the smoothness of programmed movements. The central cerebellar structures of the vermis probably deal with vestibular input and vertical gaze, whereas the lateral lobes are concerned with the maintenance of fixation and sustained conjugate gaze. Clinically, the question whether defects in the cerebellum lead directly to movement disorders, or whether the disorders are due to secondary effects on the brain stem has not been resolved.

The major oculomotor signs of cerebellar disease are as follows:

*Nystagmus.* This is usually horizontal in nature, with its fast component toward the side of the lesion. The oscillations are always greatest when the eyes are deviated toward the side of the lesion. There may be a relative position of rest with the eyes deviated 10-20° to the side opposite the lesion. This may lead to a compensatory head turn.

*Dysmetria.* This is the inability of the conjugate gaze system to damp itself at the end of a programmed movement. It can be exaggerated by having the patient move his eyes from a lateral to a straight ahead position. The eyes move past the object of regard and oscillate around it in decreasing excursions, until fixation is established. This is similar to limb dysmetria.

*Flutter-like Oscillations.* These oscillations probably represent a lack in the damping of the microsaccade system and continually correct for microdrift in fixation. This disorder is easily seen clinically, whereas, with sustained fixation, an abrupt break will occur with dysmetric type oscillations around the fixation point.

*Skew Deviation.* This sign is indicative of posterior fossa disease rather than cerebellar disease alone. It is simply a vertical deviation, which does not fit any of the characteristic findings of paretic muscle disease.

*Vestibular apparatus.* The substrate for vestibular control over extraocular movements lies in the membranous labyrinth lodged within the petrous portion of the temporal bone. The membranous labyrinth is divided functionally into three separate entities: (1) the semicircular canals, (2) the utriculus, and (3) the sacculus. The utriculus and sacculus consist of a membranous plaque of hair cells imbedded in a gelatinous material containing calcrinous crystals, the otoliths. These organs are responsible for ophthalmostatic functions. Every position of the head in space has a specified position of the eyes in the orbit with respect to the vertical. The control is exerted by the otolithic apparatus.

The semicircular canals control ophthalmokinetic functions, where the eyes respond to acceleration and tend to oppose any change with motion. The semicircular canals are three in number: (1) horizontal, (2) anterior vertical, and (3) posterior vertical, lying at right angles to each other. At one end of each canal is the ampullae, a blister-like enlargement containing sensory hair cells imbedded in a gelatinous dome. The horizontal canal is stimulated when relative endolymph flow is toward the ampullae; the other canals are stimulated when the flow is away from the ampullae. The effect of stimulation of these canals is to produce a jerk-type nystagmus in the plane of the canal. The horizontal canal lies at 30° to the horizon, and the head must be tilted 30° forward or 60° back to isolate this canal with specific tests. With the head back, we can use thermal stimulation to test the vestibular apparatus by injecting either cold or tepid water into the external auditory canal. The response is characterized by the mnemonic "COWS" with respect to the fast or corrective phase of nystagmus: cold opposite, warm same. The slow deviation of the eyes is under direct control of the vestibular apparatus, whereas the fast phase is under control of the frontal lobe. The vestibular nerve has its origin in the labyrinth and terminates in the vestibular nucleus in the flow of the fourth ventricle. There is reasonable evidence that the most anterior portion of the nuclei mediates vertical movements, the most posterior part torsional movements, and the substance between horizontal movements. Whether the horizontal movements are channeled through the pontine gaze center has not been determined, but probably they are. Lesions of the vestibular apparatus are usually accompanied by vertigo and spontaneous nystagmus in the fast phase in the direction of the involved side.

*Superior colliculus.* Retinotectal projections to the superior colliculus are well documented. Their role in pattern discrimination is still the subject of disagreement, but recent physiological evidence suggests that the superior colliculus is responsible for foveation. That is, the superior colliculus will initiate a saccadic movement to place the image of regard exactly on the fovea.

CEREBRAL CENTERS

*Frontal centers.* The left frontal center for conjugate horizontal gaze lies in Brodmann's area 8 (Fig. 6-11). It initiates all fast (saccadic) motion to the right. The fibers to the subcortical centers rise in medium-sized cells in area 8, project through the anterior limb of the anterior capsule near its knee, and run caudally with the fibers to the facial muscles. The fibers for conjugate lateral gaze decussate in the midbrain before the decussation of the facial fibers.

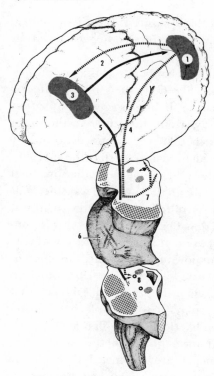

**Fig. 6-11** Theoretical gaze centers (o) and associated pathways. Occipito-parietal junction—? Brodmann's area 19 parastriate area.
1. Following movement center.
2. Association tracts—? internal sagittal striatum.
3. Saccadic frontal gaze center—Brodmann's area 8-alpha and -gamma.
4. Occipito-bulbar tract.
5. Fronto-bulbar tract.
6. Decussation of corticobulbar tracts dealing with eye movements.
7. Occipito-tectal projection.
8. Pontine gaze center.

They terminate in the pontine center for lateral gaze situated in the pontine reticular formation slightly rostral and medial to the abducent nerve nuclei. All fast phase motions (e.g., voluntary gaze, the fast phase of optokinetic nystagmus, and vestibular nystagmus) are routed through this frontal-bulbar center and pathway.

Injury to the frontal gaze center results in a loss of saccadic function to the contralateral side. This loss of function slowly fades with the assumption of this activity by the opposite frontal lobe center. Only when cortical function is depressed will a conjugate deviation of the eyes to the involved side be evident.

*Occipital lobe center.* This center probably sits at the occipitoparietal junction in or about area 19 (Fig. 6-11). It is responsible for slow movements of following, and it probably also initiates fixation movements. The projection pathways from this center to the brain stem are much less certainly known than the frontocorticobulbar pathways. At this time, the best evidence suggests that the occipito-bulbar tract courses medially along with the visual radiation, then caudally through the posterior limb of the internal capsule, and synapses in the thalamus, superior colliculus, and pons. Clinical evidence suggests that this projection decussates and controls contralateral horizontal following movements. The function of the occipito-thalamic projection is unknown at this time. An efferent connection between the occipital cortex and the superior colliculus is to be expected in face of the previously presented evidence that the superior colliculus apparently plays a role in placing the image of regard on the fovea, i.e., the fixation reflex. The fibers to the pons end in the pontine reticular formation. Whether slow movements, as well as saccadic movements, are channeled through the pontine center for lateral gaze is not firmly established, but experimental evidence indicates that they may be.

There is also an efferent connection between the occipital cortex and the frontal lobe centers for conjugate gaze. Although its location has not been established, this pathway is necessary for the initiation of microsaccades in fixation and the corrective fast phase of optokinetic nystagmus.

Lesions involving the occipital gaze center produce two clinical signs: (1) contralateral deviation of the eyes with forced lid closure (Cogan's sign), and (2) jerky microsaccadic movements rather than smooth following movements in ipsilateral gaze. These signs are explained on the basis of a spasticity phenomenon, i.e., the center is damaged and, upon recovery, becomes hyperexcitable. This, in turn, causes deviation toward the side of the normal hemisphere when fixation is broken by closing the eyes along with a jerky motion of the eyes when they are moved against the increased tone from the center.

## Vertical conjugate movements

Pure vertical movements require bilateral supranuclear input. Vertical conjugate gaze movements are represented in the cerebral cortex as part of the lateral gaze center. Their projection to bulbar centers or directly to oculomotor nuclei is not well documented. One clinical fact is well known—lesions in and around the superior and inferior colliculi are associated with vertical gaze palsies. These movement defects may involve saccadic and following functions or saccadic functions alone. Lesions in this region may also be associated with pupillary and convergence abnormalities.

## Torsional conjugate movements

These movements are unique in that they are not subject to voluntary control. They are under control of the labyrinth through the vestibular nuclei with some minor input from the "stretch receptors" in the neck muscle groups.

## Disjunctive movements

### CONVERGENCE

Convergence is the act of foveation of both eyes on the object of regard at some relatively near point. The supranuclear centers for convergence are not known, but these movements can be seen after stimulation of both frontal and occipital gaze centers. The final common pathway is funneled through the oculomotor nerve nucleus, but the exact substrate is unknown.

### DIVERGENCE

The centers for divergence are much more obscure than those of convergence. Recent evidence has proved beyond a doubt that divergence is an active process, but its substrate remains unknown.

## Summary

Figure 6-12 summarizes the pathophysiology of eye movements in man.

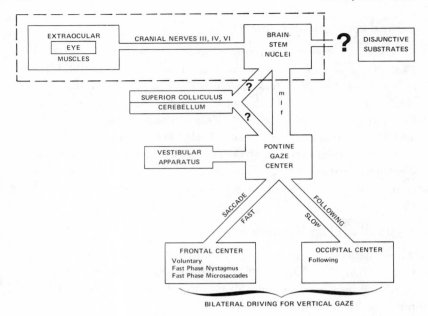

**Fig. 6-12** Pathophysiology of eye movements in man. Lesions within the dotted line, nuclear and infranuclear diplopia; lesions outside the dotted line, supranuclear loss of function; mlf, medial longitudinal fasciculus.

## References

Cogan, D. G. 1956. Neurology of the ocular muscles, 2nd ed. Charles C. Thomas, Springfield, Ill.

Walsh, F. B. and W. F. Hoyt. 1969. Clinical neuro-ophthalmology, 3rd ed. Williams & Wilkins, Baltimore.

Moses, R. A. 1970. Adler's physiology of the eye, 5th ed. Mosby, St. Louis, Mo.

## General references

Bach-y-Rita, P., C. Collins, and J. E. Hyde, eds. 1971. The control of eye movements. Academic Press, New York.

## PATHOPHYSIOLOGY OF AUDITION
### HALLOWELL DAVIS

### Classification of auditory defects

Defects of the auditory system may either be peripheral, in the sense organ and auditory nerve, or central, in the central nervous

TABLE 6-3  *Summary of Auditory Defects*

| | |
|---|---|
| PERIPHERAL | |
| Middle and External Ear | |
| Mechanical | Attenuation of sound |
| Inner Ear | |
| Mechanical | Attenuation of sound |
| Anatomical | Loss of sensory units |
| Physiological (reversible) | Elevation of thresholds |
| | Block of transmission |
| | Disorganization |
| CENTRAL | Failure of perception |
| | Failure of integration |
| | Failure of understanding |

system. These two classes of defects are entirely different in character and are handled by different medical or surgical specialties. A summary classification is given in Table 6-3. Here the peripheral defects are divided anatomically into those in the middle and external ear and those of the inner ear. The former are accessible to surgical intervention; the latter are inaccessible but raise questions of medical management or the use of a hearing aid.

The auditory defects of the middle and external ear are essentially mechanical and result in the attenuation of sound. The attenuation may be equal for all frequencies, or it may be greater for lower frequencies, as is sometimes the case in otitis media and early otosclerosis. Most often, it is more severe for the higher frequencies. The general terms for this loss of sensitivity are hearing loss or hypoacusis. More specifically, it is a conductive hearing loss.

Defects of the inner ear may represent either mechanical inefficiency, an anatomical loss of sensory cells and/or their nerve fibers, or such a reversible physiological change as temporary elevation of thresholds (threshold shift), block of transmission of nerve impulses, as by compression of the cochlear nerve, or a more subtle disorganization of the interactions between sensory units. Such inner ear defects cause a sensori-neural hearing loss.

The central defects are described in psychological terms including failure of perception, of integration, or of understanding. Here it is usually impossible to identify the structures or physiological processes at fault.

The sensitivity of hearing as a function of frequency is measured by means of a pure-tone audiometer. The results can be expressed as the sound-pressure levels at which the tones can just be heard, as illustrated by the heavy line in Fig. 6-13. More often, however, they are plotted on an audiogram as differences, in decibels, between the subject's threshold and an internationally standardized set of reference (zero) levels. These standards represent the median values for the thresholds of "otologically normal young adults." Audiometers are calibrated to read directly these differences, hear-

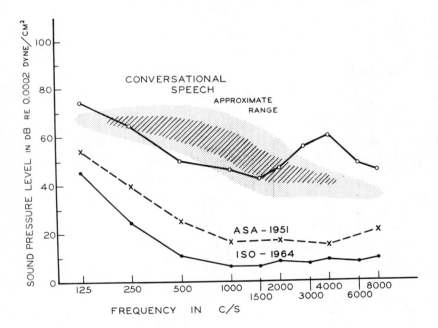

**Fig. 6-13** The lowest curve shows the International Standards Organization (ISO) reference zero levels for pure-tone audiometers (solid line and dots). The dashed line with crosses shows the old American Standards Association (ASA) levels of 1951. The upper curve (solid with open circles) is the hypothetical threshold curve of a man with impaired hearing. The shaded area shows the approximate range of the intensities and frequencies of the sounds of conversational speech at 1 m. Most of the low-frequency, but few of the high-frequency sounds would be audible to the man with the hypothetical threshold curve.

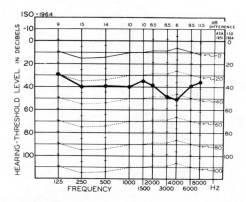

**Fig. 6-14** On this conventional audiogram blank, the ISO reference zero level is the horizontal line at 0 dB. The heavy line is an audiogram corresponding to the auditory thresholds shown in Fig. 6-13. The hearing-threshold levels, plotted downward from the ISO reference level, indicate the deviation in decibels from the reference value at each frequency. The audiometer is calibrated to read these differences directly from its dial.

The faint lines in the figure represent the coordinates of the old ASA-1951 reference levels (see Fig. 6-13) as they would appear when plotted in terms of the ISO reference system. The numerical values of the differences at each frequency are given above each frequency ordinate.

The range of normal hearing is sometimes indicated by shading the upper part of the audiogram blank from its upper edge down to roughly 20-dB hearing threshold level (ISO). The audiogram that is plotted here falls entirely outside the range of normal.

ing threshold levels, which are then plotted (Fig. 6-14). (The old ASA reference levels, Figs. 6-13 and 6-14, are no longer in use, but, in reading old audiograms, the difference between the old and new standards must be remembered.) Similar standardization has been carried out for bone-conduction audiometers, and hearing levels measured by bone conduction can be plotted on the same audiogram for comparison.

## Conductive hearing loss

The defects of conductive hearing loss are well understood, and the modern surgical procedures of tympanoplasty, fenestration, stapedectomy, etc. can alleviate much of the mechanical defect. The chief problem here is to locate the defect.

One approach is through the mobility of the eardrum and ossi-

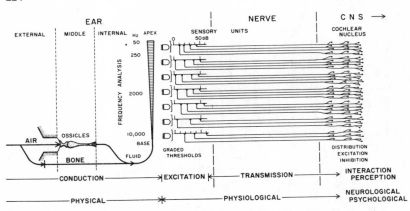

**Fig. 6-15** This summary diagram of the peripheral auditory mechanism is semi-anatomical. The air-conduction pathway shows the ossicles simplified to a sub-divided columella, disregarding their lever action. The coiled, tapering basilar membrane is represented as straight. The sensory units are represented by nerve fibers, with cell bodies omitted, running from the hair cells (arranged along the basilar membrane) to the cochlear nucleus. Each of the hair cells shown in the diagram represents a group of cells in a short segment of the organ of Corti. The sensory units from such a segment have different thresholds for any given tone. The gradation of thresholds is represented here by an arbitrary scale of decibels, 0 to 50, for each small segment. The actual range of gradation and its relation to anatomical distribution, such as inner versus outer hair cells, are not known.

cles, as observed by the pneumatic otoscope or measured in terms of acoustic impedance. Another method is through the comparison of the thresholds of hearing by air conduction and by bone conduction. The difference between them, the air-bone gap, measures the amount of middle-ear conductive hearing loss. We will not be concerned here with the details of these technical procedures.

Figure 6-15 is a diagram of the basic features of the peripheral auditory mechanism. At the left are representations of the external ear, the tympanic membrane, and the ossicles. The latter are shown as a single column across the middle ear. This is the pathway of air conduction. The pathway of bone conduction bypasses the ossicles by way of the cranial bones, but the bone-conduction and air-conduction pathways unite in the fluid-filled cochlea to produce the same movements of the semi-flexible basilar membrane that extends from the base to the apex of the cochlea.

## Sensori-neural hearing loss

Our understanding of sensori-neural hearing impairment and pathophysiology of the inner ear is not very satisfactory. We must be content at many points with tentative hypotheses and with empirical accounts of the signs and symptoms.

Returning to Fig. 6-15, note the tapering width of the basilar membrane, which causes it to be quite stiff in its narrow portion but very flexible toward the broader apical region. This gradation of stiffness makes it differentially sensitive to vibrations of different frequencies, and a basic process of mechanical frequency analysis is performed here. The result is excitation of different groups of sensory cells in the organ of Corti, depending on the frequency or frequencies in the exciting sound. Figure 6-16 will serve as a reminder of the fundamentals of the microscopic structure and the arrangement of the sensory cells (hair cells) with their cilia imbedded in the overlying tectorial membrane.

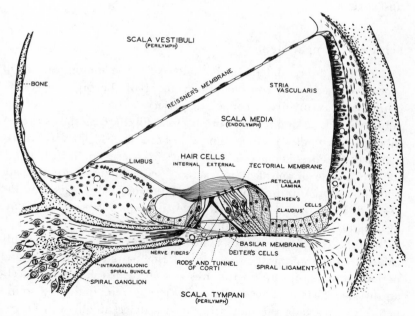

**Fig. 6-16** Cross-sectional drawing of the canal in the second turn of a guinea pig cochlea. The human cochlea is quite similar.

*Sensory unit* in Fig. 6-15 means a neuron and the sensory cells that can excite it. They are shown in groups with graded thresholds. It is a moot point at present whether there are indeed different populations of sensory units with systematically higher or lower thresholds, but it is certain that each unit is rather sharply tuned to a particular frequency, by virtue of its location on the basilar membrane, and that, as a tone becomes stronger, the mechanical movement spreads up and done the membrane and excites more neighboring units. In this sense, at least, there is a gradation of thresholds. Both frequency discrimination and the summation of loudness depend initially upon these specialized and graded sensitivities and also on complicated interactions among cooperating units in the cochlear nucleus.

We shall examine several types of impairment of this complicated mechanism and the possible basis of certain common signs and symptoms. In the discussion we shall omit entirely the efferent olivo-cochlear neural system. The synaptic endings of these fibers on the outer hair cells are large and prominent, but, for function, only a minor (inhibitory) adjustment of sensitivity has been demonstrated.

## Sense organ impairment

One of the simplest defects of the inner ear is the anatomical loss of sensory units from a considerable segment of the organ of Corti. This loss may involve a congenital defect or be the result of degeneration, as in one form of presbycusis. Figure 6-17 shows a postmortem "map" of a cochlea. The threshold at 2048 Hz was greatly elevated, and frequencies higher than this were not heard at all. This is a case of simple "subtractive" sensori-neural impairment, with no disorganization of the remaining normal portion of the organ of Corti. It is a curious fact that this type of abrupt high-tone hearing loss is quite strongly linked to the male sex.

In some conditions, notably advancing age, there are probably changes in the physical properties of the basilar membrane, and perhaps other supporting structures as well, which makes the mechanism less efficient acoustically and thereby attenuates the sound before it can excite the hair cells. Such a defect might well be frequency-selective, meaning that it might systematically depress the

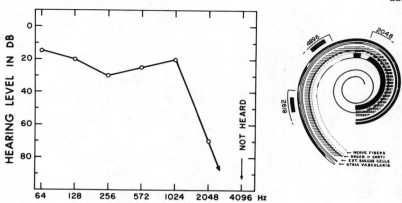

**Fig. 6-17** Audiogram and chart of postmortem findings in an ear with abrupt high-tone loss. The actual fall in sensitivity of hearing may have been even more abrupt (steeper) than shown here because no measurements were made between 1024 and 2048 Hz. Outside the spiral are indicated the zones required for the normal reception of frequencies of 2048, 4096, and 8192 Hz, based on correlation of audiograms and locations of abnormalities of 79 human ears. The shaded rectangles show the most probable locations for 4096 and 8192 Hz. (Data and chart from Crowe, Guild and Polvogt; Bull. Johns Hopkins Hospital, 54:315-739, 1934.)

sensitivity for high frequencies rather than low frequencies and thus gives the characteristic gradual high-tone hearing loss of presbycusis. This proposition is plausible, but it has not been directly confirmed experimentally.

An example of a reversible physiological change is the temporary elevation of thresholds caused by exposure to loud sound. Depending on the intensity and the duration of the exposure and the consequent severity of the threshold shift, the changes may be compared either to fatigue or to the beginning of injury. If the sound is loud enough, and the exposure long enough, recovery will be incomplete, and the condition known as permanent noise-induced threshold shift will occur. This is what used to be called boilermaker's deafness, but it occurs in other industrial situations as well. With permanent threshold shift (in experimental animals), there is almost always a loss of hair cells in the part of the organ of Corti that is "tuned" to frequency range of the hearing loss. The nature of the physiological or pathological changes associated with tem-

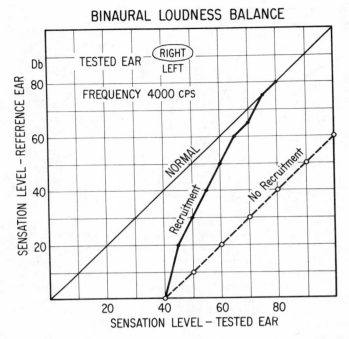

**Fig. 6-18** The results of binaural loudness balances at a given frequency may be plotted in this way. If, as in the ideal normal situation, the audiometer readings are equal for every loudness match, the points fall along the diagonal line of equality labeled normal. A hypothetical case of recruitment (unilateral sensory-neural hearing loss) is also shown. In this case, recruitment is complete at 75 dB, but convergence more often occurs at 90 dB. Recruitment is not necessarily complete. A conductive hearing loss shows displacement of all points to the right, but they still fall on a diagonal line parallel to the normal line.

porary elevation of thresholds is not yet clearly understood, but it is being vigorously examined at the present time.

A particular sign that is associated with several varieties of sense-organ impairment, including temporary and permanent noise-induced hearing loss, is recruitment of loudness. Here the threshold for hearing a particular frequency is elevated, but, when the test tone is gradually increased in intensity above the threshold, the subjective sensation of loudness increases more rapidly than normal with the increase of intensity. At a high sound-pressure level, say 90 dB above normal threshold, the test tone may sound as loud to the impaired ear as to the normal ear (see Fig. 6-18). If a patient has one normal ear it is easy to test for recruitment in the abnormal ear by giving the same test frequency alternately to the two ears and adjusting the intensity to the normal ear until it sounds equally loud to what is heard in the abnormal ear. If both ears have elevated thresholds for the frequency in question, it may still be possible to make a loudness balance in a single ear if some frequencies are heard at approximately normal threshold. In this case two different frequencies are given alternately to the same ear and are adjusted until they sound equally loud. This monaural loudness balance is a little more difficult than the binaural for the patient, but with a little encouragement most patients manage to do it quite well.

The physiological basis for recruitment is uncertain. The facts are compatible with the hypothesis that there are two populations of nerve endings and their hair cells in the organ of Corti, one of them with thresholds considerably higher than the other. The low-threshold population is assumed to be fatigued or slightly injured by the noise exposure, while the high-threshold group remains unaffected. The high-threshold group is assumed to dominate the sensory input at high sound-pressure levels, so the loss of sensitivity of the more sensitive elements is not noticed at high sound-pressure levels. Evidence from the electrochochleogram, i.e., the action potentials of the auditory nerve, which may be recorded with the help of a summating computer, strongly supports this interpretation. On the other hand, animal experiments in which the thresholds and the outputs of single auditory nerve fibers are examined have not revealed the presence of the postulated high-threshold population of sensory units. Whatever its physiological basis may be, however, the sign of loudness recruitment is strongly associated with impairment of the sense organ. It cannot be produced by conductive impairment and is present in only a minority of cases of nerve impairment due to compression by a tumor. This latter differential diagnosis is of great clinical importance.

Another type of sense-organ impairment is the syndrome, Menière's disease, which is characterized by elevation of the auditory threshold, tinnitus (ringing in the ears), dysacusis (a loss of the tonal quality of sounds), loss of speech discrimination (the ability to recognize words), and loudness recruitment. Furthermore, there is usually an involvement of the non-auditory labyrinth with the symptom of vertigo. The vertigo may be much more disabling and distressing than the auditory impairment, particularly as the disease is typically only unilateral. The characteristic pathological change in Menière's disease is distension of the membranous labyrinth. There seems to be an overproduction of endolymph or a failure of its reabsorption, and the condition is usually known as endolymphatic hydrops. This affects the non-auditory as well as the auditory labyrinth. The cause of Menière's disease is not known. It is not clear which, if any, of the symptoms are due to the hydrops. It is likely that there are chemical abnormalities in the endolymph as well as an excess of endolymph. Theories of causation range from vascular disturbances to allergy to abnormalities of salt metabolism to psychosomatic factors. Physiologically, it remains an enigma, but it is clear that the auditory disturbances express a profound disorganization of the neural input, suggestions of hyperexcitability (tinnitus), and mechanical inefficiency (elevation of threshold). Perhaps some of the symptoms, such as the loss of tonal quality and of speech discrimination, depend on the disruption of normal patterns of inhibitory interactions in the cochlear nucleus.

Certain drugs, notably some antibiotics in the mycin group (e.g., kanamycin), may cause selective degeneration of hair cells in the cochlea, particularly those in the basal turn that are sensitive to high frequencies. We can hope that the experimental study of this condition in animals will soon clarify some of the problems of peripheral pathophysiology.

Acoustic neuroma, i.e., a neuroma of the sheath of the auditory nerve in the internal auditory meatus, may compress the auditory nerve (cranial nerve VIII) and cause either auditory or labyrinthine symptoms or both. (The disturbances are considered in another chapter.) The symptoms come on gradually and continue without remission, in sharp contrast to the usual episodic character of Menière's disease. The impairment of hearing is likely to resemble that of advancing age (presbycusis) but it comes on sooner, develops more rapidly, and is unilateral. The audiological sign that is most characteristic is fast auditory fatigue. A tone, usually with a high frequency, is presented some 5 or 10 dB above threshold. Normally, such a tone will be heard indefinitely, but, with an acoustic neuroma (and in a few other conditions), the tone is no longer heard within 30 seconds or so. If the intensity is increased by 10 or 15 dB, the tone will be heard again, but again it will fade out if long continued. The basis of this sign is not clear, but it seems to resemble the so-called Wedensky inhibition that can be produced in a nerve-muscle preparation by careful local narcosis or compression of a section of the peripheral nerve or at the neuro-myal junction. One possible model for explanation is a loss of the safety factor in nerve conduction. The action potential becomes weaker, and, perhaps, the threshold for excitation at the next node of Ranvier rises, and, finally, conduction fails. A brief period of recovery restores the action potentials sufficiently to resume conduction, but exhaustion soon occurs again. This condition of rapid metabolic exhaustion would be compatible with local mechanical pressure, perhaps through the mechanism of reduced circulation.

## Central dysacusis

Central dysacusis (impairment of hearing) may be combined with peripheral impairment, as in presbycusis in which the central impairments from arteriosclerosis and senility are often the most important. A slower tempo of talking and the reduction of masking background are more helpful than amplification, although amplification may also be helpful.

Psychogenic deafness or "overlay" (hysterical) does exist, but it is rather rare. Its physiological mechanism is unknown.

Nonorganic or functional deafness (feigning) is more or less deliberate. This is fairly common.

Central dysacusis can be caused by cerebral vascular accidents, tumors, infarcts, etc., but impairment of threshold or of pitch discrimination or even of tonal quality are rare because the simple auditory functions are bilateral or subcortical or both. The comprehension (and expression) of language, however, usually depends on the left hemisphere, and certain complex auditory tasks, such as dealing with competing messages, depend chiefly on the hemisphere contralateral to the input ear.

Congenital sensory aphasia in childhood usually means a failure to learn speech, even though the audiogram is within normal limits. It can occur on the basis of bilateral impairment of the primary auditory areas. (One such case has been verified at autopsy.) A much more common condition is a difficulty in learning language (dyslogomathia). A partial impairment of peripheral hearing is usually present in the cases seen at Central Institute for the Deaf. Differential diagnoses include autism and mental retardation. Our tentative explanation for those with partial impairment of hearing is failure of normal organization of the auditory system due to the absence of an adequate patterned input (speech) during a critical period of maturation of the central nervous system.

### General references

Davis, H. and S. R. Silverman. 1970. Hearing and deafness, 3rd ed. Holt, Rinehart & Winston, New York, especially Chapters 4, 7, and 8.

Davis, H. 1962. A functional classification of auditory defects. Ann. Otol. Rhinol. Laryngol. 71:693-704.

Gloring, A. and H. Davis. 1961. Age, noise and hearing loss. Ann. Otol. Rhinol. Laryngol. 70:556-572.

Landau, W. M., R. Goldstein, and F. R. Kleffner. 1960. Congenital aphasia. Neurology 10:915-921.

## VESTIBULAR DISORDERS

PHILLIP M. GREEN AND MALCOLM H. STROUD

### Anatomy

The vestibular system includes the labyrinthine end organ of the inner ear, the auditory nerve (cranial nerve VIII), the brain-stem vestibular nuclei, and their ascending and descending connections. The purpose of the vestibular system is to signal changes in motion of the head (acceleration or deceleration) and positions of the head with respect to gravity. The labyrinthine end organ consists of a utricle and saccule, vestibule, and semicircular canals, all of which lie imbedded within the petrous portion of the temporal bone (Fig. 6-19).

The utricle connects with the end of each of the semicircular canals and, together with the saccule, contains the nervous end organ known as the macula. The macula contains sensory epithelium enclosing hair cell end organs, which are, in turn, covered by a gelatinous substance containing calcium carbonate concretions called otoliths. Gravity exerts a constant pull on the otoliths to produce an electrical potential discharged through the vestibular nerve. Changes in the position of the head cause a shift in the po-

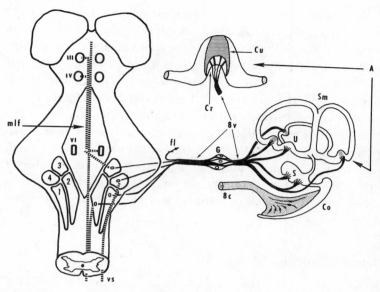

**Fig. 6-19** Diagram of the vestibular system: Left, brain stem, central nuclei, and major pathways; right, peripheral apparatus; 1,2,3, and 4, descending, medial, superior and lateral vestibular nuclei, respectively; III, IV, and VI, ocular muscle nuclei; mlf, medial longitudinal fasciculus; vs, vestibulospinal tract; fl, pathway to flocculo-nodular lobe of the cerebellum. 8v, vestibular portion of the auditory nerve, 8c, cochlear portion of the auditory nerve; G, Scarpa's ganglion; Cr, cristae; Cu, cupula; A, ampulla; Sm, semicircular canals; U, utricle; S, sacule; Co, cochlea.

sition of the otoliths and hair cells, resulting in an alteration of the discharges within the vestibular nerve.

Lying at right angles to each other within the inner ear are the three semicircular canals, each on a different plane. Each canal ends in the ampullae wherein a sensory organ detects changes of pressure or flow of endolymph within the canal. The sense organ of the semicircular canal (cristae) is a complex of supporting nervous epithelium and hair cells surrounded by a gelatinous cupola, which detects changes in movement of the head in space. Impulses from the sensory receptors of the semicircular canals join with those from the macula within the vestibular nerve to enter the medulla and the vestibular nuclei at the pontine-medullary juncture.

There are four vestibular nuclei: superior, lateral, spinal, and medial. The superior and medial vestibular nuclei project to the cerebellum. The lateral vestibular nucleus receives fibers from the cerebellum. Its primary projection is down the spinal cord to the anterior horn cells (alpha motor neurons and gamma motor neurons). The medial vestibular nucleus connects with the reticular gray substance of the brain stem, the dorsal efferent nucleus of the vagus nerve, and the spinal cord. Projections from the vestibular nuclei also ascend through pathways of uncertain location to the cerebral cortex. The vestibular system, through its connections with brain-stem nuclei, the cerebellum, and spinal cord centers, has a part in the regulation of muscular tone and the maintenance of postural reflexes. A subsidiary, but important function of the vestibular complex is the reflex coordination of extraocular movements when the head is moved.

## Evaluation of function

Clinical dysfunction of the vestibular system is usually either the result of disorders affecting the end organ (peripheral dysfunctions) or disorders affecting the brain stem (central dysfunctions). As a rule, both the gravity (static) sensor and the kinetic (movement) sensor are affected by diseases of the peripheral end organ. The two sensors, however, may be affected separately by degenerative conditions or vascular disorders. Kinetic and gravitational functions are both affected by diseases of the brain stem.

The mechanism of vestibular action is complex, but a clinically useful simplification is the assumption that vestibular input from the right ear equally opposes similar activity derived from the left. Thus, unilaterally destructive lesions result in a relative overactivity of the vestibular system of the unaffected ear, whereas irritative lesions result in unilateral hyperactivity on the affected side. Deviation of the head and eyes away from the more active ear is a consequence of unilateral disease; ocular deviation is interrupted by rapid jerking of the eye toward a mid-position (i.e., toward the more active labyrinth). If the patient is in a vertical position, there is a sense of true rotatory vertigo, a hallucination of horizontal movement in a circular fashion about the patient's head or body. In the vertical position, the hallucinated movement usually occurs toward the more active labyrinth with postural deviations and past-pointing in the opposite direction.

This simplified version depends for its veracity on the patient's head and body being approximately vertical so that the lateral semi-circular canal is the part of the vestibular organ most severely affected by the insult. The signs of unilateral vestibular disease are usually much more variable and complex and depend on the part of the vestibule affected most severely as well as the position of the head and body in space. Thus, if static sensors are predominantly affected, none of the above abnormalities may be noted, but the patient may complain of a sense of tilting or even falling in space, and, if the lesion is acute, he may actually be thrown to the ground without a sense of vertigo. The patient may describe this as a propulsive force rather than a loss of postural tone. Even in those instances where the semicircular canals are predominantly involved, modifications depending upon the position of the head and body occur. It is only when the lateral canals are predominantly stimulated that true lateral deviation of the eyes and horizontal nystagmus are seen. When there is predominant stimulation of either posterior or superior labyrinthian canals, or both, nystagmus is oblique and may have a rotatory component. The quick component of the nystagmoid movement, however, is away from the lesion. Pure vertical nystagmus is not seen with labyrinthian lesions but has a central basis. Another variation that is clinically prominent is the ability of the patient to overcome forced ocular deviation by visual fixation. Thus even during an acute episode, the eyes may remain relatively close to the midline, although rhythmic nystagmus will continue to be seen. If fixation is broken by dimming the lights, by asking the patient to close his eyes, or by having him change the direction of his gaze, both the sense of rotation and the nystagmoid movements will be increased as the eyes deviate away from the more active labyrinth.

Much of our understanding of the physiology of these clinical phenomena has come from analysis of tests of vestibular function, particularly caloric tests. Warm water instilled into one ear simulates an irritative, hyperexcitable lesion in that ear, whereas cold water simulates a destructive or hypoexcitable lesion. The standard test requires irrigation of each ear for 30 seconds at a time with at least 250 ml of water. The temperature of the water should be 7° below (30°C) or above (44°C) normal body temperature to achieve optimal results. This small change in temperature over a 30-second period is sufficient to stimulate the flow of endolymph in the semicircular canals of the tested ear. The preponderant effect occurs in the vertical plane, where gravitational pull magnifies endolymphatic currents. Thus, the position of the head and body is crucial in this test. In general, it is desirable to test the function of the lateral canal, since preponderant stimulation of this canal results in lateral deviation of the eyes with horizontal nystagmus rather than more complicated oblique movements and also produces a sense of horizontal vertigo and lateral past-pointing rather than the more complicated sensations that occur with stimulation of posterior, superior, or multiple canals. To stimulate the lateral canal, the patient must either be in the prone position with the head tilted 30° forward or seated with the head tilted 60° backward. In either of these positions, the lateral canal is now in the vertical plane with a superior orientation. In this situation, cold water causes endolymph to flow away from the ampulla, and hot water has the opposite effect. Stimulating the left ear with warm water then results in a slow deviation of eyes to the right with a quick component of nystagmus to the left. A sensation of vertigo occurs to the left with postural deviation to the right. The importance of head position can be emphasized by performing the same test with the patient seated but his head 90° to 120° forward. In this position the lateral canal is also in the vertical plane but is inferiorly oriented. Thus, endolymphatic flow is reversed. In this position nystagmus is horizontal and to the left, and the sense of vertigo is to the right. (See Fig. 6-20.)

Although the relationship of endolymphatic flow to the signs and symptoms of vestibular disease is of physiological interest, for practical purposes, tests of vestibular function are designed to discover whether there is destruction or undue sensitivity of the peripheral end organ or lesions in central vestibular pathways, particularly in the brain stem. This can best be achieved by timing the duration of nystagmus set in motion by caloric stimulation of the ear. The lateral canals are preferentially stimulated because of the greater ease in monitoring horizontal nystagmus. Under standard conditions, nystagmus should persist for $1\frac{1}{2}$ to $2\frac{1}{2}$ minutes when timed from the beginning of stimulation. In the presence of a destructive lesion of the labyrinth, there is either no reaction or the duration

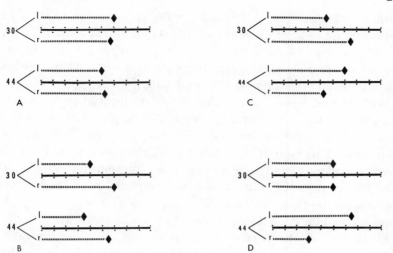

**Fig. 6-20** Graphic representation of duration nystagmus with caloric tests, using warm 44°C (44) and cold 30°C (30) to the left (l) and right (r) ears, respectively. Dots along the heavy solid line represent 20-second intervals. Dashed lines terminating in a black diamond signify duration of nystagmus. (A) Average (normal) reaction; (B) left canal paresis; (C) directional preponderance toward the left; and (D) right canal paresis plus left directional preponderance.

and the amplitude of the nystagmus is markedly reduced regardless of whether the ear is stimulated with warm or cold water.

Often central lesions will produce a different type of abnormality known as directional preponderance. To test for directional preponderance, the peripheral vestibular apparatus must be intact. It should be clear from the description of the physiology of vestibular stimulation that stimulation of the left ear with cold water with the patient supine and head 30° forward will produce deviation of the eyes to the left with a quick component of nystagmus to the right. Similarly, stimulation of the right ear with cold water and also stimulation of the left ear with warm water will produce a quick component of nystagmus to the left. In normal individuals, the duration of nystagmus to the left produced by stimulating the right, and then the left ear, appropriately, approximately equals the duration of nystagmus to the right. If the duration of nystagmus in one direction exceeds that in another by 40 seconds or more, we have what is known as directional preponderance. The site of the lesion in the brain stem is usually on the side of reduced preponderance. Thus, in lesions to the right of the midline, stimulation of the right ear with warm water and the left ear with cold water will result in a considerably shorter period of nystagmus than stimulation of the left ear with warm water and the right ear with cold water.

With central lesions, there may also be a dissociation of ocular responses to stimulation of the semicircular canals, resulting in dissociated movements of left and right eyes in either direction or amplitude. This type of dysjunctive nystagmus is often difficult to observe without electrical recording of eye movements. Nystagmus may be unassociated with subjective symptoms of vertigo, pastpointing, or postural deviation in central lesions. Pure vertical nystagmus also indicates a lesion of central vestibular pathways.

Evaluation of the normal function of the otolithic apparatus (which senses the position of the head in space) is best elicited by what is called the Bárány maneuver. The patient is seated and asked to fix his gaze at a point of the examiner's forehead. The head is turned either to the right or left and then is carried to a position 30° to 45° below the horizontal. The inner ear, which is uppermost, is differentially stimulated compared to the ear directed downward. Under normal conditions, there will be no sensation of vertigo and no nystagmus. With disease of one otolithic organ, or with asymmetrical disease affecting both otoliths, the patient develops vertigo and nystagmus, which abate within 1 to 2 minutes if he is maintained in the Bárány position. This response fatigues rapidly if the maneuver is repeated four or five times in succession. The nystagmus is generally uni-directional. The same maneuver can produce nystagmus and vertigo in patients with disease of the posterior fossa. Generally, these patients maintain the nystagmus for a much longer period of time when in the Bárány position, do not fatigue as readily, and exhibit multi-directional nystagmus, depending on head position.

The otolithic organs may also be stimulated by placing the patient in a human centrifuge and directing the centrifugal force either parallel through both ears or inward through one ear and outward via the other. Once a constant force and acceleration are obtained, the centrifuge is stopped, and the period of readjustment back to normal is measured in terms of nystagmus and deviation of posture.

A Bárány chair, in which the patient is spun at a constant rate about his own axis, and the rotation is then suddenly stopped, may also be used to test semicircular canal function. During rotation, the eyes deviate in the direction opposite to rotation. When the rotational movement ceases, nystagmus occurs with the quick component in the direction of rotation and the vertiginous movement in the opposite direction (i.e., if the patient is being rotated clockwise, when rotation ceases, the sensation of vertigo is in a counterclockwise direction). This test is used infrequently, since it is not possible to test each ear independently. It is of value, however, in testing the vestibular responses of neonates and young infants. This test can be carried out on the ward by suspending the baby above the examiner's head in a tilted position approximately 30° from the vertical. The examiner then rotates in a clockwise direction, and the infant's eyes deviate in the direction of movement. Unfortunately, the evaluation of post-rotational nystagmus is virtually impossible in this situation and requires the use of electrical and mechanical equipment unavailable in most hospitals.

## Pathophysiology

Diseases of the vestibular system generally affect end organs and central structures asymmetrically, giving rise to an imbalance that can be tested for by the clinical methods described above. Sudden acute lesions of the vestibular system produce marked symptomatology in terms of nystagmus, hallucinations of movement, deviations of posture, nausea and vomiting, and abnormal sensitivity to movement. Chronic or slowly developing lesions of the vestibular system may give rise to no symptoms whatsoever because functional adjustments can be made by the uninvolved portions of the central nervous system given sufficient time. Even so, results on the tests of function we have described will be abnormal.

Peripheral lesions that involve either the end organ or the auditory nerve usually produce canal paresis, a markedly diminished duration of nystagmus either following warm or cold water stimulation in the abnormal ear, in the presence of normal responses in the opposite ear. An abnormal response of a single canal in one ear, while other canals within the same ear respond normally, suggests that the lesion is in the inner ear rather than the auditory nerve.

Such peripheral lesions can theoretically be produced by infections, infarction, tumor, trauma, degeneration, or increased amounts of endolymphatic fluid. Damage to the vestibular nerve as a result of tumors, infection, or drugs may have similar effects. The most common disease of peripheral vestibular function in the adult is Menière's disease. Numerous theories have evolved as to the cause of this disease, including excessive amounts of endolymphatic fluid, abnormal fistulae, and degenerative changes in the ampullae. Despite considerable investigation, however, the pathophysiological mechanism of this disorder remains unknown.

Irritable lesions of one labyrinth, or of both affected to different degrees, can also yield symptoms of vertigo coupled with deviations in posture and nystagmus with nausea and vomiting. Such lesions may be caused by a local infection of the inner ear, probably, in most instances, of a viral nature, or by viral or bacterial infection of the middle ear, which results in increased pressure in the middle ear that indirectly increases hydrostatic pressure in the fluid compartment of the inner ear.

Central lesions involving the vestibular system, as we have already noted, may be without symptoms, many involve occasional attacks of vertigo, or may be associated with nystagmus sometimes accompanied by a non-rotational hallucination of movement in which the object oscillates in the direction of the nystagmus (oscillopsia). Here again, caloric tests for directional preponderance and the Bárány maneuver to elicit a postural nystagmus and a sensation of vertigo may be helpful in identifying the lesion. Lesions producing oscillopsia usually result from vascular disease and infarctions within the territory of the basilar artery, tumors of the brain stem, demyelinating disease, and encephalitis.

The tests of vestibular function we have been discussing are generally performed on conscious patients capable of verbalizing their responses. Yet these tests can be of great help in evaluating the patient in deep coma, particularly when disease of the brain stem is suspected. In the deeply comatose patient, visual and frontal motor control of extraocular movements by vestibular stimuli is thereby relatively enhanced. Since the patient's eyes do not fix, it is possible to test for a full range of eye movement by the doll's head maneuver, in which the head is moved from side to side and front to back to obtain lateral and vertical eye movements, respectively. If this stimulus is insufficient to move the eyes, a more powerful stimulus can be used if the eardrum is intact and the external canal cleared of wax—the injection of cold water into the external auditory canal. To achieve maximal results, 0°C water is often used, and the patient's head is held 30° above the supine. Under these circumstances, the eyes deviate toward the ear stimulated, and usually no nystagmus is seen. Maximal stimulation can be achieved by instilling 50 cc of ice water and then performing the doll's head maneuver immediately. Failure of the eyes to deviate in this situation may suggest considerable destruction of the brain stem, but this test has to be interpreted cautiously in the light of other clinical phenomena. As we have mentioned, for example, bilaterally dead labyrinths will put an end to ocular response. Similarly, no response will be seen with a complete paralysis of the extraocular muscles due to associated disease or possibly to herniation of the temporal lobes with paralysis of the third, fourth, and sixth cranial nerves. Lastly, certain drugs, notably the barbiturates and glutethimide, selectively depress ocular motility without damaging the brain stem. Thus, if drug ingestion is suspected, failure of the eyes to respond to caloric stimulation in a comatose patient is not compatible with complete recovery.

## General references

Cawthorne, T., M. R. Dix, and J. D. Hood. 1968. Vestibular syndromes and vertigo. Page 358 in P. P. Vinken and G. W. Bruyn, eds. Handbook of clinical neurology. Vol. 2. American Elsevier, New York.

Dix, M. R. 1969. Modern tests of vestibular function with special reference to their value in clinical practice. Brit. Med. J. 3:317.

Dix, M. R. and C. W. Hallpike. 1952. The pathology, symptomatology, and diagnosis of certain common disorders of the vestibular system. Proc. Roy. Soc. Med. 45:341.

Fisher, C. M. 1967. Vertigo in cerebrovascular disorders. Arch. Otolaryngol. 85:529.

Lindsay, S. R. 1967. Paroxysmal and positional vertigo and vestibular neuronitis. Arch. Otolaryn. 85:544.

# 7

# Disorders of Cerebral Circulation

MARCUS E. RAICHLE AND DARRYL C. DE VIVO

## Introduction

For its functional and structural integrity, the brain depends on a constant supply of glucose and oxygen and on the removal of metabolic waste, primarily in the form of carbon dioxide. This involves an intimate relationship of the cerebral blood flow, the availability of needed substrates, and the metabolic requirements of the brain. Although this relationship is protected by a number of mechanisms to be discussed in this chapter, the brain remains especially vulnerable to disturbances in its blood supply, and this is reflected in the high incidence of cerebrovascular disease in the general population.

Diseases resulting from disturbances in brain circulation are the greatest single cause of neurological disability. In the adult population, these disorders rank third in cause of death, and they are the foremost crippler of all diseases in the United States. It is estimated that over two million persons alive today have neurological manifestations of cerebrovascular disease. Many of these individuals are in the working age group of 25 to 64 years. Cerebrovascular disease is less prevalent in the children, since atherosclerosis, hypertension, and diabetes mellitus, major determinants of such disease in the adult population, are rare in children. Several diseases affecting the nervous system in children may have a vascular component, however, and this often remains unrecognized (neurofibromatosis, tuberous sclerosis, and sickle cell anemia) because of the reluctance of physicians to subject young children and infants to angiography and cerebral blood flow studies.

To understand the neurological manifestations of cerebrovascular disease one must know (1) the normal anatomy and physiology of the cerebrovascular system, (2) the effect of disturbance in this system on nervous tissue, and (3) the disease states responsible for the disturbance. This chapter will consider these three areas.

## Vascular anatomy of the central nervous system

### ARTERIAL BLOOD SUPPLY

The brain receives its blood supply from paired vertebral and internal carotid arteries as well as from anastomotic channels derived from extracranial vessels (Fig. 7-1). The two common carotid arteries lie adjacent to the internal jugular veins in the neck and bifurcate to form the right and left internal carotid arteries. These arteries supply blood to the eyes, the basal ganglia of the brain, most of the hypothalamus, and most of the areas of the frontal, parietal, and temporal lobes of the cortex. The internal carotid usually ascends from its origin in the neck into the skull without branching. It penetrates the skull in the petrous portion of the temporal bone and enters the cranium between the layers of the dura mater just beneath the Gasserian ganglion of the trigeminal nerve. It begins its subarachnoid course by perforating the dura mater and gives rise to the ophthalmic, posterior communicating, anterior choroidal, and anterior and middle cerebral arteries.

The external carotid artery begins to branch extensively just beyond its bifurcation. Blood supply to the dura mater of the brain is provided by branches from the external carotid arteries. Because of the rich vascular network supplied to the face and the orbit by the external carotid artery, it can provide appreciable and often clinically significant amounts of blood to the brain if the internal carotid artery is occluded. The primary channel for this collateral circulation is through anastomotic vessels lying within the orbit.

Most of the branches of the middle cerebral artery ramify in the

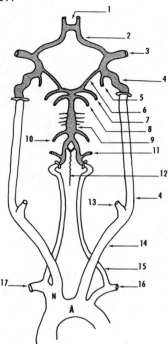

**Fig. 7-1** Anterior projected view of the arterial supply to the brain. Stippled vessels are intracranial; A, aorta; N, innominate artery (on the right side). The arteries are numbered as follows: 1, anterior communicating; 2, anterior cerebral; 3, middle cerebral; 4, internal carotid; 5, anterior choroidal; 6, posterior communicating; 7, posterior cerebral; 8, superior cerebellar; 9, basilar; 10, anterior inferior cerebellar; 11, posterior inferior cerebellar; 12, anterior spiral; 13, external carotid; 14, common carotid; 15, vertebral; 16, left subclavian; 17, right subclavian.

pia mater on the surface of the cerebral hemisphere, supplying about 80% of the blood received by the two cerebral hemispheres. The anterior cerebral artery courses medially to the longitudinal fissure of the cerebrum, and its cortical branches supply the frontal pole and the medial surface of the frontal and parietal lobes. The short anterior communicating artery joins the anterior cerebral arteries of the two hemispheres of the brain.

The brain stem and cerebellum are supplied by the two vertebral arteries, which usually arise from the subclavian arteries. These vessels reach the base of the brain through the bony tunnel formed by the adjacent transverse processes of the cervical vertebrae ($C_6$ to $C_1$). The two vertebral arteries enter the cranial cavity through the foramen magnum, follow the ventral surface of the medulla, and unite to form the basilar artery. At the rostral end of the brain stem, the basilar artery divides to form the two posterior cerebral arteries, which supply the medial and inferior surfaces and a small portion of the lateral surface of the temporal and occipital lobes.

The branches of the basilar and internal carotid arteries unite in a network of arteries to form a rough polygon, the circle of Willis. The component arteries in the circle of Willis are the two anterior cerebral arteries, the anterior communicating artery, the two posterior cerebral arteries, and the two posterior communicating arteries. This ring of connecting arteries surrounds the infundibulum and optic chiasm. Many small arteries arise directly from the vessels that comprise the circle of Willis and enter the base of the hemispheres to supply parts of the diencephalon and basal ganglia. Variations in the configuration of the circle of Willis are very common, especially in the relative sizes of its component arteries.

The anastomotic channels that comprise the circle of Willis, as well as the channels between the external and internal carotid arteries and leptomeningeal anastomoses between peripheral branches of the anterior, middle, and posterior cerebral arteries over the surface of the hemisphere, have the potential of allowing the brain to receive adequate blood flow from any one of its four major feeding arteries. The efficiency of this network can be judged from the many successful surgical ligations of the carotid artery in the neck for the treatment of intracranial aneurysm and the many well-described cases of spontaneous occlusion of one, two, and sometimes three of these arteries without serious clinical sequelae. Variations in the size of the major vessels, however (the right vertebral artery, for example, is frequently hypoplastic), and the patency of anastomotic channels, particularly those of the circle of Willis (which is frequently quite asymmetric), makes it difficult to predict the clinical effects of occlusion of a single artery. In the posterior fossa, there are anastomoses between the superior and the posterior and anterior inferior cerebellar arteries over the surface of the cerebellum. Branches arising from these circumferential arteries supply the dorsal and lateral areas of the brain stem, whereas the ventral and medial portions of the brain stem are supplied by small arteries that arise directly from the vertebral-basilar vessels and undeniably penetrate the brain. These arteries, like those that supply the branch of the diencephalon, are of less than several hundred micra in diameter.

Once arteries penetrate the pia, no significant anastomosis occurs until the capillary bed is formed, and the physiological adequacy of these capillary anastomoses can account for only millimeter variations in sizes of lesions.

VENOUS DRAINAGE

The veins of the brain drain into the dural venous sinuses and through them into the internal jugular veins. In contrast to the arteries, the surface veins of the brain have abundant anastomoses of large caliber. The ill effects of localized venous obstruction may therefore slight. The dural venous sinuses also communicate with the vascular channels in the bones of the skull, and these channels, in turn, communicate with the extracranial veins. In addition, there are emissary veins, which connect the dural venous sinuses with the

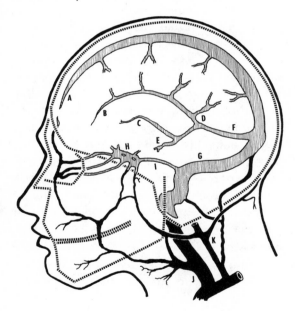

**Fig. 7-2** Lateral view of the sinuses and veins that receive blood from the brain. Dark portions are external to the skull and calvarium. A, superior sagittal sinus; B, inferior sagittal sinus; C, internal cerebral vein; D, great cerebral vein of Galen; E, basal vein of Rosenthal; F, straight sinus; G, transverse and sigmoid sinuses; H, cavernous sinus; I, superior petrosal sinus; J, internal vein; K, external jugular vein.

extracranial veins. There is enough venous capacity through the vertebral venous plexus in most healthy people to permit occlusion or removal of the external and internal jugular veins on one or both sides without producing serious intracranial hypertension. Because the veins of the central nervous system are valveless, blood may flow in or out of the skull through these vascular connections, providing a potential route for infection (Fig. 7-2).

## Physiology of the cerebral circulation

The total cerebral blood flow in a normal man averages 750 ml/minute. This is more conventionally expressed, because of the method of its derivation, as 50 ml/100 gm/minute. Further analysis of cerebral blood flow data reveals a fast flow component of approximately 70-80 ml/100 gm/minute and a slow component of 20-30 ml/100 gm/minute. The former has been related to flow through gray matter and the latter to flow through white matter.

### FACTORS AFFECTING CEREBRAL BLOOD FLOW

In a normal man, cerebral blood flow is kept very constant over a wide range of perfusion pressures. This phenomenon is known as autoregulation. Perfusion pressure in the brain represents the difference between the mean arterial blood pressure and the intracranial pressure plus the venous pressure. Under normal circumstances, the intracranial pressure and the venous pressure contribute little because of their magnitude relative to arterial blood pressure, and, thus, the mean arterial blood pressure can be viewed as the effective perfusion pressure. Autoregulation usually fails when the mean arterial blood pressure falls below 60 mm Hg. The mechanism by which cerebral vessels dilate when perfusion pressure falls and constrict when perfusion pressure rises is poorly understood. Neurogenic, myogenic, and metabolic theories have all been advanced. The practical importance of autoregulation to the central nervous system is obvious. Not only does it protect the brain from changes in perfusion pressure due to changes in body posture, but it also protects against narrowing or occlusion of major vessels in the neck, increased intracranial pressure, and decreased cardiac output (20% of which normally goes to the brain).

*Carbon dioxide.* This is the most potent stimulus known to the cerebral circulation. A 1-mm Hg change in the partial pressure of arterial carbon dioxide produces a 2% change in the cerebral blood flow. This provides a conceptual link between brain metabolism and blood flow, since the end product of the metabolism is carbon dioxide. The action of carbon dioxide on the cerebral vessels, however, appears to be mediated by changes induced in the perivascular concentration of hydrogen ions rather than by a direct action of carbon dioxide on the vascular wall. The local accumulation of such acidic metabolites as lactate and pyruvate or elevations in $P_aCO_2$ lowers the pH to produce vascular dilation. As a result, marked increases in the functional activity of the brain are associated with increased cerebral blood flow.

*Oxygen.* Although essential for the functioning and survival of the brain, oxygen has only a modest effect on cerebral circulation compared to carbon dioxide. Arterial oxygen tensions greater than 50 mm Hg have no measurable effect on cerebral circulation. Tensions below this level would appear to have a vasodilator action. When arterial oxygen tension remains above 50 mm Hg, the nervous system is able to maintain a constant supply of oxygen by adjusting the amount of oxygen extracted from the blood to changes in cerebral blood flow.

*Glucose.* This primary substrate for brain metabolism, has no effect on cerebral blood flow. A blood glucose level low enough to produce deep coma is not associated with any change in cerebral blood flow.

*Adrenergic system.* Adrenergic nerve fibers, which richly supply cerebral arterial blood vessels, travel to the intracranial vasculature via the cervical sympathetic chain. A wide variety of physiological and anatomical studies of this system have, to date, produced conflicting results, and its role in the regulation of cerebral blood flow remains an enigma.

*Blood viscosity.* Although changes in viscosity have not been convincingly shown to affect cerebral blood flow, there have been clinical observations of patients with polycythemia vera, which increases viscosity, who have a decreased cerebral blood flow. Experimentally, however, this has not been confirmed when a variety of means have been employed to change blood viscosity. Changes in blood flow in polycythemics may well be related to changes in oxygen delivery rather than blood viscosity.

*Temperature.* Changes in temperature do not affect cerebral blood flow when blood temperature remains in the range of 35° to 40°C. Below 35°C, cerebral blood flow has been shown to decrease 7%/degree change in temperature; 40° and 42°, it increases 30 to 50%. These changes in cerebral blood flow are probably related to alterations in metabolism as a consequence of changing temperature.

## Cerebral metabolism

The brain normally consumes oxygen at the rate of about 3.3 ml/100 gm/minute. This figure is remarkably constant in a normal man, both in the waking and sleeping states. The brain maintains no reserves of oxygen, and, therefore, only a few seconds of hypoxia can interfere with function. More than 10 to 15 minutes of hypoxia is almost certainly fatal to neurons. Cerebral blood flow and cerebral metabolic rate for oxygen have been studied in human brains irreversibly damaged by trauma or anoxia. As the electroencephalogram becomes isoelectric, the cerebral blood flow decreases, and the cerebral metabolic rate of $O_2$ consumption falls. At a cerebral blood flow of less than 15 ml/100 gm brain/minute and/or a cerebral metabolic rate of $O_2$ of less than 1 ml/100 gm brain/minute, irreversible brain damage will occur.

The major substrate consumed by the brain is glucose (about 5 mg/100 gm/minute). About 2 gm of glucose are usually in reserve, stored as free glucose or as glycogen. This reserve allows the organ to survive for a period of up to 90 minutes of profound hypoglycemia, in contrast to the much shorter period noted for anoxia.

Under normal circumstances, the cerebral blood flow is sufficient for the brain's metabolic needs. Sudden increases in metabolic requirements, such as those that occur with generalized seizures, are met by increases in cerebral blood flow. Conversely, when cerebral blood flow is decreased, the brain merely extracts more oxygen and glucose per unit volume of blood. The brain's metabolic rate will thus continue to be normal with decreasing blood flow, until so much oxygen has been extracted that the cerebral venous oxygen tension falls to about 20 mm Hg. To reach this value, the cerebral blood flow must fall to less than 50% of the normal value. At this point, the oxygen tension in the brain tissue remote from capillaries falls to levels that will no longer maintain metabolism. This 50% margin of safety is obviously reduced when insufficient oxygen reaches the blood, e.g., under conditions of high altitude, alveolar hypoventilation, or pulmonary disease or when the oxygen-carrying capacity of blood is reduced by anemia, methemoglobinemia, or carbon monoxide poisoning.

## Pathophysiology

As described in the preceding section, four factors protect the central nervous system against focal or generalized reduction in substrate supply: (1) increased extraction of glucose and oxygen from the perfusing blood, (2) autoregulation of blood flow in response to changes in perfusion pressure, (3) anastomosis within the artérial tree, primarily at the circle of Willis, and (4) increased cerebral blood flow. At times of generalized circulatory crises, these mechanisms are supplemented by systemic adjustments in blood flow, which favor blood flow to the central nervous system over other regions of the body. Despite this physiological insurance, cerebral blood flow and arterial concentrations of oxygen and glucose do fail to meet tissue metabolic needs under a variety of circumstances. The general consequences of this failure are discussed in this section.

The consequences of nutritional deprivation of the central nervous system, whether the result of an interference with the supply of nutrients (hypoxia or hypoglycemia) or their delivery (ischemia), are similar in many respects. Differences arise when factors related to changes in the blood vessels (i.e., rupture as contrasted with occlusion) supplying the brain add to the complexity of events. It is useful, therefore, to examine the pathophysiological events under two separate headings: infarction and hemorrhage.

### INFARCTION

When neural tissue is deprived of oxygen or glucose the functional and structural changes that can occur depend on the duration of the insult. When hypoxia persists for less than a minute, as might occur with vasodepressor syncope, postural hypotension, or decreased cardiac output (Stokes-Adams attack), clinical signs of impaired function (loss of consciousness, generalized convulsions, pupillary dilation, and loss of electroencephalographic activity) may be transient. When oxygen deprivation lasts longer than 1 to 2 minutes, neurons in the affected area undergo necrosis; those of the cerebral cortex (especially the hippocampus) and the cerebellum (the Purkinje cells) are most sensitive. Usually these changes can be recognized only by microscopy (and clinical observation, depending on the area involved). If oxygen deprivation is more severe or prolonged, as might occur with a thrombus or embolism, the cerebral cortex may appear grossly narrowed and show microscopic evidence of pseudolaminar necrosis with relative preservation of the superficial and deep cortical layers; in the white matter there may be demyelination or necrosis. If still more severe or prolonged hypoxia occurs, a relatively large area of gray and white matter will undergo complete necrosis (infarction).

When hypoxia is the result of a failure of cerebral blood flow (ischemia), experimental studies suggest that the rapidly lethal effect of the insult on brain cells is due not only to the sensitivity of these cells to hypoxia but also to the inability of the cerebrovascular bed itself to recover from a period of severe ischemia. After a period of about 4 minutes of circulatory arrest, the glial cells of the brain swell to the point of compressing capillaries, thus preventing the return of blood to the ischemic area. Experimental studies of isolated neural tissue have demonstrated that it can recover from prolonged oxygen deprivation; the retina, for instance, can be subjected to 20 minutes of complete anoxia and completely recover normal electrical activity. These studies point out the importance of local changes in circulatory dynamics in the production of lesions.

Occasionally, cerebral blood flow may be increased in or near the area of ischemia, particularly during the early stages of a lesion. This focal cerebral hyperemia has been termed "luxury perfusion" because the cerebral blood flow is presumably beyond the metabolic needs of the tissue. Autoregulation (maintenance of cerebral blood flow independent of blood pressure) frequently fails in areas of infarction, as do normal responses to acute changes in arterial carbon dioxide tension. It is postulated that luxury perfusion and loss of vascular autoregulation result from acute metabolic acidosis localized within ischemic areas of brain, but this has by no means been proved. Whatever the cause, the focal loss of normal vasomotor responses, the so-called vasoparalysis, is thought to be the basis of paradoxical responses that vasodilator and vasoconstrictor agents occasionally induce. During vasodilation induced by inhalation of carbon dioxide, for example, cerebral blood flow in the ischemic area decreases. Conversely, when generalized vasoconstriction is produced by lowering arterial carbon dioxide tension by hyperventilation, cerebral blood flow in the ischemic region can increase at a time when blood flow elsewhere decreases. These paradoxical responses presumably occur because the vessels in the diseased region, being maximally dilated, are unable to respond to changes in arterial carbon dioxide tension. As a result, with hypercapnia and consequent dilation of normal arterioles elsewhere, the blood is shunted away from the ischemic focus. With hypocapnia, the reverse occurs. All of these findings stress the importance of maintaining the systemic and cerebral circulation in the effective treatment or prevention of hypoxic brain damage.

Sometimes hemorrhage occurs in an area of infarction. These hemorrhagic infarcts may have several causes, all of which suggest that blood flowing through a damaged vascular bed is leaking into surrounding tissues. This can occur if (1) the infarction is the result of venous occlusion, (2) the capillaries are sufficiently anoxic to leak, or (3) the circulation is subsequently re-established in an infarcted area. The third alternative occurs if (1) an arterial occlusion is incomplete (an irregularly fitting thrombus or embolus), (2) there is dispersion of an embolus, (3) arterial anastomoses are sufficient to partially supply the infarcted area, or (4) there is reflux from congested veins. Only rarely are the hemorrhages large enough to increase the severity of neurological signs resulting from the infarct, but they can result in blood in the cerebrospinal fluid when the primary process is ischemic.

One additional feature of recent infarction, which has important clinical implications, is swelling of the necrotic tissue and surrounding gray matter. This edema reaches a maximum in a few days and subsides in about 2 weeks. If sufficient swelling occurs, pressure on intact adjacent neural tissue may increase the local neurological deficit. Severe edema may act as a large mass distorting the position of the brain in the intracranial cavity. The most common effect of massive cerebral edema following infarction is transtentorial herniation of the swollen cerebral hemisphere (or tonsillary herniation following cerebellar infarction) with progressive compression of the brain stem resulting in secondary infarction and hemorrhage in this area. Cerebral edema is a complication of many types of damage to the central nervous system and is discussed in more detail in Chapter 9.

### HEMORRHAGE

Two main types of spontaneous arterial hemorrhage are discussed in this chapter: hemorrhage into the subarachnoid space, usually from rupture of an aneurysm of a large artery of the circle of Willis, and hemorrhage into the substance of the brain (intracerebral), from rupture of a small penetrating artery or arteriole. Hemorrhage into the subdural and epidural spaces occurs almost exclusively as a result of trauma and, therefore, is dealt with in Chapter 9.

The consequences of subarachnoid hemorrhage are several. Acutely, this type of hemorrhage causes severe headache and, frequently, unconsciousness. Two factors are responsible for these events. First, the sudden entry of blood into the subarachnoid space leads to the obstruction of cerebrospinal fluid flow and the development of acute communicating hydrocephalus with intracranial hypertension. As a result, cerebral perfusion pressure may fall to a critically low level, causing failure of autoregulation, generalized cerebral ischemia, and unconsciousness. Second, the sudden appearance of localized blood in either the anterior or posterior fossa acts as a mass that cannot be accommodated and thus may produce shifts of the intracranial contents with distortion of pain-sensitive structures and direct compression of vital structures, leading to unconsciousness.

Within the first few hours of subarachnoid hemorrhage, a large amount of oxyhemoglobin is released into the cerebrospinal fluid because of disruption of red blood cells. This has many consequences. First, oxyhemoglobin, as well as methemoglobin and bilirubin, is highly irritating to the meninges and produces an outpouring of polymorphonuclear leukocytes (hemogenic or chemical meningitis). The clinical manifestations of meningeal irritation are neck stiffness and fever, which usually occur within several hours after the initial bleeding. Second, these products of red blood cell degradation may also directly interefere with cerebral metabolism, and this may explain the obtundation noted in patients who have no evidence of focal brain damage, intracranial hypertension, or vasospasm. Third, the introduction of whole blood and its break- down products into the subarachnoid space is often accompanied by intense localized (and sometimes generalized) arterial vasospasm that may be severe enough to produce ischemic damage to brain. We do not know what is directly responsible for this vasospasm. Fi- nally, the cellular reaction in the meninges may be sufficiently se- vere to produce an adhesive arachnoiditis of the basal leptome- ninges and a permanent obstruction to the flow and resorption of cerebrospinal fluid. This results in a chronic communicating hydro- cephalus, which becomes manifest clinically 2 to 12 weeks after the hemorrhage. The clinical picture of such hydrocephalus is variable and nonspecific, including, at times, difficulty in walking, inatten- tion, and obtundation.

Blood escaping into brain tissue (intracerebral hemorrhage) acts as a rapidly expanding mass lesion displacing and compressing ad- jacent brain tissue. The size and location of the hematoma deter- mine its clinical manifestations; in the cerebrum, hematomas of 100 ml may accumulate, whereas, in the brain stem, a hematoma of 5 ml may be fatal. Displacement of pain-sensitive structures in the surrounding meninges and vasculature leads to headache, which is a prominent and early clinical feature. Because the expanding hematoma is often close to the internal capsule, hemiplegia and hemisensory defects are prominent and frequent accompaniments to this disease. About one-half of all cerebral hemorrhages produce coma within minutes to hours of onset. There are two reasons for this. First, the rapidly expanding mass displaces and distorts struc- tures in the diencephalon and midbrain that are necessary to main- tain consciousness. In the anterior fossa, a rapidly expanding mass may lead to transtentorial herniation with diencephalic compression and secondary hemorrhages within the brain stem. In the posterior fossa, direct involvement of vital brain-stem structures by compres- sion from an expanding lesion in the cerebellum or destruction by an evolving hemorrhage originating in the pons can similarly pro- duce coma. Second, blood under high pressure may enter into the ventricular system, leading to coma and death within minutes to hours. The fatal result of blood entering the ventricular system is thought to be due to a mechanical insult transmitted to the brain stem rather than the kind of irritative effect seen in subarachnoid hemorrhage. Two observations support this first view. First, the sudden injection of saline into the lateral ventricles of dogs creates acute pressure gradients between the anterior and posterior fossa, which produce rapid medullary failure, whereas similar injections over the surface of the hemisphere have no such effect. Second, blood experimentally introduced into the ventricular system fails to elicit the prominent chemical meningitis seen with similar injections into the subarachnoid space.

## Pathogenesis

### INFARCTION

The causes of cerebral infarction can be conveniently divided into those resulting primarily from an interference with oxygen and glucose availability in the presence of normal cerebral blood flow (hypoxia and hypoglycemia) and those resulting from a failure of this flow (ischemia), either focal or generalized (Table 7-1).

### NORMAL CEREBRAL BLOOD FLOW

Brain hypoxia in the face of normal circulation can occur in two ways. First, insufficient oxygen may reach the blood so that both the oxygen content and tension are low relative to the brain's metabolic needs. Such insufficiency can result from decreased environmental oxygen tension (e.g., sudden decompression of a plane flying at high altitude); decreased ability of oxygen to cross the alveolar capillary membrane (e.g., pulmonary disease); and decreased mechanical ventilatory capacity (e.g., alveolar hypoventilation), as might be observed in such conditions affecting the neuromuscular apparatus as myasthenia gravis, infectious polyneuritis (Guillain-Barre syndrome), and poliomyelitis. Second, adequate oxygen may reach the blood, but the amount of hemoglobin available to bind and transport it may be reduced (anemic anoxia). This may result either from a loss of the hemoglobin content of blood (anemia) or chemical changes in the available hemoglobin, which reduce its ability to bind oxygen (e.g., carbon monoxide poisoning, methemoglobinemia). Under the above circumstances, the cerebral blood flow can increase but only to twice normal values. When this increase is insufficient, brain function deteriorates, and there is struc-

TABLE 7-1   *Causes of Cerebral Infarction*

| | PROBABLE DIAGNOSES |
|---|---|
| I. Normal Cerebral Blood Flow (extraction efficiency exceeded) | |
| A. Hypoxia (interference with oxygen supply to the entire brain) | |
| 1. Decreased oxygen content and tension (anoxic anoxia) | Pulmonary disease<br>Alveolar hypoventilation<br>Decreased atmospheric oxygen tension |
| 2. Decreased oxygen content, tension normal (anemic anoxia) | Anemia<br>Carbon monoxide poisoning<br>Methemoglobinemia |
| B. Hypoglycemia (interference with glucose supply to the entire brain) | Excess insulin (spontaneous, secondary to liver disease) |
| II. Reduced Cerebral Blood Flow (ischemic anemia) | |
| A. Generalized reduction<br>1. Decreased cardiac output | Stokes-Adams syndrome<br>Cardiac arrest<br>Cardiac arrhythmia<br>Myocardial infarction<br>Congestive heart failure<br>Pulmonary embolism<br>Aortic stenosis |
| 2. Decreased resistance of systemic circulation | Syncope—orthostatic vasovagal<br>Carotid sinus hypersensitivity<br>Low blood volume<br>Acquired autonomic insufficiency (idiopathic, drug induced) |
| 3. Increased cerebrovascular resistance | Hypertensive encephalopathy<br>Hyperventilation syndrome |
| 4. Widespread small vessel occlusion | Increased blood viscosity<br>  polycythemia<br>  cryoglobulinemia<br>  macroglobulinemia<br>  sickle cell anemia<br>Disseminated intravascular coagulation<br>Multiple small emboli arising from heart—bacterial and nonbacterial endocarditis, or pump oxygenator (cardiopulmonary bypass syndrome) |

TABLE 7-1   *(Continued)*

|  | PROBABLE DIAGNOSES |
|---|---|
|  | Parasitemia of malaria<br>Fat embolism<br>Decompression sickness ("bends")<br>Diseases of cerebral vessels (arteritis): systemic lupus erythematosus, polyarteritis nodosa |
| B. Focal reduction |  |
| 1. Thrombotic arterial occlusion | Arteriosclerotic disease of the intra- and extracranial vessels[a] (arteritis)<br>Infection (syphilis, tuberculous and pyogenic meningitis, typhus, schistosomiasis (*S. mansoni*), trichinosis<br>Infestation with various fungi<br>Connective tissue diseases (polyarteritis, temporal arteritis, Takayasu's disease, granulomatous arteritis, systemic lupus erythematosus)<br>Trauma<br>Metabolic disease (homocystinuria) |
| 2. Embolic arterial occlusion[b] | Valvular heart disease (rheumatic)<br>Cardiac disease with intermittent atrial fibrillation<br>Myocardial infarction with neural thrombi<br>Paradoxical emboli (patent foramen ovale) |
| 3. Venous occlusion (thrombophlebitis) | Secondary to infection of ear, paranasal sinuses, and face<br>Secondary to intracranial infection (meningitis, subdural empyema)<br>Debilitating states<br>Postpartum states<br>Post-operative states<br>Hematological disease (polycythemia, sickle cell disease)<br>Undetermined etiology |
| 4. Vasospasm (focal) | Subarachnoid hemorrhage<br>Migraine<br>Trauma<br>Bacterial meningitis |

[a] Largest single cause of focal cerebral ischemia and infarction in the adult.
[b] Probably the most common cause of focal cerebral ischemia in children.

tural damage that varies according to the duration and severity of the hypoxia.

Hypoglycemia is a frequent cause of coma in all age groups. In the adult, it most often results from the improper use of insulin. It may also occur in association with a variety of metabolic diseases in children, in association with liver disease in both children and adults, and spontaneously. In contrast to hypoxia, hypoglycemia does not appear to trigger an increase in cerebral blood flow. As a result, when the brain's efficiency in extracting glucose is exceeded, and its stores of glucose are depleted, signs of impaired function appear.

REDUCED CEREBRAL BLOOD FLOW

Brain ischemia and infarction may result from a general reduction in cerebral blood flow, which exceeds the brain's ability to extract needed nutrients. This usually follows a failure of autoregulation to maintain blood flow in the face of a precipitous fall in perfusion pressure resulting from decreased cardiac output (e.g., myocardial infarction), decreased peripheral resistance (e.g., acquired autonomic insufficiency), or both. The paradigm of this group of diseases is vasovagal syncope, which usually occurs without sequelae. A more serious and infrequently recognized member of this group of diseases, particularly in hospital patients, is pulmonary embolism, which can produce a sudden fall in cerebral blood flow secondary to a reduction in cardiac output.

Two other disease mechanisms may reduce over-all cerebral blood flow to the point of cerebral ischemia and infarction: increased cerebrovascular resistance and widespread small vessel occlusion. Cerebrovascular resistance may increase as the result of a generalized constriction of resistance vessels. This is most commonly seen in the hyperventilation syndrome with reduced cerebral blood flow secondary to an acute fall in arterial carbon dioxide tension. Hypocarbia, although symptomatically troublesome, rarely leads to the significant cerebral damage that often accompanies hypertensive encephalopathy, the other and much rarer condition associated with a severe increase in cerebrovascular resistance. This condition, with its severe attendant cerebral vasospasm, is usually seen in known hypertensives who have experienced a sudden rise in blood pressure. The degree of arterial spasm can be appreciated in the retinal vessels, which appear threadlike.

The over-all cerebral blood flow may also be significantly reduced as a result of widespread small vessel occlusion (precluded anastomotic flow). This may result from changes in the rheological or clotting properties of the blood, the presence of small emboli (e.g., detritus from heart valves, gas bubbles, fat globules, parasites), or an inflammatory vascular disease (e.g., polyarteritis).

## FOCAL REDUCTION IN CEREBRAL BLOOD FLOW

By far the most common cause of focal cerebral infarction in adults is arterial thrombosis associated with arteriosclerotic disease of the intra- and extracranial vessels. Significant atherosclerotic changes are usually evident in the major cerebral arteries of persons dying from other causes as early as the second or third decade of life. The sites most frequently involved are the internal carotid arteries at their origin in the neck or as they traverse the syphon, the origin of the middle cerebral arteries, the vertebral arteries just after they enter the skull, and the entire course of the basilar artery. The degenerative process is similar to that seen elsewhere in the vascular system: lipid deposition in the intima, fibrous tissue overgrowth, hemorrhage into the plaques, and ulceration of the plaques. The severity of the process is greater and its development earlier in patients with either diabetes mellitus or hypertension, and there is thus a higher incidence of brain infarction (often at an earlier age) in patients with these disorders.

The presence of atherosclerotic disease, even with marked vascular narrowing, does not necessarily produce brain ischemia and infarction. It can, however, lead to cerebral infarction in two ways. First, detritus from an atherosclerotic plaque in the form of cholesterol crystals and platelet aggregates may disseminate downstream (arterial emboli) to produce either transient (transient ischemic attacks) or permanent (completed stroke) cerebral ischemia and infarction. Second, the plaque can serve as a nidus for the development of a thrombus, which eventually occludes the vessel. The mechanism by which a thrombus is precipitated upon a given plaque is not understood. The rate of thrombus formation is quite variable, taking from minutes to weeks to produce occlusion, and this probably explains the variable clinical course before cerebral thrombotic infarction occurs.

Thrombotic occlusion of major cerebral vessels has been well documented in children but differs in its pathogenesis from the disease in adults. Rather than being the result of atherosclerosis, thrombotic occlusions in children result from direct trauma to the carotid artery by objects carried in the mouth or blows to the neck, from perivascular inflammatory reactions secondary to localized infections of the head and neck, or from intracranial sepsis and such pediatric illnesses that produce polycythemia and intravascular sludging as sickle cell anemia and congenital cyanotic heart disease. An example of the latter condition is tetralogy of Fallot, in which silent or symptomatic occlusions of the internal carotid artery are frequently identified. Embolic arterial occlusion may be even more common than thrombotic disease in children with cyanotic heart disease.

The problems resulting from cerebrovascular disease *in utero* or during the neonatal period (at the time of birth) are unique and are treated in some detail in Chapter 1.

Occlusion of the cerebral veins or venous sinuses, in children as well as adults, is most frequently seen in association with infectious diseases of the face, paranasal sinuses, and meninges. A variety of other conditions primarily affecting blood rheology or clotting characteristics, particularly severe dehydration, have been implicated without clear evidence.

Focal cerebral vasospasm can be sufficiently severe to produce infarction. In its mildest form, it produces the focal neurological signs of classic migraine headache, and the deficit is rarely permanent. Severe focal spasm with infarction is commonly associated with subarachnoid hemorrhage from an intracranial aneurysm, severe head trauma, and, occasionally, bacterial meningitis. The cause of this stereotyped vascular phenomenon in these diverse circumstances is not known.

HEMORRHAGE

Intracranial hemorrhage may be roughly classified on the basis of location into epidural, subdural, subarachnoid, and intracerebral hemorrhage. Some overlap does exist in this classification, and we will deal only with subarachnoid and intracerebral hemorrhage. Epidural and subdural hemorrhage are discussed in Chapter 9.

In adults, the most frequent cause of subarachnoid hemorrhage is the rupture of an aneurysm (congenital or saccular) in a large artery of the circle of Willis.

The available information on the pathogenesis of these aneurysms, although incomplete, may be summarized as follows. Large arteries in the subarachnoid space develop aneurysms in the crotch of their bifurcation, probably because of the superimposition of two lesions: (1) a congenital absence of the media, which occurs at this site in about one-half of all bifurcations, and (2) a degeneration of the internal elastic lamina, which normally contributes significantly to the strength of the cerebral arterial wall. This requirement for the combination of two lesions may account for the relative rarity of aneurysms (they occur in about 2% of the general population). Atherosclerosis is usually considered the most common disease that destroys the elastic lamina, but typical atherosclerotic plaques are not as common in aneurysms as are irregular fibromuscular scars. Such scars may represent the final stage of an entirely different type of arteriosclerosis, one beginning even before birth and characterized by degeneration of the musculo-elastic pads. The random overlapping of these two anatomical lesions (fibromuscular scars and absence of media) may still not be sufficient to produce an aneurysm without further degenerative changes. These may occur with age as a result of further splitting of the elastica of the musculo-elastic pads due to hemodynamic stresses resulting from turbulent flow within the aneurysmal sac and increasing blood pressure. This concept of the disease would account for the extreme rarity of aneurysms in children.

Most aneurysms occur on the circle of Willis. They commonly appear adjacent to the anterior communicating artery, at the juncture of the posterior communicating and internal carotid arteries, at the origin of the anterior cerebral arteries, and at the first major bifurcation of the middle cerebral artery. In from 10 to 15% of patients, more than one aneurysm exists.

*Saccular aneurysms.* These may present pathologically in four ways: (1) as an incidental finding (present in about 2% of routine autopsies); (2) as an expanding mass lesion (aneurysms vary from small 1-mm blebs to huge sacs 3 to 4 cm in diameter) compressing and displacing surrounding structures; (3) as a subarachnoid hemorrhage; and, occasionally, (4) as a rapidly expanding mass after the aneurysm has hemorrhaged into brain tissue. When aneurysms associated with the anterior communicating artery rupture posteriorly into the third ventricle and aqueduct, sudden death occurs.

*Mycotic aneurysms.* Associated with bacterial endocarditis, they occur when septic emboli lodge distally in the smaller branches of the major cerebral vessels (usually the middle cerebral artery), producing a local necrotic vasculitis. These lesions tend to be multiple. Although they may lead to hemorrhage, they can also be associated with infarction resulting from arterial occlusion caused by the associated vasculitis. A brain abscess may form at or near the site where such a septic embolus lodges.

*Arteriovenous malformations.* Accounting for cases of subarachnoid (as well as intracerebral) hemorrhage in both children and adults, these thin-walled vascular channels representing connections between arteries and veins without intervening capillaries may be microscopic or huge, covering an entire hemisphere. Thus, patients with arteriovenous malformations may initially present with the symptoms and signs of hemorrhage, as a mass with focal signs, particularly seizures, or, rarely, with progressive deterioration of neurological function of unknown etiology possibly related to shunting of blood from surrounding tissue. A rather common form of clinical manifestation in infants is high output congestive failure, since a relatively large proportion of the infant's blood volume may rapidly circulate through the malformation.

In contrast to subarachnoid hemorrhage, the lesion responsible for the majority of intracerebral hemorrhages in adults is poorly understood. The most common lesion observed in the cerebral vessels of patients with intracerebral hemorrhages is a micro or miliary aneurysm (Charcot-Bouchard aneurysm) resulting from hyalin degeneration of small arteries and arterioles. These changes are thought to result from long-standing hypertension. It is believed by some that rupture of these aneurysms may be the cause of the hemorrhage. This view, however, has been challenged for several reasons. First, it is difficult if not impossible to evaluate small vessels in the area of recent hemorrhage. As a result, ruptured aneurysm has rarely been demonstrated in association with intracerebral hemorrhage. Second, micro and miliary aneurysms are seen in areas of the brain (e.g., cortex) where hypertensive hemorrhage does not usually occur. Hypertensive intracerebral hemorrhages have an unexplained predilection for certain areas of the brain. They occur most commonly in the striatum (50 to 60% of all cases) and, in decreasing order of frequency, in the subcortical white matter (about 15%), thalamus (about 12%), brain stem (about 10%), and cerebellum (about 10%).

A variety of hematological disturbances predispose adults and children to intracerebral hemorrhage. These include leukemia, hemophilia, thrombotic thrombocytopenic purpura, and improperly controlled anticoagulation. Hemorrhage is occasionally seen in association with cerebral infarction (usually embolic), but in this case it is rarely of major clinical significance. Finally, there may be hemorrhage into a primary or metastatic brain tumor, but again, particularly in the former, it is not usually of clinical significance. Significant hemorrhages have occasionally been associated with metastatic tumor nodules, particularly malignant melanoma.

## Clinical features of cerebral circulatory disorders

Based on an understanding of pathophysiology, it is possible to formulate a general picture of the more common clinical syndromes that arise when the brain's vascular system fails and its metabolic needs are not met.

*Acute diffuse anoxia.* Such anoxia of the brain produces a diffuse and symmetrical neurological picture. Consciousness is lost in less than 10 seconds, and, depending on the duration of the anoxia, generalized convulsions, pupillary dilation, and bilateral extensor plantar responses follow. In the mildest and most common example of this group of diseases, vasovagal syncope, consciousness is usually regained immediately after assuming a recumbent position. When the erect posture is maintained, either by well-meaning friends or environmental props, generalized convulsions may result and the return of normal consciousness is delayed. This sometimes makes it difficult in retrospect to distinguish syncope from epilepsy.

When diffuse anoxia is the result of a generalized increase in cerebrovascular resistance (e.g., hypertensive encephalopathy) or widespread small vessel occlusion, the clinical picture is one of progressive diffuse and focal neurological signs. Impaired consciousness (delirium, stupor, or coma) is frequently combined with generalized or focal seizures and multifocal neurological signs, which may be transient. This is to be contrasted with the diffuse and symmetrical neurological signs seen in the other anoxic encephalopathies.

*Hypoglycemia.* Here an altered state of consciousness, varying from agitated delirium to stupor and coma, is produced. It may also present as a stroke-like illness with prominent focal neurological signs and sometimes coma. The pathogenesis of these focal neurological signs is not clear. It is attractive to postulate that they occur in areas of marginal blood supply where the extraction efficiency of the brain is already taxed to the limit (cerebral blood flow does not increase with hypoglycemia). This hypothesis, however, fails to account for the shifting nature of the focal deficit or its occurrence in children, where vascular disease presumably is not a factor. Finally, hypoglycemia may produce single or multiple generalized convulsions resistant to any form of treatment other than restoration and maintenance of normal levels of blood glucose.

*Arterial occlusion (stroke).* Thrombotic arterial occlusion is frequently heralded by brief, transient neurological symptomatology (transient ischemic attacks) in the days, weeks, or months preceding the onset of the fixed neurological deficit. These brief early warnings tend to be identical. This is to be contrasted with the multifocal and changing nature of the transient deficit seen with hypoglycemia and widespread small vessel occlusion. The fixed deficit usually develops in a stepwise fashion over a period ranging from minutes to hours (a stroke in evolution). Once the thrombosis is secure, the syndrome stabilizes (a completed stroke). When the area of infarction is large, the apparent neurological deficit may increase as a result of surrounding edema. This gradually clears in 1 to 2 weeks. Cerebral thrombotic infarction in adults may occur at any time, but a disproportionately large number seem to appear at night, while patients are sleeping. The reason for this is unknown.

Embolic arterial occlusion presents signs of cerebral infarction, which occur abruptly (seconds to minutes) and are usually maximal at the time of onset. Unlike thrombotic occlusion, there are no warnings. Rapid improvement is frequently seen, presumably due to the disintegration and passage of the obstructive clot.

The precise form of the neurological syndrome associated with either thrombotic or embolic arterial occlusion depends on the particular vessel occluded. Occlusion of the internal carotid artery or any of its branches may be characterized by one or more of the following: contralateral motor and/or sensory dysfunction, contralateral visual field impairment, impairment of language function with dominant hemisphere involvement, and, occasionally, transient or permanent loss of vision in the ipsilateral eye due to involvement of the ophthalmic artery. Arterial occlusion in the vertebral-basilar system can produce an array of neurological abnormalities because of the concentration of function in this area. These abnormalities may include diplopia, dysarthria, and ataxia; motor and sensory disturbances, often affecting one side of the face and the opposite side of the body; vertigo; unilateral or bilateral visual field disturbances; hiccoughs; single or multiple cranial nerve palsies; and dysphagia.

About one-fifth of adult patients with either thrombotic or embolic infarction die when the first attack occurs. The mortality rate is greatly influenced by the patient's age, the extent of the vascular disease, the degree of neurological disability, and the cardiac status. For those surviving the first attack, the threat to life is not so much recurrent cerebral infarction (about 20% in 2 years) as cardiac disease; fully one-half of these patients ultimately die of myocardial infarction.

The clinical picture of cerebral infarction caused by cerebral vein or venous sinus occlusion is ordinarily influenced by symptoms of the predisposing illness. This illness is usually infection of the face, paranasal sinuses, mastoid air cells, or meninges. In addition to a focal neurological deficit, other features prominently seen are seizures, periorbital edema with occlusion of the cavernous sinus, and increased intracranial pressure secondary to obstruction of cerebrospinal fluid flow and the development of acute communicating hydrocephalus.

*Intracerebral hemorrhage.* Here, the hemorrhage usually occurs without warning, while the patient is active. Severe headache, often with nausea and vomiting, precedes the development of focal neurological signs. Because of the disorder's unexplained predilection for the region of the basal ganglia and subcortical white matter (50 to

60% of cases), hemiparesis and hemianesthesia usually appear early and are frequently followed by stupor, coma, and death. With hemorrhage into the pons, early coma, quadriplegia, external and internal ophthalmoplegia are common, whereas, with cerebellar hemorrhage, vertigo, vomiting, ataxia, and coma can occur without paralysis being a prominent feature. The cerebrospinal fluid in most cases is under increased pressure and is grossly bloody.

The over-all mortality of patients with intracerebral hemorrhage is about 50%. Mortality is much higher in patients who are in coma when first seen. In contrast to subarachnoid hemorrhage, recurrence is uncommon in this disease. Recovery is slow and variable. A collection of blood within brain parenchyma is removed slowly, so that symptoms and signs due to mass also resolve slowly. Because of the propensity for an intracerebral hemorrhage to dissect between structures rather than destroy them, as occurs in infarction, recovery from an intracerebral hemorrhage may be surprisingly complete once the mass of blood has been cleared.

*Subarachnoid hemorrhage.* The symptoms of subarachnoid hemorrhage—excruciating headache, nausea, and vomiting—usually begin without warning. A reasonable degree of alertness is often maintained, but occasionally unconsciousness, either sustained or transient, or a single seizure, may mark the onset of the bleeding. Signs of meningeal irritation (stiff neck) usually appear within the first several hours. Focal neurological signs, less prominent than those with intracerebral hemorrhage and infarction, may appear as a consequence of vasospasm. The first hemorrhage from an aneurysm may be massive and fatal, but frequently it ceases and then recurs several days later. The greatest incidence of recurrent bleeding occurs in the first 2 weeks after the initial hemorrhage. This tendency to recur is not understood, and it contrasts with primary intracerebral hemorrhage, in which recurrent bleeding from the same site appears to be rare.

The mortality rate from ruptured aneurysms within 2 weeks of the initial hemorrhage is approximately 50% and is exponential: about 25% of the death occur before the hospital is reached, about 25% in the first day or so after hospitalization, and the remaining 50% over the next 13 days. If a patient survives such an insult for 2 months without a recurrence, it is extremely unlikely that he will again suffer rupture of an intracranial aneurysm.

## General references

Banker, B. Q. 1961. Cerebral vascular disease in infancy and childhood. 1. Occlusive vascular diseases. J. Neuropath. Exp. Neurol. 20:127.

Bickerstaff, E. R. 1964. Aetiology of acute hemiplegia in childhood. Brit. Med. J. 2:82.

Brierly, J. B. and B. S. Meldrum, eds. 1971. Brain hypoxia. Clinics in developmental medicine, Nos. 39/40, Spastics International Medical Publications, Lippincott, Philadelphia.

Kalberg, R. M. and A. L. Woolf. 1967. Cerebral venous thrombosis. Oxford University Press, London.

Marshall, J. 1956. The management of cerebrovascular disease. Little, Brown, Boston.

Pool, J. L. and D. G. Potts. 1965. Aneurysms and arteriovenous anomalies of the brain: Diagnosis and treatment. Hoeber/Harper & Row, New York.

Reivich, M. 1969. Regulation of the cerebral circulation. Clinical Neurosurg. 16:378.

Soloman, G. E., S. K. Hilal, A. P. Gold, and S. Carter. 1970. Natural history of acute hemiplegia in childhood. Brain 93:107.

Taveras, J. 1969. Multiple progressive intracranial arterial occlusions in children and young adults. Caldwell Lecture at American Roentgen Ray Society, 1968. Amer. J. Roentgen. 106:235.

Tyler, H. R. and D. B. Clark. 1957. Cerebrovascular accidents in patients with congenital heart disease. Arch. Neurol. Psychiat. 77:483.

Walton, J. 1956. Subarachnoid hemorrhage. E. and S. Livingston, Ltd., Edinburgh.

# 8
# Intracranial Tumors

WILLIAM S. COXE

Insight into the pathophysiology of intracranial tumors requires awareness of their variety, particularly from two standpoints, tumor location and tissue origin. Broadly categorized, tumors may occur in extra-axial, intra-axial, or both intra- and extra-axial locations. The cell types from which the tumor originates are often anticipated from knowledge of its anatomical position. Extra-axial tumors originate in skull (osteoma, sarcoma, and hemangioma), meninges (meningioma), cranial nerves (neurinomas), and brain appendages (pituitary tumors) or from congenital cell rests (craniopharyngioma, epidermoid cysts, teratomas, and colloid cysts) and produce physiological alterations by impressing themselves against the brain and/or neighboring cranial nerves. Certain of the tumors listed above (choroid plexus papillomas, colloid cysts, and rare meningiomas) arise within the ventricular system and technically might be considered intra-axial but, in fact, are not within the brain substance. The majority of primary intra-axial tumors originate from glial cells, cells that exhibit a wide range of pathological behavior. Included are the most malignant of brain tumors (glioblastoma multiforme and medulloblastoma), less malignant varieties (oligodendroglioma, astro-

cytoma, and ependymoma), and relatively benign forms of the latter two cell types, which sometimes are completely cured by surgical
excision. Hemangioblastomas are peculiar vascular tumors occurring most commonly in the cerebellum as single or multiple lesions;
they may also arise in the medulla or cerebral hemisphere. They
are especially interesting by virtue of their extraordinary genetic
linkage. Metastatic tumors also make up a large percentage of intracranial tumors and are found in any of the positions mentioned. As
with certain malignant gliomas, they may also metastasize diffusely
within the subarachnoid space (meningeal carcinomatosis). Arteriovenous malformations, although involving brain parenchyma, sometimes cause effects similar to tumors, but they are not true neoplasms.

The pathophysiological mechanisms by which tumors produce
symptoms may include one or a combination of all of the following
factors:

1. Increased intracranial pressure resulting from tumor encroachment upon normal intracranial structures or by obstruction of circulation and absorption of cerebrospinal fluid by virtue of strategic
location near or within the ventricular system or subarachnoid
pathways.

2. Abnormal neuronal activity (epileptic seizure) resulting from
alterations of synaptic input or metabolism of neurons by pressure,
invasion, or edema.

3. Loss of neuronal function by invasion and/or replacement of
neurons and tracts by tumor tissue, edema, etc.

4. Endocrine abnormalities causing changes in growth, metabolism, and sexual function, either by increased endocrine activity or
destruction of normal structures having to do with these functions.

## Increased intracranial pressure

Among the earliest and most frequent symptoms of intracranial tumors are headaches, nausea, and vomiting, symptoms usually attributed to increased intracranial pressure. In this connection, it is important to note first, that wide fluctuations in pressure from normal
to high may be recorded in patients experiencing these symptoms
from brain tumors and second, that marked pressure increases ar-
tifically produced by subarachnoid injections of normal saline in

human volunteers do not produce these symptoms. It therefore seems likely that headache is caused by distortion or deflection of dura, falx, and vascular walls of the larger arteries and veins by the tumor mass or edema rather than simply a diffuse increase of pressure. Trigeminal nerve (cranial nerve V) afferents in these structures are thought to mediate pain sensations to the brain. Headache and vomiting are more common in the morning shortly after awaking and may relate to increased venous pressure associated with the supine position. Furthermore, sleep may be associated with a reduction in ventilation leading to an increase in $PCO_2$, increased cerebral blood volume, and, in turn, increased intracranial pressure. In special situations, as when tumors arise from the floor or within the fourth ventricle, sudden vomiting from irritation of vagal centers may occur before hydrocephalus and increased pressure develop.

Impairment of sensorium and blunting of intellectual functions may occur without signs of increased pressure, progressing to stupor and coma if the tumor is allowed to enlarge. The time course may vary from a few weeks to years, depending on the type of tumor and its location. The following brief discussion of pathological and physiological changes associated with intracranial mass lesions causing increased pressure is applicable to any space-occupying lesion. The terminal neurological changes to be mentioned are less likely to be seen during the initial encounter with patients harboring brain tumors as compared to those with hemorrhagic or traumatic lesions, since tumor detection usually occurs much earlier.

The Monro-Kellie doctrine put forth in 1824 described the cranial vault as an unyielding structure with a fixed volume of brain, blood, and fluid. Since these structures are relatively incompressible, the blood volume within the cranium was thought to remain relatively constant. Subsequently, this doctrine required modification, and it is now obvious that displacement of blood and cerebrospinal fluid volumes occurs with intracranial masses without increasing pressure until the limits of displacement are reached.

The physiological correlates of increased pressure were first studied extensively by Cushing and Kocher and more recently by Langfitt and his associates. Both described four stages of cerebral compression, and, in general, their observations are in agreement. The first stage is one of compensation during which a minimal rise of intracranial pressure is associated with the enlarging mass, but, during stage two, relatively small changes in size of mass cause increasingly greater rises of intracranial pressure since all possible compensatory displacement of cerebrospinal fluid and blood has occurred. During stage three, intracranial pressure may approach arterial blood pressure and is associated with marked deterioration in consciousness, irregular breathing, and bradycardia. Prior to stages two and three, hypoxia or hypercapnia would produce dilation of cerebral vessels, causing small increases in intracranial pressure, but when most of the available cerebrospinal fluid has been displaced, small increases in cerebral blood volume produce sharp increases in intracranial pressure. Therefore, mild respiratory insufficiency in the obtunded patient with brain swelling or intracranial mass may produce a dramatic increase in pressure, and ultimately, a severe reduction in cerebral blood flow. This leads to the last stage, when arterial and intracranial pressure become the same and effective cerebral blood flow ceases. If not relieved immediately, both respiration and electroencephalographic activity cease. Alterations in $PCO_2$ no longer effect changes in blood flow (loss of autoregulation) and, secondarily, intracranial pressure.

Depending upon the location of the tumor (or other expanding mass), shifts of brain occur within the cranium and are associated with a variety of herniations of brain relative to dural structures. With slowly expanding lesions, the brain may accommodate the mass for long periods of time without any increase in intracranial pressure, even though herniations of brain beneath the falx or through the tentorium may have occurred. Eventually, as the limits of accommodation are reached, increased pressure will develop, and symptoms of this state become obvious. The commonest space-occupying lesions occur above the tentorium either within or pressing upon one of the cerebral hemispheres. After reaching a certain size, brain tissue is pushed from one cranial compartment to another. Subfalcine herniation is quite common with the cingulate gyrus ipsilateral to the mass being displaced beneath the falx, particularly if the mass is pushing downward or from the high convex surface. Rarely, this may compromise the circulation through the anterior cerebral arteries, which are displaced together with brain tissue, resulting in infarction of portions of the mesial cortex. Of greater significance is transtentorial herniation of the mesial temporal lobe (uncus and hippocampal gyrus). As the mesial temporal lobe is displaced over the free edge of the tentorium, the midbrain and diencephalon are compressed, and the ipsilateral oculomotor nerve may be stretched or compressed, causing ipsilateral pupillary dilation. The uncal syndrome usually begins with restlessness, deteriorating consciousness, confusion, contralateral weakness, and, as lateral diencephalic pressure increases, midbrain decompensation occurs. Coma, hyperventilation, dilation of pupils, and decorticate or decerebrate posturing ensue, and eye movements incident to caloric stimulation may be impaired or cease. As the rostrocaudal disintegration progresses to ponto-medullary centers, respirations become irregular and ataxic, ocular movements cease, and body tone changes from decerebration to flaccidity.

Concomitant with lateral transtentorial herniation, or occurring as a separate category of intracranial herniation, is caudal displacement of the diencephalon and rostral midbrain (central transtentorial herniation). In most such herniations associated with brain tumors, some elements of the lateral transtentorial syndrome must precede shifts of this magnitude. These displacements usually result from lesions in frontal, parietal, and occipital locations and, particularly, in large, bilaterally positioned tumors. Impairment of upward gaze from tectal pressure or kinking of midbrain structures may appear to be followed later by further oculomotor dysfunction. Impairment of circulation in one or both posterior cerebral arteries may occur as mesial temporal lobe and hippocampal gyrus herniation stretches and compresses them, leading to infarction of the mesial hemispheric cortex back to the occipital poles, a finding more common with lateral transtentorial herniation.

If herniation is unabated, hemorrhage and infarction proceed in the midbrain and upper pons. Two mechanisms for this are proposed, one secondary to venous congestion and the other, a tearing of perforating arteries from the brain stem as a result of shearing strains between the brain and the relatively immobile vertebrobasilar arterial system. As Plum has emphasized, one may predict an orderly rostrocaudal pattern of neural disintegration beginning with drowsiness, lethargy, small reactive pupils, and increased muscle tone in the early diencephalic stage progressing, with increasing lethargy, to coma, irregular or Cheyne-Stokes respirations, reduced oculocephalic reflexes, decorticate and decerebrate posturing, and, finally, proceeding to the ponto-medullary preparation described before.

Cerebellar tonsil herniation may result from transmission of pressure below the tentorium from a supratentorial lesion, with or without significant transtentorial herniation of the hippocampus, depending, to some extent, on anatomical variations at the tentorial hiatus. In addition to caudad displacement of the midbrain and pons, the cerebellar hemispheres may be compressed in vertical dimensions with impaction of the tonsils against the foramen magnum or underlying medulla. Langfitt and others have emphasized that intracranial pressure may not be uniform from one compartment to the other as a result of obstructions at the tentorial hiatus or foramen magnum produced by the herniations mentioned above. Therefore, measurements of lumbar spinal fluid pressure will not necessarily reflect pressures within the head and is not only inaccurate but may aggravate herniations further, causing death.

Hydrocephalus is the other major cause of increased pressure from intracranial tumors. This may result from obstruction of any portion of the lateral ventricular system, third ventricle, aqueduct of Sylvius, fourth ventricle, or posterior and basilar cisterns. The large majority of neoplasms that cause hydrocephalus occur within the posterior fossa or posterior third ventricle and are more common in children (excepting metastatic tumors).

In spite of many clinical and experimental observations, much remains to be learned about cerebrospinal fluid production and absorption (discussed in detail in Chapter 12), particularly in pathological situations. Most agree that the choroid plexuses of the lateral, third, and fourth ventricles produce the bulk of the cerebrospinal fluid, although some may arise from interstitial fluid of the brain and pass across the ependymal surfaces or into the subarachnoid spaces adjacent to the pial surfaces of the brain and spinal cord. The rate of formation in normal persons ranges from 0.35 to 0.40 ml/minute. The bulk of that produced within the ventricles circulates out by way of the fourth ventricle foramina to the basilar cisterns, upward around the brain stem at the tentorial hiatus, and thence to the subarachnoid spaces and arachnoid villi, where most of the fluid is probably absorbed. Fluid may also be absorbed across the ependymal lining of the ventricles and perineural sheaths of cranial and spinal nerves. Whatever the mechanism, as obstruction commences, intracranial pressure increases as ventricular distention takes place. The lateral ventricles seem to enlarge first, and later, the third ventricle and aqueduct. Arterial pressure waves transmitted from the pulsatile and richly vascularized choroid plexus are thought to contribute to this. If ventricular distention is sufficiently great, tears in the ependymal lining may appear, allowing fluid access to surrounding white matter. As pressure increases and ventricular enlargement continues, compression of subarachnoid pathways may impair cerebrospinal fluid circulation and absorption, further aggravating the problem. Cerebral blood flow may decrease as a result of greater resistance within cerebral capillary beds.

Hydrocephalus, as demonstrated by ventriculography or pneumoencephalography, occurs without complete obstruction of cerebrospinal fluid pathways when only encroachment upon or distortion of the system is seen. This suggests that partial or intermittent obstruction can be responsible or that products of the tumor that have access to cerebrospinal fluid pathways may impair absorption in the subarachnoid pathways. Such blocks of air passage at the tentorial hiatus or over the cerebral hemispheres are sometimes demonstrated in addition to the more obvious distortions produced elsewhere by the tumor itself. Furthermore, tumors remote from the cranium, lying within the lumbar canal, may increase the intracranial pressure with papilledema and hydrocephalus (notably neural sheath tumors and ependymomas). It is postulated that increased cerebrospinal fluid protein content and/or "arachnoiditis" result when tumor products gain access to the subarachnoid fluid pathways. In either case, impairment of circulation and absorption via arachnoid villi have been invoked as possible mechanisms. Removal of the spinal tumor may reverse the process within the cranium.

From the foregoing discussion, it is evident that increases in intracranial pressure from mass lesions or hydrocephalus might produce certain indirect effects upon the brain and/or cranial nerves, to cause signs that are sometimes called "false" localizing signs. The term is unfortunate, since the signs are not truly "false," but they do require an understanding of how they come about. Several of the more common ones are described below.

As mentioned previously, herniation of the hippocampus through the tentorial notch may produce oculomotor-nerve palsy. In addition, compression of the ipsilateral cerebral peduncle produces contralateral hemiparesis, but, on rare occasions, the midbrain is displaced so much that the contralateral peduncle is impaled against the opposite tentorial edge, causing hemiparesis ipsilateral to the lesion. In the same manner, infarction of the occipital pole by compression of the posterior cerebral artery has been mentioned. If the patient is responsive, homonymous hemianopsia may be detected. It is evident that this group of signs results most often from unilateral supratentorial masses.

Another common "false" sign is abducent-nerve paralysis, either unilateral or bilateral, which may result from hydrocephalus, supratentorial masses, or benign intracranial hypertension (pseudotumor cerebri). In the first two instances, downward stretching of the abducent nerve (cranial nerve VI) at its point of dural penetration ventral to the pons is the usual explanation. When this occurs as a result of diffuse increased pressure without displacement of cerebral structures (pseudotumor syndrome), this explanation leaves much to be desired.

Unilateral or bilateral trigeminal-nerve (cranial nerve V) deficits are very rare signs of rostrocaudal brain-stem displacement. Stretching of the nerve (or nerves) as it passes over the petrous apex into its dural sleeve (Meckel's cavity) is considered the cause. Treatment of the lesion causing these signs usually leads to early resolution of these deficits.

## Neuronal dysfunction

The hallmark of the next two pathophysiological mechanisms, epilepsy and loss of neuronal function of various sorts, is the focality of neurological symptoms. By careful analysis of symptoms and neurological findings, a clear indication of the site and, quite frequently, the type of tumor may be apparent. It is obvious that this is not invariably true, and a variety of studies are usually required to establish the diagnosis. Because of the great number and combination of focal symptoms and signs tumors produce, they cannot be detailed in this chapter, and the reader must consult texts of clinical neurology and neurological surgery.

The pathophysiological mechanisms of epilepsy are considered in Chapter 5, but a brief discussion here seems in order. Since the advent of elegant electrophysiological and anatomical techniques, a vast amount of study has been devoted to the mechanisms of epilepsy, both in experimental animals and man. Some of the evidence derived suggests that neuronal input to the epileptic neurons is altered by partial denervation of normal synaptic connections. Reduction of such input results in hyperactivity of neurons and renders them more susceptible to abnormal paroxysmal discharge. Experimental studies upon slabs of isolated cortex have demonstrated that the neurons contained therein are more prone to paroxysmal discharge. Modification of input by subcortical and cortical infiltration of tumor may then enhance the occurrence of seizures. Tumor infiltration or direct impingement upon the cortex by extracerebral tumors, or marked edema accumulation adjacent to the tumor, may produce physical distortion and altered permeability of neurons and their dendritic trees both of which are factors of probable importance in the evolution of seizures. These mechanisms have not been demonstrated in humans with brain tumor but are inferred from data obtained in studies of experimental animals and cases of human epilepsy.

Seizures may be grand mal (generalized) in type, occurring without warning or identifiable aura, and are of no localizing value. On the other hand, focal seizures are often helpful in determining the region of the cortex affected by the tumor. Several examples of focal seizures may help illustrate this principle. A focal motor seizure, i.e., one beginning in the hand and spreading to the face or a leg, points to the primary motor-sensory cortex. Similarly, seizures characterized primarily by sensory phenomena (spreading numbness, tingling, and paresthesias) are indicative of paracentral cortex involvement. Temporal lobe seizures, although focal, are of less value in indicating the side of the lesion. A variety of symptoms may occur including feelings of fear, unreality, visual distortion, déjà vu, vertigo, lip smacking, head turning, and violent behavior. Olfactory auras, usually of foul, unpleasant odors, are often associated with tumors of the mesial temporal lobe (amygdaloid-hippocampal region). Visual auras are of some value in that formed visual hallucinations are more characteristic of temporal lobe lesions, and unformed hallucinations (flashes of light, jagged visual images, etc.) are said to be more typical of occipital lobe lesions.

## Tumor expansion

Interruption of neuronal connections with loss of neurological function may be the first evidence of a tumor. This may be coincident with seizure onset or develop later after other signs of tumor growth are apparent. Such changes result from direct invasion of the cortex or subcortical tracts by a tumor or from edema and a subsequent alteration in local blood flow around the tumor. A brief consideration of these factors seems appropriate.

A tumor may enlarge as an encapsulated mass, compressing surrounding or underlying brain or cranial nerves or occluding cerebrospinal fluid pathways. The tumor will grow as a roughly spherical mass until its surface abuts a more rigid structure such as falx or cranial bone. In addition to growth by cell proliferation, some tumors, depending on cell type, malignancy, etc., may enlarge as a result of necrosis and hemorrhage within the tumor. For instance, meningiomas are usually well contained and show little evidence of internal degeneration or hemorrhage; whereas metastatic lesions, also clearly demarcated from surrounding brain, may contain fluid and extensive degenerative and hemorrhagic products.

Infiltration is characterized by the spread of tumor cells through interstices of neighboring brain and is most characteristic of gliomas and some metastatic lesions. Extensive spread through brain tissue may take place before a significant interruption of function is apparent. Aggregates of tumor cells may be found distant from the main tumor, raising the question of a multicentric origin of tumor or an increased mobility of neoplastic cells from the primary source. It is also recognized that brain neoplasms may infiltrate tissue spaces widely, becoming diffuse without forming a single obvious mass. Gliomatosis cerebri is one term used to describe such tumors. Within the optic tracts and brain stem, this growth pattern is characteristic of glial tumors (spongioblastoma polare) causing marked, diffuse enlargement of these structures before the function of the neural matrix is impaired. In the brain stem, multiple nuclei of cranial nerves may be "picked off" as the tumor elongates. Usually, "long tract" signs (corticospinal and ascending sensory tracts) develop, signaling an intra-axial position of the tumor. Gliomas of the cerebral hemisphere produce interruptions of neural function early if strategically located. For instance, in the great majority of individuals, the left hemisphere is dominant for speech and language functions. Tumors arising in the left posterior frontal, parietal, and temporal lobe junctures often interfere with speech or language function, resulting in one of a variety of aphasic disorders. Similarly, lesions within the posterior frontal or anterior parietal area, or in a parasagittal or high convexity position, impair functions in the arm, leg, or face of a motor or sensory nature or both. Lesions within the temporal, parietal, or occipital lobes affect vision by interrupting the optic radiations in well-defined patterns.

These same processes associated with intra-axial tumors of the cerebellum give rise to symptoms that are anatomically less specific. Lateralization to one side or the other, or to the midline position, is often possible based on the pattern of neurological dysfunction (ataxia, dysmetria, dysdiodokokinesis, gait disturbance, nystagmus, etc.), but the clear focal symptoms often displayed by telencephalic tumors are not seen, at least when the tumor is small. Quite frequently, cerebellar tumors come to the patient's attention only when the circulation of cerebrospinal fluid is compromised, and hydrocephalus with increased intracranial pressure develops (vida supra).

Edema incident to tumors varies greatly with the type of tumor and its position. It may damage the brain by interfering with metabolism and blood flow either regionally or generally. Small metastatic tumors may induce widespread edema in an entire hemisphere by unknown mechanisms. On the other hand, a meningioma may attain an enormous size without edema until interference with metabolism from vascular congestion and circulatory injury takes place. Appropriate therapy with steroids or dehydrating agents sometimes reverses a neurological deficit within hours, even though the size of the neoplasm itself remains unaltered. Edema occurs both intra- and extracellularly and is greater in white than in gray matter. There is evidence that, in gray matter, edema fluid first accumulates intracellularly and, if the cell membranes rupture, in extracellular spaces as well. On the other hand, in white matter, edema appears in extracellular positions first and later accumulates in glial processes (primarily astroglia). This raises questions as to whether glial cells behave differently in these two locations and whether edema fluid reaches the cells through capillary cell walls or through their junctures. Studies of edema from brain neoplasms induced in experimental animals show swelling of glial processes, and, with the rupture of these processes, an increase of fluid in extracellular spaces. An analysis of this fluid may show cellular debris if cell membranes are ruptured, increased protein, increased sodium and chloride content of both gray and white matter, decreased potassium content, and increased water content. Creatine phosphate and adenosine triphosphate are decreased, whereas adenosine diphosphate and adenosine monophosphate and inorganic phosphate are increased in areas of increased water uptake. Such studies have not identified any process within the tumor tissue itself that generates edema. Furthermore, no clear distinctions have been observed between edema fluid produced by neoplasm, hematoma, and abscess.

In addition to the loss of neuronal function associated with an intra-axial tumor of the cerebral hemispheres and cerebellum, another important effect of pressure is cranial nerve dysfunction from direct compression by extra-axially positioned tumors. It is worth noting again that certain types of tumors are predominantly associated with specific cranial nerves; for example, olfactory nerve and meningioma; optic nerves and primary pituitary tumors, craniopharyngioma, and meningioma; and auditory nerves and neurilemoma. The cause of impaired function in the various nerves is a subject of debate. At least two mechanisms are considered of primary importance: stretching and compression of the nerve fibers and/or impairment of circulation to these same structures by tumor growth or sudden expansion within the tumor by hemorrhage and necrosis. The latter events are of particular significance with pituitary tumors (pituitary apoplexy) and are characterized not only by sudden visual deterioration but, frequently, by endocrine incompetence from the destruction of the remaining pituitary function. In the majority of examples of cranial nerve dysfunction resulting from extra-axial tumors, however, the loss of function is so insidious that it escapes early detection by the patient and often by the physician. As a result, serious permanent residua may remain after proper therapy.

Those portions of the olfactory and optic nerves (cranial nerves I and II) commonly affected by tumors are composed of tissues of the central, not the peripheral nervous system. They may recover from the effects of pressure upon, but not interruption of, their component fibers. The patterns of visual loss from the optic nerve, chiasm, and tract compression are considered in Chapter 6. The motor cranial nerves (III, IV, VI, and XII and portions of V, VII, IX, and X) all have the capacity to regenerate, even if they have been functionally interrupted for a time. Fiber regeneration, however, may not be anatomically precise (aberrant regeneration) so that normal patterns of motor function are not recovered. Damage to the sensory portions of the nerves, central to the ganglion cells, is more likely to incur permanent deficit (V and VIII for example), since regeneration does not take place. As is frequently noted with auditory nerve tumors, function of both divisions (acoustic and vestibular) may be completely interrupted, while the juxtaposed motor facial nerve (cranial nerve VII) continues to work even though equally distorted and stretched. For description of the clinical syndromes related to cranial nerves and the host of tumors that may involve them, the reader should consult other sources.

## Metabolic effects

Endocrine and metabolic malfunction constitute the last major manifestation of tumor pathophysiology. The vast majority of tumors of endocrine significance arise in the region of the pituitary gland or adjacent hypothalamus. Most are "extra-axial" in position, but a few take origin within the brain substance. The pituitary gland originates from ectoderm of the primitive buccal pouch, which develops into the anterior lobe, or adenohypophysis, and from buccal ectoderm of the infundibular extension of the brain, which forms the posterior lobe, or pars nervosa. The vast majority of pituitary tumors arise from the anterior lobe, though both portions of the gland may be severely damaged by tumors of primary or parasella origin. For instance, craniopharyngiomas, one of the more common intracranial tumors of childhood, are thought to arise from embryonic cell nests of buccal epithelium forming either cystic or solid tumors either within or above the sella, which may produce panhypopituitarism of both lobes of the gland. It is important also to keep in mind that associated with the endocrine abnormalities to be mentioned are a variety of other pathological changes, which frequently occur and have been mentioned earlier in this chapter. Examples include compression of the optic nerves, chiasm, or tracts; compression of the extra-ocular nerves; obstruction of the third ventricle, or aqueduct, causing hydrocephalus; or extensions of tumor mass or cyst into adjacent frontal or temporal lobes, causing general symptoms of increased pressure or irritative phenomena.

The endocrine changes may be ascribed to increased production of hormones typical of secreting adenomas of the pituitary or impairment by destruction of normal glandular function. The most common clinical manifestation of increased function is gigantism or acromegaly associated with the so-called eosinophilic adenomas. Acromegaly results from an increased production of growth hormone by the tumor, which, in turn, produces gigantism, if present before puberty, and enlargement of the hands, feet, and face, as well as the viscera after puberty and the closure of the epiphyses. Headaches, joint pains, diabetes mellitus, and cardiac enlargement and failure may ensue, shortening the life span of the victim by 15 to 20 years.

Increased production of adrenocorticotropic hormone (ACTH) by the pituitary occurs with the so-called basophilic adenomas, which usually are associated with adrenal cortical hyperplasia and manifested clinically by Cushing's syndrome. This is characterized by facial swelling (moon face); increased weight about the neck, thorax, and abdomen; stria about the abdomen and hips; thin limbs and increased hair growth; hypertension; and diabetes. It is debatable whether or not a pituitary adenoma is always present or if bilateral adrenal hyperplasia alone is responsible. In only about 10% of these cases is enlargement of the sella turcica found, but it is quite probable that micro-adenomas of the pituitary are present in all patients.

In both instances, it is becoming evident that the fundamental disturbance may reside in the hypothalamus and not in the anterior lobe of the pituitary. In a rapidly evolving field of study, it has been established that for some, and probably all, of the pituitary hormones the hypothalamus elaborates chemo-transmitters or releasing hormones, which, in turn, effect the production and release of hormones from the anterior lobe. These are CRF (corticotropin releasing factor), FRF (follicle releasing factor), LRF (luteinizing hormone releasing factor), TRH (thyrotropin releasing hormone, which is the only one chemically characterized and synthesized), and GRF (growth hormone releasing factor). With regard to prolactin, growth hormone, and melanocyte stimulating hormone, there is evidence that both releasing and inhibiting factors accomplish regulation of hormone release to further complicate these concepts.

Signs and symptoms of growth hormone hypersecretion accompanied by elevated serum growth hormone levels may precede, by long periods of time, any evidence of pituitary adenoma. As stated before, this is often observed in Cushing's syndrome, suggesting that increased or inappropriate secretion of GRF and CRF at the hypothalamic level may induce hyperplasia within the responsive cells of the anterior lobe, which ultimately develop into adenomas. This theory by no means is proved.

Astrocytomas of the hypothalamus or optic chiasm are very rarely responsible for a condition found in early infancy, the diencephalic syndrome, which is characterized by failure to gain weight, absence of body fat, and emaciation. Yet, growth hormone levels may be quite elevated suggesting that inhibition of growth hormone release is impaired by anterior hypothalamic involvement.

On the other side of the coin, and much more common, are states of hypopituitarism from tumors arising from, or near the pituitary gland (chromophobe adenomas, craniopharyngioma—occasionally meningiomas) and from aneurysms. These lesions are more frequently associated with compression of the optic nerves and chiasm. Secretion of the various hormones produced in the anterior lobe, mentioned earlier, may be severely impaired but to differing degrees. One of the earliest signs is amenorrhea in the female and diminished libido or impotence in the male. Symptoms of hypothyroidism are common, and eventually hypofunction of all main target glands, gonads, adrenals, and thyroid becomes evident. In youngsters, marked impairment of growth often occurs associated with fatigue, fine hair, and smooth delicate skin. If subjected to sudden stress, such as a major injury or operation, these patients may develop adrenal failure.

Impairment of posterior pituitary function, or involvement of the supraoptic nuclei of the ventral hypothalamus, produces diabetes insipidus and thermoregulatory disorders. These are more common accompaniments of craniopharyngiomas, granulomas, histocytosis, and primary hypothalamic tumors rather than pituitary adenomas.

Very rarely, astrocytomas of the medulla cause paroxysmal hypertension in association with increased blood levels of catecholamines similar to those seen with pheochromocytoma. It is postulated that neurogenic hypertension results from excitation of vasomotor centers within the posterior hypothalamus and medulla oblongata leading to excitation of sympathetic adrenal pathways with increased secretion of catecholamines. This hypothesis is supported by the fact that treatment of the brain tumor reverses these changes and that abdominal exploration for pheochromocytoma proves negative.

## General references

Critchley, M., J. L. O'Leary, and B. Jennett. 1972. Scientific foundations of neurology. Heinemann Medical Books, London.

Evans, C. H., V. Westfall, and N. O. Atuk. 1972. Astrocytomas mimicking the features of pheochromocytoma. New Eng. J. Med. 286:1397-1399.

Frohman, L. A. 1972. Clinical neuropharmacology of hypothalamic releasing factors, New Eng. J. Med. 286:1391-1397.

Martin, J. B. 1973. Neural regulations of growth hormone secretion. New Eng. J. Med. 288:1384-1393.

Youmans, J. R. 1973. Neurological surgery. Saunders, Philadelphia.

# 9

# Trauma to the Central Nervous System

## CENTRAL NERVOUS SYSTEM TRAUMA: SPINAL

WILLIAM S. COXE AND ROBERT L. GRUBB

### Spinal trauma

Whereas some of the principles in the discussion of cranial injury apply to the spine, there are obvious differences that relate to the complex anatomy of the vertebral column, the great concentration of important neural tracts in a structure of small cross-sectional area, and numerous variables peculiar to the bony spine that do not apply to the skull and brain. These variables include age and the flexibility of the body, the size of the bony canal as influenced by heredity, degenerative changes of joints and intervertebral discs, the thickness of both the posterior longitudinal ligament and the yellow ligament, congenital anomalies, and variations in blood supply.

The spinal levels most commonly involved with injury are the lower cervical spine ($C_4$, $C_5$, $C_6$, $C_7$, and $T_1$) and the thoracolumbar juncture ($T_{12}$, $L_1$, and $L_2$), the areas of greatest mobility. The thoracic spine is less subject to violent injury because of the rigidity imparted to it by the rib cage.

MECHANISMS OF INJURY

*Vertebral injury.* Injuries to the spine (and spinal cord) may be caused either by direct or indirect forces. Force applied directly to

284

the back of the neck or trunk may cause fractures of spinous processes of laminal arches, concussion of the spinal cord, or direct compression of neural tissue by depressed bone fragments.

Indirect injury is a more common mechanism resulting from forces applied to the head and trunk or from movements that exceed the normal range (hyperflexion, hyperextension, or excessive lateral or rotatory movements). These excessive movements may occur when the head is suddenly accelerated or decelerated in relation to the trunk, or when the trunk is decelerated with respect to the lumbar spine, as might occur in a car accident when the lower body is restrained by a seat belt. Compression or disruptive injuries result from forces acting along the axis of the spine. Depending upon a slight variation in the direction of lines of force, such injuries may also have extension or flexion components. For instance, in diving accidents, the force is directed against the top of the head in slight flexion, resulting in a compression-flexion injury that may cause a compression fracture of a cervical vertebral body with displacement of the posterior part of the body against the cord and possible sub-

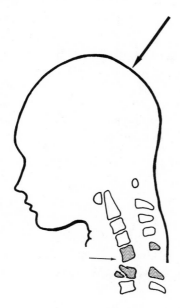

**Fig. 9-1** Force (arrow) typical of diving injury causing compression fracture C5 and cord damage from posterior displacement of portion of C5 body.

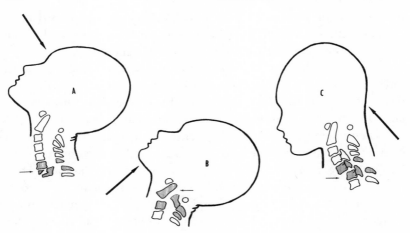

**Fig. 9-2** Three types of vertebral injuries (A, B, C), resulting from forces acting in different directions.

luxation at this level (Fig. 9-1). A blow striking the head more posteriorly would produce increased flexion together with disruption of spine and ligaments resulting in vertebral dislocation with locked articular facets at the affected interspace (Fig. 9-2C). Although the lower vertebra ($C_5$, $C_6$, and $C_7$) are most often involved, higher vertebral levels may be affected as well.

*Neural elements.* The most important consideration in spinal trauma is, of course, the effect on the spinal cord and nerve roots. These structures are injured by (1) compression from bone, ligaments, extruded disc material, and hematoma; (2) disruption or overstretching of neural tissues; (3) edema following compression or concussion; and (4) disturbance of circulation. The resulting neurological syndromes vary from complete loss of function below the injured segments to temporary loss of cord function followed by complete recovery. Between these extremes are a variety of syndromes, some of which are characteristic of a particular mechanism of injury.

The most severe damage is caused by bony compression, commonly resulting from flexion luxation with locked facets, compression from a posteriorly displaced vertebral body fragment, and hyperextension injuries. If the neural arches of vertebra remain attached to the body following luxation, the spinal cord is almost invariably compressed between the laminal arch of the superior ver-

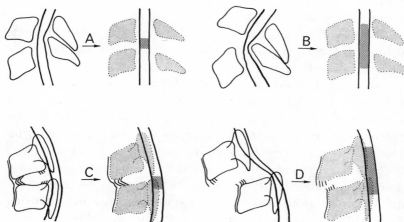

**Fig. 9-3** Cord injury produced by hyperextension (A) mild and (B) severe and hyperflexion (C) mild and (D) severe. Cross-notched areas emphasize the length as well as the cross-sectional dimension of possible cord damage. The clear and shaded vertebral outlines show, respectively, the position of vertebra at the time of injury and shortly afterwards, illustrating that films may not reflect the dynamics or extent of injury.

tebra and the posterior edge of the inferior vertebral body. If the laminal arch separates from its body, serious injury to the cord may be averted. In hyperextension injury, the cord may be crushed between the body and the laminal arch of adjacent vertebra without producing dislocation (Fig. 9-3A and B). In the latter group, radiographic abnormalities of the spine are often absent. Younger patients may experience only transient neurological changes, but complete or severe partial cord damage may occur in older patients with spondylosis and a congenitally narrow spinal canal. With hyperextension, the anterior longitudinal ligaments may be torn, the disc torn from the vertebral body, and the cord pinched between the inferior posterior border of the dislocating body and the leading edge of the laminal arch of the vertebra below it. After the injury, the relationship of these vertebral structures returns to normal, yet the cord may be severely injured.

Overstretching, causing disruption of cord tissue, usually follows hyperflexion injuries (Fig. 9-3). The tensile properties of the cord are not precisely known nor is the part age plays, but the fact that relatively minor injuries may cause neurological damage in the aged suggests that stretch tolerance decreases with age. Gross cord destruction is more likely in thoracic spine dislocations, probably because mobility is limited, and the dimensions of the canal relative to the cord size are less.

Cord edema may develop soon after injury and last several weeks. This may contribute further to tissue compression from other sources and to impairment of capillary circulation and venous return. Experimental studies on cord trauma, using a standard injury, have shown that within a few minutes after injury few changes can be seen microscopically. Within a few hours, however, leakage of red blood cells around vessels in the central gray matter occurs and later extends into coalescent hemorrhagic areas; accompanying this swelling, chromatolytic neuronal damage probably related to ischemia occurs. As swelling from hemorrhage and edema increases, compression of the surrounding white matter, axonal swelling, thinning of the myelin sheath, or disruption and enlargement of the periaxonal spaces are seen. Fluorescent microscopy reveals edema in central gray matter within 1 hour after injury and reduction in perfusion in central gray and, to a lesser extent, white matter. The perfusion pattern returns to normal in white matter within 24 hours, while remaining altered in gray.

Studies of changes in the metabolism and chemistry of the injured areas have shown a rapid decrease in oxygen tension within 30 minutes after injury, a transitory increase in tissue lactate, and an increased concentration of norepinephrine in the injured areas.

Local ischemia of cord tissue may result from the compression of the anterior or posterior arteries by angulation over bone or herniated disc material. In rare instances, the vertebral artery may be damaged as it courses through the transverse canal; if its contribution to radicular arteries and the anterior spinal artery is compromised, there may be severe cord ischemia. Hemorrhage involving the spinal cord, other than the microscopic hemorrhage associated with edema and contusion, rarely is the cause of significant impairment of neural function. Although epidural and subdural hematomas are found, they rarely are of sufficient size to produce serious compression, unlike these same entities within the cranium. Subarachnoid bleeding is common but of little clinical significance. Occasionally, larger intramedullary hematomas may develop, extending up and down the spinal cord from the point of injury and producing a true hematomyelia (tubular hematomyelia), which may cause complete or partial interruption of cord function.

A classification of cord lesions may be based on morphological change or functional deficit. The latter is more useful, since there is no strict correlation between the two. For instance, complete functional transection may occur either with obvious destruction of cord tissue or with minimal evidence of gross structural damage. The victim experiences immediate flaccid paralysis and loss of reflexes and sensation below the injured level. The cremasteric reflex may persist, and, in some cases, ankle jerks, plantar response, and sphincter and bulbocavernous reflexes persist only to disappear within a few days. After this period of spinal shock, which may last days or weeks, reflexes return and flaccidity may change to spasticity. If complete motor and sensory paralysis is present for a day or so after injury, recovery of any function is extremely rare.

The anterior cord syndrome is characterized by immediate paralysis, hypesthesia, and hypalgesia below the level of damage but with some preservation of touch, motion, position, and, occasionally, vibratory sensibilities. These injuries commonly follow fractures in which a displaced bone fragment and/or prolapsed disc material compresses the anterior cord surface, but they may also follow hyperextension injuries. The central cord syndrome is characterized by a greater motor weakness in the upper extremities as compared to the lower extremities, with variable sensory deficits, depending on the severity of the injury. The discrepancy in motor deficit may be explained by damage to the anterior horn cells destined for the arms and hands or damage to the more medially placed fibers of the corticospinal tract, which are passing off to the central gray matter to synapse within anterior horn cells. The softness and relative vascularity of central gray matter may allow edema and hemorrhage to extend more easily both longitudinally and transversely.

The Brown-Sequard syndrome results from injury to one-half of the spinal cord, causing ipsilateral paresis and loss of proprioception and contralateral loss of pain and temperature sense. This syndrome, in pure form, is rarely seen in cord injuries caused by blunt trauma but occurs more often following penetrating injuries (stab wounds, gunshot wounds, etc.). The term is generally used when a relative difference in function is noted in patients suffering bilateral cord damage.

The term contusio cervicalis posterior refers to a reversible syndrome characterized by pains and dysesthesias in the neck, arms, or trunk, which may be accompanied by mild motor and sensory dysfunction of arms and hands and mild long tract findings (hyperreflexia, extensor toe signs). The causative injury is usually hyperextension.

Cord concussion implies a momentary disturbance of cord function. Since the duration is so short, the physician rarely has the opportunity to observe it.

Injuries to the lower spinal cord, conus medullaris, and cauda equina may produce damage to long tracts, anterior horn cells, and nerve roots separately or in combination so that patients may show features characteristic of both upper and lower motor neuron dysfunction. Though less frequent, significant root lesions may also be seen with cervical injuries.

Delayed loss of neurological function after injury may occur within a few days or many years. Losses occurring shortly after injury are frequently a result of unrecognized vertebral injury, either because the initial symptoms were not impressive or because of inadequate X-ray examination of the spine, particularly of the $C_7$ to $T_1$ level, an area quite difficult to visualize in obese or heavily muscled patients. Progressive epidural hematoma or disc prolapse may also be responsible for such functional losses. Intramedullary cysts or syringomyelia in upper thoracic and cervical cord may form many years after cord injury at lower thoracic levels or at levels immediately adjacent to the injury site. This has been ascribed to vascular insufficiency from pressure on anterior spinal arteries or arachnoid scarring at the site of injury, producing a tethering effect upon the cord above it. Angulation of cord over a kyphotic spine or protruded disc may, over a period of years, cause similar progressive changes in the cord.

Fractures and dislocations involving the upper two cervical vertebra, although fairly common, rarely produce immediate neurological symptoms, since, if serious damage is done to the spinal cord at this level, the patient does not survive long enough to receive medical attention. The most common spinal injury is fracture of

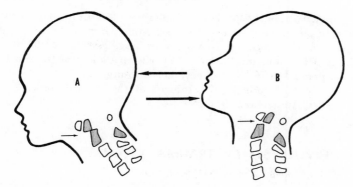

**Fig. 9-4** Direction of the force that produces odontoid fractures.

the odontoid process of the axis ($C_2$). This is thought to result from shearing forces delivered by blows to the head directed either from front or back or by violent flexion of the head on a neck held rigidly erect.

Most patients surviving such injuries have no neurological deficits immediately. If healing in normal position does not occur, either because the fracture was not recognized or union did not take place after reduction, late onset of spastic quadriparesis with a variety of sensory syndromes may occur as a result of instability in this area. The atlas is usually displaced forward, pinching the cord between its arch and the odontoid process in front of the cord, but, occasionally, the loose odontoid process and arch of $C_1$ may be displaced posteriorly on $C_2$, compressing the anterior surface of the cord (Fig. 9-4).

## General references

Assenmacher, D. R., and T. B. Ducker. 1971. Experimental traumatic paraplegia: The vascular and pathological changes seen in reversible and irreversible spinal cord lesions. J. Bone Joint Surg. 53 Am:671-680.

Barnett, H. J. M., E. H. Botterell, A. T. Jousse, and M. Wynn-Jones. 1966. Progressive myelopathy as a sequel to traumatic paraplegia. Brain 89: 159-174.

Fairholm, D. J. and I. M. Turnbull. 1971. Microangiographic study of experimental spinal cord injuries. J. Neurosurg. 36:277-286.

Locke, G., D. Yashon, R. A. Feldman, and W. E. Hunt. 1971. Ischemia in primate spinal cord injury. J. Neurosurg. 34:614-617.

Rossier, A. B., A. Werner, E. Wildi, and J. Berney. 1968. Contribution to
    the study of late cervical syringomyelic syndromes after dorsal or lum-
    bar traumatic paraplegia. J. Neurol. Neurosurg. Psychiat. 31:99-105.
Wagner, F., G. Dohrmann, and P. Bucy. 1971. Histopathology of transitory
    traumatic paraplegia in the monkey. J. Neurosurg. 35:272-276.
Braakman, R. and L. Penning. 1971. Injuries of the cervical spine. Ex-
    cerpta Medica, Amsterdam, 1971.

# CENTRAL NERVOUS SYSTEM TRAUMA: CRANIAL

ROBERT L. GRUBB AND WILLIAM S. COXE

## Mechanisms of head injury

The mechanical causes of head injury can be broadly grouped into
three main categories: impact loading, impulsive loading, and static
loading. An *impact* is defined as the collision of two solid objects
at a considerable velocity and is illustrated by collision of the skull
with a hammer, bullet, or an automobile windshield. An impulsive
load produces sudden motion of the head in the absence of significant effects from direct physical contact. Such injuries are produced
when the body is suddenly arrested, while the head is unrestrained
and free to continue moving. A static loading injury is produced by
a vice-like crushing force such as might occur when the head of the
victim is compressed between a wall and heavy machinery. As a result of these various injury mechanisms, the tissues of the cranium
are subject to strains, which can be defined as states of elongation,
compaction, or angular distortion produced by tensile, compressive,
or shear stresses, respectively.

Following an impact, two distinct types of effects are produced
in both the striking object and the object struck. Stress waves are
initiated and propagated, eventually encompassing the entire volume of the colliding objects. At the impact point there occurs a
relative indentation of both the striker and the target, which may
be either temporary or permanent. Depending on the velocity and
mass of the object striking the head, the resulting force may cause
a linear, comminuted, depressed, or perforated fracture of the skull.
A high velocity impact tends to produce depression or perforation
of the skull at the site of impact with laceration of the dura and
brain beneath, whereas a lower velocity impact tends to produce
skull distortion and linear fractures of the skull; the latter com-

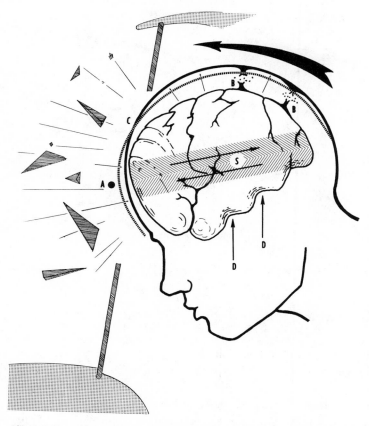

**Fig. 9-5** Closed blunt injury. Skull molding occurs at the site of impact. (A) Stippled line, pre-injury contour; (C) solid line, contour moments after impact with in-bending at (A), outbending at vertex. (B) Subdural veins torn as brain rotates forward. (S) Shearing strains throughout the brain. (D) Direct trauma to inferior temporal and frontal lobes over floors of middle and anterior fossae.

prises 70% of skull fractures. Studies of skull fracture demonstrate that an impact of low velocity causes an area of inbending at the point of injury with simultaneous outbending around the region of impact. The inbent area rebounds outward, creating an area of stress concentration. In the areas of outbending, tensile stresses initiate fracture lines that extend toward the point of impact and toward the base of the skull. Buttresses of the skull help direct the fracture toward the base of the skull (Fig. 9-5). Using stress coat

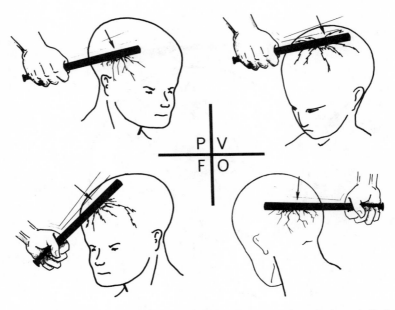

**Fig. 9-6** Linear fracture lines. Lower velocity impacts tend to produce skull distortion and linear skull fractures. Fracture lines originate in areas of outbending around the inbending produced by the impact, with radiation of fracture line toward the site of impact and the base of the skull.

techniques on human cadaver skulls, it has been demonstrated that the location and direction of linear fractures can be predicted (Fig. 9-6). An anterior impact to the skull produces linear fractures of the orbit with extension into the cribiform plate and pituitary fossa. Occipital impacts usually produce transverse parietal fractures and/or fractures extending into the petrous portion of the temporal bone and middle fossa. A midline interparietal blow producing a depressed fracture at the area of impact might cause an isolated fracture of the cribiform plate or lesser wing of the sphenoid.

Important sequelae of base fractures involving air sinuses or the structures of the ear are bleeding or leakage of cerebrospinal fluid from the nose and/or external auditory canal, providing a route for meningeal infection. Blood vessels running through foramina or in close contact with the skull may be damaged, and an extradural hematoma may subsequently develop. Injury to the internal carotid artery as it passes through the floor of the skull may result in severe hemorrhage, thrombosis, or arteriovenous fistula if the tear occurs where the artery courses through the cavernous sinus. Similarly, cranial nerves passing through the skull floor may be damaged. Of the cranial nerves, the auditory (VIII) and facial (VII) nerves may be involved by fractures of the temporal bone, the optic (II) and olfactory (I) nerves by fractures in anterior cranial fossa, whereas the lower cranial nerves are rarely damaged by base fractures.

The great variety of injuries caused by gunshot wounds of the head (Fig. 9-7) depends upon where the skull is struck, the speed and size of the bullet, and whether or not the bullet changes shape after the impact. A bullet that strikes the head tangentially may only lacerate the scalp, but it may have an impact sufficient to cause concussion or contusion of the brain immediately beneath the point of injury. Soft-nosed bullets flatten on impact and lacerate the tissues more than harder bullets, which do not lose shape. A penetrating missile wound not only destroys the structures in its pathway, but it produces expansion effects transmitted throughout the brain.

A closed, blunt head injury tends to produce contusions and disrupts brain tissue. A contusion directly below the site of an impact is called a coup lesion, those on the side of the brain opposite the impact are called contre-coup, and those in between intermediate coup. Blows to the front of the head usually produce coup lesions

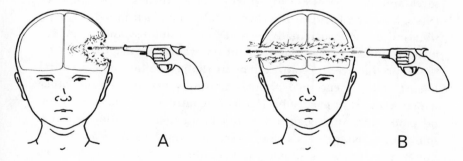

**Fig. 9-7** Bullet wounds of the head. (A) Soft, low velocity bullets cause compound (open) penetrating wounds of the skull and dura and local laceration of the brain. (B) A high velocity bullet causes a compound, penetrating wound of the skull and dura with severe laceration of the brain in its path. Expansion effects are transmitted throughout the brain.

alone, but blows to the back of the head produce both coup and contre-coup lesions. Blows to the side of the head produce either coup or contre-coup lesions in approximately equal proportion. The most common sites of cerebral contusions after head injury are in the temporal and frontal lobes, which occupy the middle and anterior fossae, respectively.

The mechanisms of brain injury after blunt head trauma are a source of debate. Two main hypotheses of injury have been proposed: (1) head translation (or linear acceleration) with cavitation and (2) skull distortion and/or head rotation. In mathematical models of simulated skulls containing idealized "brain," areas of significantly decreased pressure are present at different times adjacent to both coup and contre-coup zones, with maximum underpressure near the contre-coup area. Several types of phenomena could be associated with cavitation: release of dissolved gases from such fluids as blood and cerebrospinal fluid, and from brain tissue to produce bubbles, causing lesions primarily proximate to blood vessels and cerebrospinal fluid pathways. This selective association, however, has not been seen. This could produce extensive disruption of the brain tissue, but this is not ordinarily seen without associated severe compound fractures of the skull. Another mode of cavitation might occur when the force of underpressure exceeds the tensile strength of the tissue, forming small vacuum cavities. The subsequent collapse of these cavities would generate enormous pressures and shear stresses with disruption of tissues. A discrepancy exists, however, between the theoretically predicted areas of cavitation and the lesions actually seen at human autopsy and in experimental animals. The cavitation theory would predict that frontal blows produce contre-coup lesions in the cerebellum and occipital lobes, but, as mentioned above, this rarely occurs. On the other hand, occipital impact often results in contre-coup damage to frontal poles. This discrepancy does not mean that cavitation is not a source of cerebral lesions under certain conditions of head impact but that it does not appear to be as significant as other mechanisms in the production of many coup and contre-coup lesions.

One then turns to the theory of skull distortion and/or head rotation. It has been proposed that rotation of the head is the major factor in the production of brain injury and that severe injuries to the brain could thus be explained by its physical properties, especially the fact that, although the brain is easily deformed, it is extremely incompressible. Lying within the rigid skull, it responds to distorting forces by gliding and rotating. Acceleration of the head sets up rotational forces that are transmitted to the brain, causing it to move within its dural sheath to produce shearing strains and distortion of brain tissue (Fig. 9-5). More recent models of this mechanism have shown that large shear stresses maximal at the brain surface and extending halfway to the center of rotation in the "brain" can occur. Such bony and dural protuberances as the floors of the anterior and middle fossae, the sharp wings of the sphenoid ridge, and the falx prevent movement of the brain and enhance such stresses. These stresses would also be increased at such large exit foramina as the foramen magnum, where disruption of the brain as well as damage to blood vessels may occur. This theory received support from high speed movies of head trauma to monkeys in which the calvarium had been replaced by a transparent Lucite dome. When the head was set in motion by a blow, even of sub-concussive force, the brain rotated and moved within the dura, especially in the parietal and occipital areas, where the skull has a smooth convexity. There was less motion in the frontal and temporal regions, where the irregular anterior and middle fossae floors and the sphenoid ridge restrain brain movements. A large amount of brain movement occurred only when the head was freely mobile, and little or no rotational movements occurred when the head was fixed. The areas of greatest injury in these experiments were the frontal and temporal lobes.

Both head rotation and skull distortion thus play important roles in brain injury. Skull distortion is most important when head movement is restricted; head rotation becomes important when an impact moves the head. Skull distortion can be highly localized and produce mainly coup lesions, especially if a fracture is produced. A non-fracturing blow produces more generalized skull distortion and causes greater brain distortion in both coup and contre-coup sites where the brain is stopped by bony irregularities. Although the specific way in which skull distortion causes cerebral lesions is not known, it is probably related to change in intracranial volume, enhancement of structural irregularities at the base of the brain, and strains caused by stress waves passing through the brain. Thus, energy entering the head after an impact seems to be portioned in three ways: (1) skull distortion (contact phenomenon of impact); (2) translation of the head (movement in a straight line); (3) rotation of the head (hyperflexion, hyperextension, lateral bending, and twisting of the head on the neck). The relationship of these three modes of energy distribution is not known, but translation of the head seems to be the least important.

## Concussion

Concussion occurs when the function of the nervous system is disrupted by trauma, the most dramatic manifestation being loss of consciousness. Clinically, concussion is recognized when head injury produces loss of consciousness and loss of memory, i.e., traumatic amnesia. The duration of both losses has been used as an index of the severity of concussion. In human patients dying after a head injury and prolonged coma, there is usually evidence of brain damage in the form of contusions, hematoma, and edema. Death shortly after an uncomplicated concussion is rare. Therefore, most of the information on cerebral concussion has come from experimental work in which a standardized impact has been used to produce unconsciousness of different degrees and duration in different animals. From a bio-mechanical viewpoint, the experiments done on such primates as monkeys and chimpanzees have the most relevance to the problems of concussion in humans.

In experiments by Ommaya and his co-workers on monkeys, the site of the impact to the skull was not as important as the efficiency of the impact. In these experiments, there was no statistically significant relationship between changes in the intracranial pressure produced at the time of the impact and concussion, although others believe intracranial pressure does play a role. Acceleration of the head was statistically significant when related to the onset of concussion. If the animal's head were fixed during the impact, either rigidly or by use of a cervical collar, a greater impact was required to produce concussion. Ommaya also found that acceleration of the unrestrained head could produce concussion in the absence of an impact to the head, but it required approximately twice as much head rotational velocity to produce unconsciousness as compared to the force required after direct impact.

After experimental concussive impact definite changes in the respiration, blood pressure, electrocardiogram, electroencephalogram, and cerebrospinal fluid pressure are noted. A period of apnea lasting for a few seconds is followed by a change in respiratory rhythm and/or amplitude. In animals not surviving the concussive impact, permanent apnea may ensue or follow a period of respiratory gasps. In most animals, there is a sudden fall in blood pressure, which lasts from 30 seconds to 10 minutes and which may be followed by a secondary rise of blood pressure, particularly in those succumbing to injury. In addition to bradycardia, which is almost invariably present, significant electrocardiogram changes follow experimental cerebral concussion. Dropped beats, extrasystoles, elevated T waves, and increased amplitude of the QRS complex may occur, and, if they persist, they signal a poor prognosis. In concussed animals, the electroencephalogram shows an immediate onset of high amplitude slow wave activity, especially in the parietal areas, which disappears as consciousness is regained. At impact the cerebrospinal fluid pressure momentarily rises as high as 600 mm $H_2O$, but a persistent increase is not seen except in fatally concussed animals. The changes in respiration, electroencephalogram and electrocardiogram readings, and blood pressure last until the animal regains consciousness.

What are the anatomical and physiological changes in the brain that produce concussion? Since the discovery of the role of the reticular formation of the brain stem in the maintenance of consciousness, there have been several reports correlating concussion with histological changes in the brain stem. Groat found chromatolysis and destruction of neurons in the reticular formation of the pons, the red nucleus, and the vestibular nucleus in concussed monkeys. Ommaya demonstrated that intravenously administered sodium fluorescein leaked into the brain stem and upper cervical spinal cord of some, but not all, concussed monkeys. With nonconcussive trauma, there was no fluorescence of the brain stem. Electrophysiological studies of concussed monkeys showed that cessation of spontaneous activity measured from electrodes placed in the reticular formation was more striking than the often observed slowing of the cortical electroencephalogram. Immediately after concussion, electrical responses in the medial lemniscus to peripheral stimulation were unchanged, while responses in the reticular formation were absent. Anatomical evidence to support the hypothesis that changes in the reticular formation are the only mechanism of concussion in humans has been difficult to find. Widespread changes in cortical and brain-stem neurons have been demonstrated after head injury in man, but it is not clear whether these changes were primary or secondary to such other processes as hemorrhage, brain swelling, and hypoxia. Interference with the reticular formation may explain short periods of unconsciousness in man but not prolonged coma, since most of these cases show widespread cerebral damage at autopsy.

Another theory of how unconsciousness and amnesia are produced by concussion was proposed by Holbourn. He suggested that brain damage and dysfunction result from shearing strains secondary to skull distortion and rotational acceleration of the head. He predicted that, depending on the degree and direction, shearing strains could produce either extensive laceration of the brain or only tearing of nerve fibers without gross evidence of injury. It is possible that mild shearing strains could produce temporary dysfunction of neuronal transmission. A study of patients who died after head trauma and remained unconscious until death showed no evidence of increased intracranial pressure. Diffuse degeneration of the white matter in the cerebral hemispheres and brain stem was found with "retraction balls" on many nerve fibers, indicating severance of these fibers.

On a theoretical and experimental basis, Ommaya has proposed that shear stresses and strains produced by inertial loading of the brain are the crucial factors for the production of cerebral concussion as well as for some, but not all the visible brain lesions. Amnesia and traumatic coma are thought to be responses of the brain to increasing degrees of these stresses, which functionally disconnect first the diencephalon and then the midbrain structures from the cerebral cortex. Amnesia would be produced by functional disconnection of the temporal lobes from the diencephalon, whereas disconnection of the rostral midbrain reticular formation from the cerebral cortex would produce coma. Structural disconnection of the same structures might explain permanent memory defects, coma vigil, and death with increasingly severe primary injuries to the brain. It should be noted that, in this hypothesis, the brain stem is considered to be the most resistant part of the brain to trauma.

## Rapidly expanding intracranial lesions

The following course is characteristic of rapidly expanding hematomas and masses. After an impact, which may or may not cause loss of consciousness, a lucid or symptom-free interval may follow during which the patient is regarded as having a minor injury. But, in a few hours, the patient becomes restless, and then confused and stuporous, and finally comatose. In reality, this picture is seen in only 50% of patients with epidural hematomas, the rest of the patients being unconscious from the time of injury. In patients already comatose, the coma may deepen if they have an acute expanding epidural hematoma. The space available for expansion of a hematoma is represented mainly by fluid displacement from the subarachnoid space and the ventricular system. As the limit of this displacement is reached, the inferior medial part of the uncus and hippocampus is pushed medially through the tentorial hiatus, compressing the midbrain, and may impale the opposite cerebral peduncle against the contralateral tentorial edge. The ipsilateral oculomotor nerve (cranial nerve III) is also compressed by the herniation. Irritation of this nerve by herniating temporal lobe may initially constrict the ipsilateral pupil, but this is soon followed by dilation and fixation of the ipsilateral pupil and later by paralysis of the extraocular muscles supplied by the oculomotor nerve. While the ipsilateral pupil dilates, the patient is rapidly becoming comatose and may develop a bradycardia secondary to the increasing brain-stem compression. Compression of the posterior cerebral artery at this time may produce infarction of the occipital and inferior temporal lobes. As the condition progresses, and intracranial pressure and brain-stem compression increase, a secondary rise in blood pressure may occur (Cushing response). This reflex increase in the blood pressure is an ominous sign of impending irreversible brain-stem damage. It should be noted that a slow pulse rate and a rising blood pressure are not always seen with expanding supratentorial masses. Concomitantly, as the hematoma enlarges, a contralateral hemiparesis may develop from pressure on the hemisphere or cerebral peduncle. Less frequently, ipsilateral hemiplegia may develop if the contralateral cerebral peduncle is compressed against the contralateral tentorial edge (Kernohan's notch). If the hematoma is not evacuated by this time, irreversible brain-stem decompensation develops not only from lateral compression of brain structures but from rostrocaudal displacement of the stem as well. Brain-stem, pontine, and diencephalic hemorrhage and ischemia may occur, probably because of compression and stretching of both arteries and veins supplying these structures. The opposite pupil dilates and then becomes fixed, oculovestibular responses are lost, hyperventilation is present, and bilateral decerebrate posturing appears. As the brain-stem decompensation progresses into the lower pons and upper medulla, regular, but shallow respirations appear, the extremities become flaccid, and, finally, the medulla is damaged with ensuing slow, irregular respirations, an irregular pulse, and falling blood pressure.

Lesions lying over the vertex or the frontal pole may not compress the diencephalon and midbrain laterally but rather result in a rostrocaudal degeneration of the brain stem. Clinically, there is decreasing alertness progressing to drowsiness, stupor, and coma as the cerebral hemispheres displace the diencephalon caudally. Early in this syndrome many patients will exhibit periodic respirations of the Cheyne-Stokes type. The pupils become small but remain reactive. This pupillary response may represent hypothalamic sympathetic damage or functional decortication. The eye movements remain full on Doll's head maneuver and caloric testing. Motor dysfunction may begin unilaterally with hemiparesis contralateral to the supratentorial lesion producing the syndrome, while the ipsilateral extremities show paratonic resistance, or gegenhalten, but continue to respond appropriately to painful stimulation. As the syndrome progresses, bilateral decorticate responses appear. The signs of the "diencephalic" stage of the transtentorial herniation syndrome may result from diffuse bilateral cerebral hemisphere dysfunction or functional derangement of the upper midbrain and diencephalon. If the syndrome progresses to involve the midbrain, the pupils become fixed in a midposition. Other signs and symptoms resemble those already described for the uncal herniation syndrome as it progressively damages the brain stem rostrocaudally.

## Epidural hematoma

Epidural hemorrhage develops between the dura and the inner table of the skull, occurring in 0.4% to 3% of head injuries in the various series reported. Early recognition is most important, since death usually results if treatment is delayed. The hematoma usually forms in the middle fossa where a skull fracture may lacerate the middle meningeal artery, which is imbedded in or closely attached to the temporal bone. Tearing of other meningeal arteries or of the dural sinuses or veins can lead to the formation of epidural hematomas in other locations. Those incident to arterial injury enlarge rapidly, forming a significant intracranial mass in a few hours and producing a rapidly progressing uncal herniation syndrome.

## Subdural hematomas

Subdural hematomas are usually classified as acute, subacute, or chronic, depending on the delay in onset of clinical symptoms following the precipitating injury. The clinical symptoms of all three types are due to mass effects with resultant displacement of the cerebral hemispheres. The bleeding in the subdural space is nearly always of venous origin, and the hematomas usually lie over the convexities of the frontal and parietal lobes. Acute subdural hematomas become symptomatic in the first 2 to 3 days after injury, subacute subdural hematomas appear clinically a few days to 1 to 2 weeks after injury, and chronic subdural hematomas do not become clinically evident for several weeks after an injury. These hematomas differ pathologically and prognostically.

### ACUTE SUBDURAL HEMATOMA

These hematomas may follow relatively mild trauma in which the head is accelerated or decelerated. As mentioned earlier, an impact producing acceleration of the head would cause the brain to glide within the dura, and the greatest motion would be in the parietal and occipital areas. Whereas the smooth interior of the skull in these regions tends to prevent lacerations of the brain, bridging veins between the cortical surface and the dural sinuses are torn, allowing blood to diffuse freely and quickly throughout the subdural space. More commonly, acute subdural hematomas are seen after more severe head trauma and may be associated with serious cerebral contusions, lacerations, and intracerebral hematomas. In these injuries, blood can enter the subdural space from torn vessels in the subdural space and/or lacerated vessels on the brain surface. The clinical picture is determined not only by the mass effects of the expanding extracerebral mass but also by parenchymatous damage, which may be extensive. As the hematoma enlarges, one can see the transtentorial herniation syndrome or the uncal herniation syndrome as previously described for epidural hematomas. Because of the frequent location of subdural hematomas over both convexities of the brain, the transtentorial herniation syndrome is perhaps more common.

### SUBACUTE SUBDURAL HEMATOMA

These hematomas are less often accompanied by immediate underlying brain damage. The blood in the subdural space may be liquid or gelatinous, and early membrane organization on the periphery of the hematoma may occur. The clinical course following trauma is usually one of decreasing responsiveness to stimuli, although there is often a lucid interval before the level of consciousness deteriorates. As the hematoma enlarges and compresses the brain, the clinical signs and symptoms resemble those previously described for intracranial hematomas.

### CHRONIC SUBDURAL HEMATOMA

These hematomas frequently follow trivial trauma to the head. In many instances, no definite history of injury to the head can be established. Symptoms may not appear for weeks or months after the formation of the hematoma begins. They are usually located on the antero-fronto-parietal surface of the hemisphere, are frequently bilateral, and are composed of decomposed blood, blood pigments, and proteins in the subdural space. The hematoma contents are surrounded by a fibrous membrane, which is thicker and more vascular on the outer (subdural) side and quite thin and avascular on the brain surface. Watanabe and his associates found that, in order to produce chronic subdural hematomas in experimental animals, blood must be mixed with cerebrospinal fluid. They noted that the fibrin formed by this combination differed markedly from regular fibrin. The membrane thus formed is not semi-permeable but allows free flow of hemolyzed red blood cells and proteinaceous material through it. These investigators believe that the continued enlargement of the hematoma can be attributed to continuous oozing of the extravasated blood from the fibrous capsule, especially the numerous macrocapillaries in the sinusoid layer of the outer membrane. The rate at which symptoms appear is much slower than that seen with more acute hematomas, since the brain can tolerate significant molding and displacement without producing clinical signs of a mass lesion. Again, clouding of consciousness, confusion, and memory loss are the presenting clinical signs and may be followed by hemiparesis, sensory loss, dysphasia, or other signs of cerebral hemisphere dysfunction. If the lesion is permitted to continue to enlarge, transtentorial or uncal herniation syndromes will ensue. Subdural hematomas do not always continue to expand but may be reabsorbed, leaving thickened membranes in the subdural space. Rarely, they become calcified and remain asymptomatic.

### SUBDURAL HYGROMA

This is a collection of clear or yellowish cerebrospinal fluid in the subdural space, producing the same symptoms and signs as a subdural hematoma. It is presumed that a tear in the arachnoid membrane permits the leakage of cerebrospinal fluid into the subdural space, which is then unable to return to the subarachnoid space because of a "flap valve" mechanism. As a result, increasing amounts of fluid accumulate in the subdural space. These cases are rarely associated with severe brain damage.

## Contusions, lacerations, intracerebral hematomas, and subarachnoid hemorrhage

The most common form of traumatic intracranial hemorrhage occurs within the subarachnoid space. It usually arises from surface lacerations or contusions of the brain and is often associated with skull fractures. With contusions, the pial covering of the cortical surface remains intact, but underlying cortex and white matter may be hemorrhagic and necrotic (pulped). A laceration is a traumatic tearing of the cortical surface of the brain. Contusions and lacerations are commonly found beneath depressed skull fractures and around penetrating wounds caused by sharp objects or missiles. A small object of low velocity penetrating the brain may produce only localized injury and no loss of consciousness, but one moving at high velocity causes massive destruction and hemorrhage in its path as well as remote damage secondary to blast effects. Rotational movements of the brain cause shearing strains in the cerebral tissue and may produce unconsciousness. Major vessels may be damaged, leading to ischemia of the area of brain supplied by these vessels. Intracranial and subdural hematomas may be formed. Massive blunt trauma, with or without fracture, often causes contusions and lacerations beneath the site of impact, particularly in the anterior temporal lobes and frontal lobes, where shearing strains are maximal. At sites of injury, further hemorrhage and cerebral edema may develop, adding to brain bulk and further increasing intracranial pressure. Such lesions also destroy neurons, glial elements, and nerve fibers.

Massive intracerebral hematomas after trauma are uncommon, being found in about 1% of severe head injuries. They occur most frequently in the frontal and temporal lobes, either beneath fractures or as a contre-coup lesion. Such hematomas probably arise from injury to a deeply placed cerebral vessel. Multiple small hemorrhages occur in the corpus callosum, thalamus, and basal ganglia, especially after blows to the vertex that displace the brain downward against the base of the skull. Bleeding may also arise from ependymal tears in the ventricular system and, though infrequent, may fill the ventricular system with a blood clot and lead to death.

## Cerebral edema

Cerebral edema after trauma to the head is usually associated with contusions and lacerations of the brain. Edema usually appears in the white matter around or beneath contusions, lacerations, hematomas, and ischemic lesions. Widespread cerebral edema may also be associated with large epidural or subdural hematomas, both before and after they have been removed. The pressure of the extracerebral hematoma probably obstructs venous blood outflow with resultant escape of edema fluid from the capillaries.

Edema and increased intracranial pressure following head injury is usually proportional to the severity of the injury. Among several mechanisms proposed for the production of cerebral edema by head traums, two merit attention.

A mechanical injury to the brain tissue may abolish cerebral autoregulation and reduce the resting tone of the cerebral resistance vessels (arteries and arterioles) with a resultant increase in the cerebral blood flow. This is called the vasogenic theory. The dilation of the cerebral resistance vessels and the increased cerebral blood flow increases the pressure in the cerebral capillaries and venules (the cerebral capacitance vessels). Under Starling's hypothesis, this causes a net exchange of fluid toward the cerebral tissues, producing cerebral edema. The increase in brain volume leads to an increase in the intracranial pressure.

Another proposed mechanism is that injury primarily affects the cerebral capacitance vessels, with resultant venous dilation and stasis. The cerebral blood flow decreases, and cerebral hypoxia occurs secondary to insufficient cerebral perfusion, while $CO_2$ accumulates in the brain, and glial cells swell secondary to hypoxia and hypercarbia. It has been shown that reducing the perfusion pressure of the brain by increasing the intracranial pressure to levels that do not change the cerebral blood flow can increase the tissue concentrations of lactate. Siesjo and his colleagues think this is a result of tissue hypoxia in focal areas. The fluid balance of cells depends on the active extrusion of Na (cation pumps), a process that requires the expenditure of energy in the form of oxygen, ATP, ADP, and phosphocreatine. When the brain is deprived of oxygen, ATP, ADP, and phosphocreatine stores are depleted rapidly. The cation pumps cease to function properly, allowing sodium chloride and water to accumulate in glial cells. This mechanism is the more commonly accepted explanation of intracellular edema. Hypoxia and hypercarbia impair the function of the cerebral resistance vessels, leading to defective autoregulation and, in turn, to vasogenic edema. Thus, both mechanisms of edema formation may play a role in traumatic cerebral edema. As cerebral edema increases, the intracranial pressure rises, further reducing cerebral perfusion, increasing cerebral hypoxia, and causing more edema. This vicious cycle is often fatal if not interrupted by appropriate therapy.

## General references

Benedict, J. V. 1969. An analysis of an impact-loaded fluid-filled thin spherical shell as a mathematical model for investigation of the cavitation theory of brain damage. Ph.D. Thesis. Department of Mechanical Engineering, Tulane University.

Chasen, J. L., W. D. Hardy, J. E. Webster, and E. S. Gurdjian. 1958. Alterations in cell structure of the brain associated with experimental concussion. J. Neurosurg. 15:135-142.

Echlin, F. 1949. Traumatic subdural hematoma—acute, subacute and chronic. An analysis of seventy operated cases. J. Neurosurg. 6:294-303.

Engin, A. E. 1968. The axisymmetric response of a fluid-filled spherical shell. Ph.D. Thesis. Department of Engineering Mechanics, University of Michigan.

Freytag, E. 1963. Autopsy findings in head injuries from blunt forces: Statistical evaluation of 1,367 cases. Arch. Path. 75:402-413.

Foltz, E. L. and R. P. Schmidt. 1956. The role of the reticular formation in the coma of head injury. J. Neurosurg. 10:342-352.

Goldsmith, W. 1966. The physical processes producing head injury. Pages 350-382 in W. F. Caveness and A. E. Walker, eds. Head injury: Conference proceedings. Lippincott, Philadelphia.

Groat, R. A., W. F. Windle, and H. W. Magoun. 1945. Function and structural changes in the monkey's brain during and after concussion. J. Neurosurg. 2:26-35.

Gurdjian, E. S., J. E. Webster, and H. R. Lissner. 1953. Observations on the prediction of fracture sites in head injury. Radiology 60:226-239.

Gurdjian, E. S. and J. E. Webster. 1958. Head injuries. Churchill, London.

Gurdjian, E. S. 1966. Mechanism of head injury. Pages 112-128 in J. Shillito, W. C. Cotter, S. Flanigan, R. Ojemann, and J. Stoll, eds. 1966. Clinical neurosurgery. Williams & Wilkins, Baltimore.

Gurdjian, E. S. 1972. Recent advances in the study of the mechanism of impact injury of the head—a summary. Pages 1-42 in G. T. Tindell, R. H. Wilkins, E. B. Keener, and G. A. Meyer, eds. Clinical neurosurgery, Williams & Wilkins, Baltimore.

Holbourn, A. H. S. 1943. Mechanics of head injuries. Lancet II:438-441.

Holbourn, A. H. S. 1943. The mechanics of brain injuries. Brit. Med. Bull. 3:147-149.

Langfitt, T. W. 1972. The pathophysiology of the cerebral circulation in head injury. Pages 84-97 in G. T. Tindell, R. H. Wilkins, E. G. Keener, and G. A. Meyer, eds. Clinical neurosurgery. Williams & Wilkins, Baltimore.

Lee, Y. C. and S. H. Adveni. 1970. Transient response of a sphere to torsional loading—a head injury model. Math. Biosciences 6:473-486.

Ommaya, A. K., S. D. Rockoff, and M. Baldwin. 1964. Experimental concussion—a first report. J. Neurosurg. 21:249-265.

Ommaya, A. K. 1966. Trauma to the nervous system. Ann. Royal College Surg. (England). 39:317-347.

Ommaya, A. K., F. Faas, and P. Yarnell. 1968. Whiplash injury and brain damage. JAMA 204:285-289.

Ommaya, A. K., R. L. Grubb, Jr., and R. A. Naumann. 1971. Coup and contre-coup injury: Observations on the mechanics of visible brain injuries in the rhesus monkey. J. Neurosurg. 35:503-516.

Plum, F., and J. B. Posner. 1972. The diagnosis of stupor and coma. F. A. Davis, Philadelphia.

Pudenz, R. H. and C. H. Shelden. 1946. The lucite calcarium—a method for direct observation of the brain. II. Cranial trauma and brain movement. J. Neurosurg. 3:487-505.

Rand, C. W. and C. B. Courville. 1946. Histologic changes in the brain in cases of fatal injury to the head. VII. Alterations in nerve cells. Arch. Neurol. Psychiat. 55:79-110.

Rowbotham, G. F. 1946. The mechanisms of injuries of the head. Pages 55-92 in G. F. Rowbotham, ed. Acute injuries of the head. Williams & Wilkins, Baltimore.

Sano, K., N. Nakamura, K. Hirakawa, et al. 1967. Mechanisms and dynamics of closed head injury. Neurol. Medicochir. (Tokyo) 9:21-23.

Siesjo, B. K. and N. N. Zewetnow. 1970. Effects of increased cerebrospinal fluid pressure upon adenine nucleatides and upon lactate and pyruvate in rat brain tissue. Acta Neurol. Scand. 46:187-202.

Strich, S. J. 1961. Shearing of nerve fibers as a cause of brain damage due to head injury. Lancet II:443-448.

Unterharnscheidt, F. and K. Sellier. 1966. Head injury: Conference proceedings. Pages 321-341 in W. F. Caveness and A. E. Walker, eds. Mechanics and pathomorphology of closed brain injuries. J. B. Lippincott, Philadelphia.

Watanabe, S., H. Shimada, and S. Ishii. 1972. Production of the clinical form of chronic subdural hematoma in experimental animals. J. Neurosurg. 37:552-561.

# 10

# Central Nervous System Infections

RALPH FEIGIN AND PHILIP DODGE

## Introduction

A number of terms are used to describe infections of the central nervous system and its coverings. Meningitis denotes inflammation of the meninges but does not indicate that the dura mater is involved, whereas leptomeningitis denotes inflammation of the arachnoid and pia mater, the usual distribution of meningitis. Such noninfectious causes of meningitis as leukemia involving the central nervous system, chemical irritation of the meninges, or hypersensitivity reactions will not be considered further. The term parameningeal infection encompasses those infectious processes adjacent to the meninges and includes brain abscess, epidural abscess, subdural empyema, and encephalitis. In many cases, parameningeal and meningeal infection occur concurrently. Encephalitis denotes inflammation of the brain itself; if there is some associated meningitis, then the term meningoencephalitis is commonly employed.

## Organisms encountered

A wide variety of pathogens, including bacterial, mycobacterial, rickettsial, fungal, and viral agents, may produce central nervous system inflammation. Infection of the nervous system with spiro-chetes, bedsoniae and metazoan and protozoan parasites, as well as mycoplasma, has been well documented. Although meningeal or parameningeal inflammation may result from infection with any of these organisms, sites of predilection can be delineated. These sites depend to some extent upon the specific type of infectious agent and upon the route by which infection is acquired.

## Routes of infection

The most common route by which infectious microorganisms reach the central nervous system is via the bloodstream; hence, bacter-emia, viremia, fungemia, rickettsemia, and so on frequently precede or occur concomitantly with central nervous system infection. Infec-tion of the nervous system from a contiguous focus of disease such as infection of the paranasal sinuses, middle ear, or mastoids is not an infrequent occurrence. Direct invasion of the central nervous system by microorganisms (usually bacteria or fungi) may occur as a result of congenital defects, as in patients with a myelomeningo-cele or a dermoid sinus tract, or may follow trauma that permits contact between the environment and the meninges. For example, a compound fracture of the skull with wound contamination or a craniotomy wound infection may produce meningeal infection with organisms commonly encountered on the skin. In contrast, a frac-ture through one of the frontal sinuses may produce meningitis or a brain abscess with organisms commonly harbored in the sinuses or nasopharynx.

The fetus may be infected *in utero* with organisms that cross the placenta from the mother. Infection of the central nervous system with such viruses as an RNA virus (rubella) or cytomegalovirus, and with the protozoan, *Toxoplasma gondii,* have been well docu-mented. The effects of these agents upon the fetus are most devas-tating when infection occurs during the first trimester of pregnancy. Syphilis, due to a spirochete, may also be transmitted *in utero;* this organism, however, rarely, if ever, crosses the placenta before the second trimester of pregnancy. Transplacental infection with bac-terial organisms is difficult to prove in most cases, but documenta-tion exists in the case of *Listeria monocytogenes.*

Neonatal bacterial infection may be acquired by aspiration of in-

fected amniotic fluid during the course of delivery of a septic
mother or may result from infection by organisms found normally
in the birth canal. Group B, beta hemolytic streptococci are normal
inhabitants of the vagina. The pathogenic potential of these organisms has gone unrecognized in standard textbooks despite increasing evidence of their importance as a cause of clinical disease.
In many institutions, they have become the leading cause of meningitis due to Gram-positive organisms during the first 3 months of
life. In some series, a vaginal carrier rate for group B, beta hemolytic streptococci of 5 to 6% has been documented, and infectious
complications in the newborn have been described in up to 30%
of the children born to mothers who carry this organism. Similarly,
viral infection may be acquired during the process of delivery, as in
the case of neonatal herpes simplex due to infection with the geni-
tal strain (type II) herpes simplex virus. Finally, the neonate may
be infected from the environment as in cases where heavy coloniza-
tion with *Staphylococcus aureus* occurs. A resurgence of diseases of
this type may follow recent decisions to prohibit routine hexa-
chlorophene bathing of the newborn infant. Neonates, and particularly premature infants placed in a humidified environment, may
develop septicemia and meningitis due to organisms that prolifer-
ate within the moist atmosphere. Under these conditions, an increased incidence of meningitis due to *Pseudomonas aeruginosa* or
*Serratia marascens* would be anticipated.

## Factors predisposing to central nervous system infection

Many of the factors that predispose to infections of the central
nervous system are similar or identical to those that predispose to
infection at other sites. These factors may be related to the host, to
the organism, to the environment, or to some critical interrelationship among the three. Although we shall attempt to discuss these
factors separately, their interdependence will become apparent.

## Host factors

There is substantial evidence that males suffer central nervous system infections more frequently than females at all ages. In the
neonate, where septicemia is frequently accompanied by meningitis, the male to female predilection has been placed at 1.7 to 1.

There is an increased incidence of central nervous system disease in the very young and the very elderly, and, in these patients, the disease process tends to be of increased severity as well. Premature infants are more susceptible than full term infants, as highlighted by the fact that premature infants account for 48% of all infected neonates, although they comprise but 8% of all live births.

Additional factors, that have been implicated as predisposing factors to neonatal sepsis or meningitis include premature rupture of the fetal membranes, prolonged labor, excessive manipulation during labor, with attendant risk to contamination of amniotic fluid, and overt infection in the mother during the last week of pregnancy. Some investigators have noted an increased incidence of placenta praevia and placenta abruptio in mothers of infants with neonatal sepsis, but the relationship of these conditions to the development of neonatal sepsis remains ill defined. The presence of congenital (physiological or pathological) or acquired deficiencies in the immunological response of the host to infection are important factors predisposing to the occurrence of central nervous system disease.

Defense mechanisms involved in protecting the host against infectious illness have been subjected to extensive study. Congenital deficiency of the three major classes of immunoglobulins (agammaglobulinemia or dysgammaglobulinemia) predispose to serious bacterial infection. A physiological deficiency of immunoglobulin is noted in the normal newborn infant. Placental transport of immunoglobulin G (IgG) provides the neonate with antibodies present in maternal IgG. There is little or no transport immunoglobulin A (IgA) and M (IgM) across the placenta; thus, the neonate lacks the bactericidal antibodies to Gram-negative enteric organisms. These antibodies are, for the most part, in the IgM globulin serum fraction. Although this deficiency has been suggested as the cause of an increased frequency of Gram-negative sepsis and meningitis in the newborn infant, the rarity of such infection in infants who uniformly lack this material suggests that other host defenses play a more important role in protecting the neonate from invasion by enteric organisms. Moreover, an increased incidence of meningitis and septicemia due to Gram-negative organisms is noted in elderly patients, even though a deficiency of IgM has not been documented in these individuals.

Congenital defects involving thymic-dependent small lymphocyte function as documented in Di George's syndrome (absent thymus and parathyroid gland), Nezelof's syndrome (absent thymus), ataxia telangiectasia (dysplastic thymus, reduced serum IgA, neurological pathophysiology, and cutaneous telangiectasia), and Wiskott-Aldrich syndrome (eczema, thrombocytopenia, and recurrent infection) are known to predispose the patient to overwhelming viral infection. Indeed, central nervous system involvement due to the administration of live attenuated oral polio vaccine has been well documented in patients with defects in thymic-dependent small lymphocyte function. Severe combined immunodeficiency disease (deficits in both humoral and cellular function) also predisposes to serious infection, including disease of the central nervous system. It has been suggested that congenital or acquired defects in polymorphonuclear leukocyte function may predispose to central nervous system infection. Miller has demonstrated that the phagocytes of the normal neonate are less efficient than those of adults and that there is a deficiency in the opsonizing ability of plasma of the neonate compared to the normal adult. Coen and his associates have reported decreased bactericidal activity in the leukocytes of some full term newborn infants within the first 12 hours of life, despite normal phagocytic activity. The importance of these observations as regards the increased incidence of meningitis in the neonate remains to be determined. In chronic granulomatous disease of childhood, phagocytosis proceeds unimpaired but bactericidal function is disturbed. In particular, hydrogen peroxide production by the leukocyte is impaired. Bacteria that lack the ability to produce hydrogen peroxide or that produce catalase, e.g., *Staphylococcus aureus*, lead to severe infection in these patients. Despite these findings, an increased incidence of central nervous system infection in patients with this disorder has not been documented.

Congenital asplenia has been associated with an increased incidence of septicemia and meningitis, and infection with *Diplococcus pneumoniae* has been particularly prominent. An increased incidence of overwhelming sepsis, in some cases with meningitis, has been associated with removal of the spleen, but the predilection of the host for infections under these conditions depends upon the age at the time the spleen was removed, the indication for splenectomy, and the number of years elapsed since splenectomy was performed. It has been suggested that the increased incidence of sepsis and meningitis following splenectomy may be more closely related to the disease process that necessitated removal of the spleen than to its absence per se. Removal of the spleen for thalassemia major has been followed by sepsis in up to 33% of patients, whereas removal necessitated by trauma produced no increased risk of septicemia. It has also been suggested that the difference between patients with splenectomy and the normal population may be less the frequency of infection than the rapidity with which they succumb to what under other circumstances should not have been a fatal infection.

Other hereditary and acquired diseases of man that are not primary defects in the immune system also predispose to an increased severity and incidence of central nervous system infection. Malignancy of the reticuloendothelial system is associated with a significant increase in central nervous system infection. The reason for this has been documented. Such diseases as leukemia, lymphoma, multiple myeloma, and Hodgkins' disease have been associated with decreased production of normal immunoglobulins, delayed and defective antibody response to antigenic stimuli, production of abnormal immunoglobulin, depression in the clearing mechanism of the reticuloendothelial system, and depression of cellular immunity.

The use of irradiation or immunosuppressive agents and antimetabolites also predisposes the host to central nervous system infection. In some cases, it is difficult to attribute the occurrence of central nervous system infection specifically to the use of one of these agents, for the underlying disorder may be of prime importance in predisposing the host to infection.

The debilitated host is more susceptible to infection, including infection of the central nervous system. Many of the factors that contribute to a debilitated state, including old age, chronic illness, and malignancy, have been noted already. Malnutrition must be included as an important world-wide cause of debility in the host.

The concept that malnutrition can make man more susceptible to infectious diseases and also alter the course and outcome of the resulting illness is time honored. Although circumstantial evidence is plentiful, it is principally based on clinical experience, and well-controlled studies have been few and slow to accumulate. It has been much easier to demonstrate that infection is often directly responsible for lowering the state of nutrition. The fact that infectious diseases are widespread in areas of the world where malnutrition prevails suggests that the two phenomena are interrelated.

It is now apparent that various combinations of immunological deficiency may exist in malnourished individuals. A number of investigators have described occasional low levels of gammaglobulin, impairment in cell-mediated immunity, low levels of serum complement, impaired phagocytic activity of the leukocytes, and perhaps even decreased levels of transferrin, a factor that possesses bacteriostatic properties. These factors may act alone or in concert to predispose the malnourished individual to severe infection. Although the picture is far from complete, recent developments appear to support the concept that malnutrition is an important factor in poor response to infection.

Central nervous system infection also occurs with increased incidence and severity in alcoholics and in patients with diabetes mellitus and renal failure. Although such illness may be characterized by serious derangements in metabolic balance, no single mechanism has yet been identified to explain the increased susceptibility to infection in these disorders. It should be noted that acidosis, which sometimes accompanies diabetes and renal insufficiency, may result in a sluggish polymorphonuclear response of reduced intensity, ineffective phagocytosis, and defective bactericidal function.

The presence of infection in the otherwise healthy host at sites outside the central nervous system is also associated with an increased incidence of central nervous system infection. This may be bloodborne, as in concurrent venous thrombophlebitis, bacterial endocarditis, and pneumonia, or, by more direct extension, as in otitis media and osteomyelitis of the skull or facial bones.

## Factors related to the infecting organism

An increased incidence of infection with Gram-negative organisms in the very young and very old has been mentioned. Specific mechanisms responsible for this predilection remain undefined.

Meningitis due to *Hemophilus influenzae* occurs most frequently but not exclusively in hosts between 3 months and 3 years of age. On the basis of data collected by Fothergill and Wright in 1933, it has been assumed that 100% of normal adults and most normal newborn infants have bactericidal antibody to *H. influenzae,* type B. Thus, meningitis with *H. influenzae* in the adult was usually attributed to a defect in immunological function of the afflicted adult host. Similarly, the rare cases of neonatal infection with *H. influenzae,* type B were assumed to be the result of failure of the neonate to acquire antibody from a mother who lacked *H. influenzae,* type B antibody. During the past decade, numerous epidemiological studies have documented an increased prevalence of *H. influenzae* infection throughout the United States, Canada, and England. Despite the increased prevalence of this disease, the peak incidence remains between 3 months and 3 years of age. In addition, recent studies have documented that as many as 30% of normal neonates and 28% of normal adults lack bactercidal antibody to this organism. Although these data suggest a distinct change from the pattern of antibody to *H. influenzae* in the population studied by Fothergill and Wright, statistical comparisons of their data with those obtained within the past few years fail to confirm a statistically significant difference. Moreover, the stimulus that prompts the development of antibodies to *H. influenzae* by the human host has been carefully scrutinized. Failure to acquire serum bactericidal antibody has been documented in as many as 76% of children under 2 years of age following *H. influenzae* meningitis, although they were otherwise normal. In contrast, prolonged nasopharyngeal carriage of this organism in the absence of clinical disease has been associated with the development of high titers of *H. influenzae* bactericidal antibody.

Although it is impossible to place each of these observations in proper perspective, one can predict that meningitis due to *H. influenzae* will be seen in an increasing number of patients less than 3 months and more than 3 years of age. The increased number of cases in these age groups may be a reflection of a general increase in the prevalence of the disease rather than a change in the age-specific pattern of acquisition of bactericidal antibody to *H. influenzae.*

Certain organisms rarely produce central nervous system infection except under conditions where the host has been compromised. Neurosurgical treatment of hydrocephalus in which a ventriculo-atrial shunt has been placed may be followed by meningitis due to *Staphylococcus epidermidis.* This organism is generally not pathogenic and is part of the normal flora of the skin. The host whose reticuloendothelial or lymphoid system has been compromised by disease is more likely to be infected with such bacterial microorganisms as *Corynebacterium diphtheriae, L. monocytogenes, P. aeruginosa, S. marcescens,* and *Staphylococcus.* In addition, central nervous system infection with such organisms as *Nocardia, Aspergillus, Candida, Cryptococcus* and *Mucor,* or such viruses as cytomegalovirus or herpes, has been well documented.

Central nervous system infection with diphtheroids, staphylococci, aspergilli, or candida occurs more frequently following cardiac surgery, and prolonged intravenous catheterization may be followed by septicemia and meningitis with mimeae, candida, cryptococci, or staphylococci.

## Environmental influences

Environmental influences are important in a consideration of the pathogenesis of central nervous system infection. Perhaps the most widely publicized association between the environment and the occurrence of meningitis has been that involving *Neisseria meningitidis.* Although meningococcal meningitis can occur at any age in the normal host, its incidence increases markedly in situations where individuals are in close contact with one another. Thus, recruits living in close contact in a military camp may become nasopharyngeal carriers of this organism and pass it to one another. It has been well documented that under conditions where the number of carriers of *N. meningitidis* is increased, an increase in the incidence of meningococcal septicemia and meningitis will usually follow.

Syphilis, with its potential for central nervous system involvement when untreated, is primarily spread by venereal contact.

Contact of the human host with non-human vectors may also be important in predisposing to central nervous system infection with certain organisms. Encephalitis produced by arboviruses is only possible when the appropriate reservoir host (e.g., a farm animal) is infected, and an arthropod vector is available to transmit the disease to man. Similarly, rickettsial diseases, which produce central nervous system involvement as part of a diffuse vasculitis, are acquired by contact with infected ticks, fleas, lice, or mites. Contact with birds may suggest central nervous system infection with such an organism as *Chlamydia psittaci,* which produces ornithosis. Meningitis following human contact with mice or dogs may suggest leptospirosis or, with cats, toxoplasmosis.

Residence in or travel to particular regions of endemic disease is of anamnestic import. Travelers in Central and South America or in parts of Europe and Asia may acquire cerebral cysticercosis (usually solitary cysts containing the larval form of the pork tapeworm, *Taenia soleum*). In Africa or Southeast Asia, echinococcal cysts of the brain, cerebral malaria, and cerebral schistosomiasis should be considered as possible causes of focal or generalized neurological symptoms.

## Factors influencing morbidity and mortality

Each of the factors related to the host, the organism, or the environment may influence, to a greater or lesser extent, the morbidity or mortality of central nervous system infection. The single most important determinant of morbidity and mortality, however, is delay in the institution of appropriate therapy following onset of the disease. The more prolonged the illness prior to diagnosis and institution of effective therapy, the more likely it is that death or permanent defects will follow. The fact that specific therapy is now available for most bacterial, mycobacterial, spirochetal, fungal, and rickettsial microorganisms serves to underscore the important role of the physician in ameliorating the effects of central nervous system infection. Recently, agents effective against certain viruses *in vitro* have been applied to the treatment of viral infection of central nervous system. Although their effect in altering the course of these infections has been variable, more convincing evidence of their potential values has been suggested by reports in which patients were treated shortly after the onset of their disease.

## Clinical syndromes and pathogenetic factors

### MENINGITIS

Regardless of etiology, inflammation of the meninges is associated with a set of symptoms and signs that includes headache, pain in the back, and stiff neck with resistance to anterior flexion (rotation and side to side bending may be unrestricted). Often, when an attempt to flex the neck is made, the legs will flex at the knees (Brudzinski's sign); when the hip is flexed at a 90° angle, complete extension of the knee is restricted (Kernig's sign). This latter maneuver may be associated with involuntary flexion of the contralateral leg at the knee and hip (Brudzinski's crossed flexion response). These signs are protective reflexes, the result of inflammation of sensory fibers. The patient with meningitis frequently complains of photophobia, but the pathophysiology of this symptom is obscure.

All these findings may be minimal or absent in the neonate and young infant. Signs of meningeal irritation in the infant, however, may include inhibition of normal neck flexion best demonstrated when the non-supported head of the recumbent patient is extended over the edge of the examining table. Some of the general irritability and restlessness of the infant with meningitis may also relate to meningeal irritation.

Increased intracranial pressure is the rule in meningitis. This can be documented by measuring cerebrospinal fluid pressure in a patient of any age. In the infant, this increased pressure is reflected by a full or bulging fontanel, which often loses its normal pulsation. In the neonate, this sign may be absent, although diastasis of the cranial sutures may be found. It is probable that this diastasis permits rapid enlargement of the head thereby minimizing the degree of bulging of the fontanel. Vomiting occurs frequently. Headache almost certainly is partially explained by the elevated intracranial pressure distorting pain-sensitive nerves of the dura and related structures. The brain itself and the leptomeninges are insensitive to pain. Even though the recorded cerebrospinal fluid pressures may exceed 500 to 600 mm of $H_2O$, and are frequently in excess of 300 mm of $H_2O$, papilledema is rare in meningitis, probably because of the relatively brief duration of pressure elevation (a few days only). When papilledema is noted, associated conditions including brain abscess, subdural empyema, or venous sinus occlusion should be considered.

The pathogenesis of the increased intracranial tension can only be surmised. Accumulation of purulent material about the base of the brain impeding the circulation of cerebrospinal fluid, and especially through the cisterns to result in a communicating hydrocephalus, has been demonstrated. Non-communicating hydrocephalus occurs rarely from obstruction within the ventricular system at the foramen of Monro, the aqueduct, or at the level of exits of cerebrospinal fluid from the fourth ventricle.

Theoretically, inflammation of the choroid plexus and ependyma could increase cerebrospinal fluid production, but, to our knowledge, this has not been demonstrated. Impaired absorption of cerebrospinal fluid has not been shown or inferred except when the major venous sinuses are occluded simultaneously. With effective therapy, significant meningeal exudate persists for a few days. When the initiation of therapy is delayed, the natural reaction to meningeal inflammation (fibrosis) is excessive; in cases where the choice of therapy has been inappropriate, or the organism is resistant to the antibiotic utilized for treatment, permanent and progressive hydrocephalus may develop.

There is some evidence to suggest that, in meningitis, there may be an excessive release of antidiuretic hormone with consequent water retention and sodium dumping by the kidney. This combination places the patient at risk of further increased intracranial pressure, especially if excessive amounts of free water are administered during the course of therapy. Brain swelling may be extreme in meningococcal disease, particularly in cases of meningococcemia. Curiously, the cerebrospinal fluid may reflect minimal inflammatory changes in these patients, even though the fluid is teeming with meningococci. The mechanism of brain swelling in such instances is obscure, but an altered blood-brain barrier in response to endotoxin has been suggested.

Because the cranial and spinal nerves must course through the subarachnoid space, they often become irritated. Transient or permanent paralysis of neural function is unusual in meningitis. Deafness and vestibular disturbances are well-recognized complications of meningitis, and visual loss from optic nerve involvement occurs rarely. One suspects that vasculitis contributes to this; the optic nerve is a central nervous system tissue and reacts as does the rest of the brain to disease. Involvement of the auditory nerve complex is suspected by some to occur at the cochlear and vestibular end-organ level as the result of accompanying inner ear infection or toxic reactions to drugs (e.g., streptomycin, kanamycin). Factors in addition to a direct involvement of the nerves as they course through the infected meningeal spaces must be considered when extraocular and facial nerve functions are compromised. For example, increased intracranial pressure may result in uncal herniation and compression of the extraocular nerves. The facial as well as the auditory nerves are at risk as they pass through the infected temporal bone. Their ability to swell without compromising the vascular supply is limited. Were direct inflammation of the nerves in the infected meninges the only consideration, one would expect that cranial nerve abnormalities would be more common and also that peripheral motor deficits from spinal root involvement would be found occasionally; such spinal root paralysis, rarely, if ever, obtains.

Obtundation, stupor, and, rarely, coma are encountered in patients with meningitis. As indicated above, irritability and restlessness also may be seen, especially in infants and children. These findings relate to cerebral dysfunction, and, although increased intracranial pressure may partially explain them, the predominant cause of the neuronal dysfunction is almost certainly a bacterial encephalopathy related to the infection itself. Pathological changes in the cerebral cortex tend to support this conclusion. Signs of focal cerebral disease may also reflect encephalopathy or result from cerebral infarction, a consequence of an accompanying vasculitis in which veins and arteries are involved about equally. The incidence of vasculitis is greater when treatment is delayed or when it is ineffective. Although signs of this complication may be witnessed during the early hours of disease, they can be delayed for several days. Seizures are the most common manifestation of cerebral cortical dysfunction, but visual field defects and motor and somatosensory abnormalities are also observed. Some of these findings may be postictal (e.g., Todd's paralysis) and clear rapidly, whereas others persist. A general deficit in intellectual functions leading to permanent mental retardation may be related not only to inflammation of the meninges but also to the shock and hypoxia that may accompany the acute illness. All of these findings are more common in children than in adults, but they can occur at any age. During the first year of life, up to 40% of patients with meningitis exhibit seizures, which carry with them no particular prognostic significance unless they are persistent and difficult to control. In such circumstances, significant and often permanent damage to the brain may occur. Because of the known liability of infants to convulse with fever from any cause, it seems probable that fever, rather than a disturbance in cerebral function as a direct consequence of the meningeal infection, could explain this high incidence of seizures with meningitis under a year of age. Both factors could operate synergistically to the detriment of the infant. Epilepsy complicates meningitis in 2 to 3% of pediatric cases; it occurs less frequently in adults.

*Subdural effusions.* Collections of fluid in the subdural space can be demonstrated in approximately 50% of infants with meningitis during the acute illness. This subdural fluid may or may not be grossly infected. The pathogenesis is unclear, but the effusions are probably secondary to dural inflammation, if not to actual infection, which can lead to the formation of fibrovascular membranes that eventually encapsulate the effusions. Distortion and stretching of veins transversing the subdural space, as in trauma, may result in secondary bleeding. In most instances, these subdural effusions are asymptomatic, and they disappear spontaneously over a few days or weeks. Large subdural effusions, however, may increase intracranial pressure and produce a full fontanel as well as enlargement of the head, vomiting, and, at times, obtundation and irritability. Seizures and striking focal neurological deficits almost certainly relate to one or the other pathogenetic mechanisms discussed and not to the subdural collection itself. Periodic tapping of the subdural collection to relieve signs of increased intracranial pressure is indicated, but otherwise these lesions can be ignored. It is probable that they occur beyond the age of infancy, but because the subdural space is inaccessible their frequency is unknown. Surgery is rarely if ever necessary to treat these lesions, unless gross infection (subdural empyema) is present. Subdural empyema can also occur in the absence of meningitis and is discussed below. It should be noted that subdural membranes and large fluid collections have been found many years later in patients who suffered from meningitis in infancy. Careful analysis of such cases indicates that the cerebrum was severely damaged early in the course of the disease by meningitis and/or the accompanying shock or hypoxia. Brain atrophy occurs secondarily, and, under such circumstances, subdural collections persist because of a disparity between brain size and cranial volume.

## PARAMENINGEAL INFECTIONS

As indicated above, this term may denote a number of infectious processes including brain abscess; subdural empyema; epidural,

cerebral, and spinal abscesses; thrombophlebitis; arteritis; and mycotic aneurysms secondary to septic emboli.

Clearly, the neurological expression of these several disorders depends upon the site of the lesion(s). The location of the pathology
is determined by the route through which the intracranial or intraspinal infection is established. Thus, otitic infections produce epidural abscess, subdural empyema, or parenchymatous abscess in the
adjacent temporal lobe or cerebellum. Lateral sinus occlusion can
also occur, and, on occasion, the thrombosis extends to other venous
sinuses and cerebral veins. Similarly, infections about the face spread
in a retrograde fashion by way of the orbital plexus of veins to the
cavernous sinus or beyond. Most commonly, however, the signs of
cavernous sinus occlusion predominate. Frontal lobe involvement
(cerebral abscess, corticothrombophlebitis, or subdural empyema)
results most often from infection of the frontal sinus and less often
from infection of other air sinuses. The infection spreads here, as in
the case of otitic infections, by way of the bone (osteomyelitis) or of
phlebitis of small penetrating veins or both. Metastatic cerebral lesions may be solitary or multiple and occur usually in the distribution of the middle cerebral artery regardless of the source or origin
of the infectious process. Abscess formation from a septic focus in
the lung, or associated with a right to left shunt in congenital heart
disease, usually is not accompanied by bacterial endocarditis. Bacterial endocarditis itself leads most often to embolic occlusion of
medium-sized vessels and consequent infarction, which may secondarily undergo abscess formation, or lead to the development of
a mycotic aneurysm, which can rupture causing a subarchnoid hemorrhage. These complications develop more often when the endocarditis is acute and the organism is *S. aureus.*

Epidural abscess may occur intracranially, and at any level of the
spine, and is caused most often by *S. aureus,* although many other
organisms have been incriminated. Intracranial epidural abscess
produces no neurological symptoms. In spinal epidural abscess,
the source is often furunculosis with transient bacteremia. Seem-
ingly minor injury to the back often precedes the development of
symptoms by several days to weeks. This suggests that local injury
to tissues can form a nidus in which the organisms, once lodged, can
multiply readily. The adjacent vertebrae may harbor infection, but,
surprisingly, evidence of osteomyelitis is usually lacking in radio-

graphs. The epidural pus can extend widely and not only act as a compressive mass but produce symptoms because of associated vasculitis. The spinal level of the pathology determines the clinical syndrome.

## ENCEPHALITIS

A non-suppurative, parenchymatous inflammation of the brain, encephalitis, can result from infection with a wide range of microorganisms. Although most are bloodborne, some microorganisms (e.g., the herpes simplex virus) also reach the central nervous system by coursing along peripheral and cranial nerves. Because the meninges are inflamed in most forms of encephalitis the descriptive term meningo-encephalitis is often employed. Most encephalitides tend to be generalized in distribution, although some show a predilection for gray (polio encephalitis) or white (leukoencephalitis) matter. The clinical syndromes include disturbances in behavior, alterations in consciousness, and bilateral deficits in motor and sensory functions. Seizures are a common manifestation of most varieties of encephalitis. Asymmetry of involvement is not unusual, however, and some forms of encephalitis show a particular preference for certain regions. Thus, for example, the herpes simplex virus is often localized to the temporal lobes.

Some agents have a necrotizing effect on central nervous system tissue, others produce little tissue disruption, and still others evoke a striking reactivity of tissue. The usual forms of encephalitis have an acute or subacute course, but syphilis, for example, may be a very chronic infection. So-called slow or temperate viruses have been frequently incriminated in diseases that have a latent period of many years and minimal, if any inflammatory pathological features. Kuru, an exotic disease of New Guinea natives, and Creutzfeldt-Jakob disease, a dementing illness of middle age, are transmitted by unidentified agents, which are probably viruses. The rubeola virus has been identified as the probable cause of subacute sclerosing panencephalitis. In the past, this has been called subacute sclerosing encephalitis and subacute inclusion body encephalitis (Dawson's disease). This disease characteristically develops many years after the patient's infection with rubeola. The virus appears to lie dormant before symptoms of the devastating and almost always fatal illness become manifest.

## Differential diagnosis

The seriously ill patient whose symptoms suggest central nervous system infection presents a challenging diagnostic problem. It is important to ascertain whether involvement of the meninges is primary, as in bacterial meningitis, or secondary, as in a number of parameningeal infections (encephalitis, brain abscess, subdural empyema, etc.). Of equal importance in treating the patient is the determination, if possible, of the specific etiology of the infection. Central to both these problems is the presence, or absence, of pleocytosis within the cerbrospinal fluid and the degree thereof. Although most infective microorganisms elicit a cerebrospinal fluid response, a similar reaction may be produced by a variety of noninfectious processes including chemical irritation, hypersensitivity reactions, and tumors.

CEREBROSPINAL FLUID EXAMINATION

The diagnosis of central nervous system infection is most readily made by documentation of changes within the cerebrospinal fluid. The importance of a carefully performed lumbar puncture and meticulous study of the cerebrospinal fluid cannot be overemphasized. Cerebrospinal fluid findings characteristic of various inflammatory diseases of the central nervous system are outlined in Table 10-1. Measurement of the initial pressure is an essential part of every cerebrospinal fluid examination, although accurate pressure measurements may be difficult to obtain in the young struggling child. In the presence of extremely high pressure, just enough fluid should be removed to allow for an accurate examination. Compression of the jugular vein should be avoided except in cases of suspected spinal cord compression. Xanthochromic (deeply yellow) fluid derives its color primarily from bilirubin pigment. In the absence of hemorrhage, this is most frequently associated with elevated protein concentration of the cerebrospinal fluid and may be seen when cerebrospinal fluid circulation has been impaired. Bilirubin staining of the cerebrospinal fluid may also occur in jaundiced patients with meningitis, as in the case of neonatal sepsis or leptospirosis.

As few as 200 to 300 leukocytes/cu mm impart an opalescence to the fluid, whereas fluid containing thousands of cells may be frankly purulent. Cerebrospinal fluid should be promptly examined for cells in a counting chamber, and a differential cell count should be performed on a Wright-stained smear of the sediment after centrifugation. In the case of a traumatic lumbar puncture, care must be exercised to ensure that an underlying pleocytosis is not missed. This can be accomplished by obtaining a total cell count in a counting chamber and then adding acetic acid to the fluid and repeating the cell count. Acetic acid will lyse the red blood cells and permit an accurate count of the remaining white blood cells. If the number of white blood cells compared to the number of red blood cells is in excess of that in whole blood, one may assume that pleocytosis within the cerebrospinal fluid exists. A separate smear should be made and Gram-stained for bacteria. Quellung and agglutination reactions with type-specific antisera can occasionally provide an immediate etiological diagnosis, when the appropriate antisera are available. Most recently, the use of countercurrent immunoelectrophoresis utilizing the specific antibodies for *H. influenzae*, type B, for *D. pneumoniae*, and for *N. meningitidis* has permitted the detection of bacterial antigen in the cerebrospinal fluid within 1 hour following receipt of the specimen in the laboratory. With this new technique for demonstrating antigen, bacterial infection can be detected even in patients who have been pretreated with the appropriate antibiotic agents; thus, a definitive diagnosis may be made in cases in which cultures of spinal fluid fail to grow a microorganism. On the other hand, there may be some cross reactivity between the antigens, and a precise diagnosis is not always possible. When tuberculous meningitis is a possible diagnosis, a Ziehl-Neelsen stain or Kinyoun stain should be performed on the sediment and on the protein coagulum or pellet that frequently forms on standing. Examination of the cerebrospinal fluid utilizing the India ink technique may outline *Cryptococcus neoformans* in cases where cryptococcal meningitis is suspected. The presence of budding forms of the yeast in cerebrospinal fluid will help distinguish cryptococci from lymphocytes. Even the most experienced examiners, however, have found this technique somewhat less than precise.

The cerebrospinal fluid should be cultured whenever a lumbar puncture is performed for a suspected infection. The absence of cells does not invariably exclude the possibility of bacterial meningitis. Cerebrospinal fluid should be inoculated onto a variety of

TABLE 10-1  *Initial Cerebrospinal Fluid Findings in Suppurative Diseases of the Central Nervous System and Meninges*

| | PRESSURE (mm $H_2O$) | LEUKOCYTES/CU MM | PROTEIN (mg/100 ml) | SUGAR (mg/100 ml) | SPECIFIC FINDINGS |
|---|---|---|---|---|---|
| Acute bacterial meningitis | Usually elevated; average, 300 | Several hundred to more than 60,000; usually a few thousand; occasionally less than 100 (especially meningococcal or early in disease); polymorphonuclears predominate | Usually 100 to 500, occasionally more than 1000 | Less than 40 in more than half the cases | Organism usually seen on smear or recovered on culture in more than 90% of cases |
| Subdural empyema | Usually elevated; average, 300 | Less than 100 to a few thousand; polymorphonuclears predominate | Usually 100 to 500 | Normal | No organisms on smear or by culture unless concurrent meningitis |
| Brain abscess | Usually elevated | Usually 10 to 200; fluid is rarely acellular; lymphocytes predominate | Usually 75 to 400 | Normal | No organisms on smear or by culture |
| Ventricular empyema (rupture of brain abscess) | Considerably elevated | Several thousand to 100,000; usually more than 90% polymorphonuclears | Usually several hundred | Usually less than 40 | Organism may be cultured or seen on smear |
| Cerebral epidural abscess | Slight to modest elevation | Few to several hundred or more cells; lymphocytes predominate | Usually 50 to 200 | Normal | No organisms on smear or by culture |
| Spinal epidural abscess | Usually reduced with spinal block | Usually 10 to 100; lymphocytes predominate | Usually several hundred | Normal | No organisms on smear or by culture |
| Thrombophlebitis (often associated with subdural | Often elevated | Few to several hundred; polymorphonuclears and lymphocytes | Slight to moderately elevated | Normal | No organisms on smear or by culture |

| Disease | Pressure | Cells | Protein | Glucose | Smear / Culture findings |
|---|---|---|---|---|---|
| carditis (with embolism) | elevated | lymphocytes and polymorphonuclears | | | ...or by culture |
| Acute hemorrhagic encephalitis | Usually elevated | Few to more than 1000; polymorphonuclears predominate | Moderately elevated | Normal | No organisms on smear or by culture |
| Tuberculous infection | Usually elevated; may be low with dynamic block in advanced stages | Usually 25 to 100, rarely more than 500; lymphocytes predominate except in early stages when polymorphonuclears may account for 80% of cells | Nearly always elevated, usually 100 to 200; may be much higher if dynamic block | Usually reduced; less than 50 in 75% of cases | Acid-fast organisms may be seen on smear of protein coagulum (pellicle) or recovered from inoculated guinea pig or by culture |
| Cryptococcal infection | Usually elevated; average, 225 | Average, 50 (0 to 800); lymphocytes predominate | Average, 100; usually 20 to 500 | Reduced in more than 1/2 of cases; average, 30; often higher in patients with concomitant diabetes mellitus | Organisms may be seen in India ink preparation and on culture (Sabouraud's medium); will usually grow on blood agar; may produce alcohol in cerebrospinal fluid from fermentation of glucose |
| Syphilis (acute) | Usually elevated | Averages 500; usually lymphocytes; rarely polymorphonuclears | Average, 100; gamma-globulin often high, with abnormal colloidal gold curve | Normal (rarely reduced) | Positive reagin test for syphilis; spirochete not demonstrable by usual techniques of smear or by culture |
| Sarcoidosis | Normal to considerably elevated | Zero to less than 100 mononuclear cells | Slight to moderate elevation | Normal | No specific findings |

media capable of growing all the pathogens known to be associated with meningitis. These might include blood agar plates, chocolate agar plates, special *H. influenzae* media, and thioglycolate broth. In addition, various environmental conditions including reduced oxygen tension and increased carbon dioxide tension are utilized routinely. Special media (Saboraud's or mycocell) are available for the recovery of fungi, whereas Petrognani's media can be utilized for recovery of *Mycobacterium tuberculosis*. In addition, *M. tuberculosis* may be isolated following inoculation of guinea pigs. Tissue culture techniques and inoculation of mice and embryonated eggs are used for viral isolation.

The concentration of protein in the cerebrospinal fluid increases whenever there is interference with the blood-cerebrospinal fluid barrier as seen in inflammation. In bacterial, tuberculous, mycotic, and carcinomatous meningitis, as well as in some cases of subarachnoid hemorrhages or when epithelial cells from such tumors as a dermoid appear in the cerebrospinal fluid, the glucose concentration may be reduced (hypoglycorrhachia). Although the mechanism of hypoglychorrhachia is not well understood, the metabolic activity of rapidly growing cells, phagocytosis, proliferation of a variety of microorganisms, and impaired glucose transport into and out of cerebrospinal fluid are all probably involved. In some cases, viral infection, in particular, mumps may be associated with hypoglycorrhachia. The gammaglobulin concentration may be increased compared with other protein constituents in such inflammatory disorders as syphilis, subacute sclerosing panencephalitis, and certain demyelinating disorders.

A variety of fluorescent antibody techniques are available for the specific detection of a number of microorganisms in cerebrospinal fluids and other tissues. Fluorescent antibody procedures are difficult to standardize and should only be performed in laboratories where a special interest in the technique is maintained.

## ANCILLARY CLINICAL AND LABORATORY DATA

*Immunochemistry.* An immediate etiological diagnosis is only possible when the responsible agent can be identified by the use of a specific immunochemical or fluorescent antibody technique. The clinical and cerebrospinal fluid data can help exclude certain disorders early in the diagnostic study. When the signs and symptoms reflect involvement of the meninges, and there is no evidence of cerebral or spinal cord disease, primary meningitis is probable. If, in addition, the cerebrospinal fluid contains about 100 or so lymphocytes per cubic millimeter, a normal quantity of sugar, and a slightly increased protein concentration, then bacterial, tuberculous, or fungal meningitis is less likely, and some form of aseptic or viral meningitis should be suspected. It should again be emphasized, however, that bacterial meningitis is possible despite limited pleocytosis. The cerebrospinal fluid cell count may also be normal on initial examination of patients with tuberculous meningitis. History of exposure to mumps in the presence of parotitis makes the diagnosis of mumps meningitis probable. If this diagnosis is suspected, a specific complement fixation test for the determination of mumps S, or soluble antigen, and V, or viral antigen, should be performed. The S antibody rises early during the course of mumps, remains elevated for several weeks, and then declines. The V antibody titer rises 4 to 6 weeks after exposure and remains elevated for long periods of time. Thus, a high S titer in the face of a negligible V titer indicates acute infection with mumps. Signs of cerebellar ataxia in a patient recovering from varicella should suggest a diagnosis of post-infectious varicella encephalitis. This is presumed to be an immunological reaction rather than a primary viral encephalitis. A similar pathological process can complicate rubeola, rubella, and other viral illnesses, but cerebellar signs are less prominent.

In addition to primary meningeal disease, parameningeal infections can produce cerebrospinal fluid abnormalities similar to those described. The co-existence of a progressive dysphasia, a superior quadrantanopsia, and hemiparesis on the right side associated with a history of a chronic draining left ear indicate a left temporal lobe abscess.

*Microbiology.* A definite diagnosis unfortunately cannot be made from either the initial clinical or cerebrospinal fluid findings in many cases. Nevertheless, every attempt should be made to amplify the immediate and remote history, including epidemiological data, for such historical information may suggest the right diagnosis. A thorough search for foci of infection adjacent to or remote from the meninges must be performed. The extent of dysfunction of the nervous system must be defined by repeated neurological examinations and appropriate laboratory studies. In addition to culturing cerebrospinal fluid, blood cultures should be obtained because bacteria are present in blood in more than one-half the cases of primary bacterial meningitis. Secretions of the upper and lower respiratory tract should be cultured for bacteria and fungi. Viral cultures, particularly for the enteroviruses that cause aseptic meningitis and encephalitis, should be made from the stools and pharyngeal washings of patients. The development of specific neutralizing and complement-fixing antibodies will help confirm the diagnosis. Acute phase sera should be obtained on admission and a convalescent sera two or three weeks later. A four-fold rise in complement-fixing or neutralizing antibody is usually considered to be evidence of a recent infection.

Septicemia or viremia is frequently heralded by the occurrence of petechial or purpuric lesions of the body. A smear of one of the petechial lesions following puncture by a small lancet may reveal microorganisms on Gram stain. This procedure has been especially helpful in cases of meningococcal, streptococcal, and pneumococcal septicemia. When the concentration of bacteria within the bloodstream is very high, a smear and Gram stain of a buffy coat obtained from the blood may be helpful in identifying the microorganism.

*Roentgenology.* Roentgenograms of the skull, sinuses, chest, or spine may be helpful in establishing a diagnosis by disclosing a focus of disease. An electroencephalogram or isotope scan may reveal discrete areas of infection within the brain, even when these foci have been clinically silent. Roentgenographic contrast studies, including myelography, pneumoencephalography, ventriculography, and angiography, are reserved for the more precise localization of a focal lesion that has already been suspected on clinical grounds.

*Biopsy.* Occasionally, one must resort to a tissue biopsy. This procedure has been used to demonstrate granulomatous lesions of sarcoidosis in a lymph node or in the liver and also has been useful in defining such disorders as trichinosis or toxoplasmosis or hypersensitivity diseases following appropriate microscopic examination of muscle tissue. Biopsies of the meninges or brain are made only rarely, but they will, at times, help establish the diagnosis in certain central nervous system infections. The availability of such antiviral compounds as idoxuridine and cytosine arabinoside for the treatment of herpes simplex encephalitis have made it essential to establish the diagnosis as early as possible. In such cases, brain biopsy may be done because the histological picture is specific enough to permit an exact diagnosis. Similarly, brain biopsy may be used for the diagnosis of subacute sclerosing panencephalitis and acute necrotizing hemorrhagic encephalitis. Whenever tissue is obtained for routine histological study, appropriate methods for the recovery of an infectious agent should be employed and, where facilities permit, electron microscopy for visual identification of an infectious agent should be utilized.

## General references

Adair, C. V., R. L. Gauld, and J. E. Smadel. 1953. Aseptic meningitis, a disease of diverse etiology: Clinical and etiologic studies on 854 cases. Ann. Intern. Med. 39:675-704.

Dodge, P. R. and M. N. Swartz. 1965. Medical Progress. Bacterial meningitis—a review of selected aspects. II. Special neurologic problems, postmeningitic complications and clinicopathologic correlations. New Eng. J. Med. 272:954, 1003.

Gotoff, S. P. and R. E. Behrman. 1972. Neonatal septicemia. J. Pediatr. 76: 142-153.

Lepon, M. L., D. H. Carver, H. T. Wright et al. 1962. A clinical epidemiologic and laboratory investigation of aseptic meningitis during the four year period, 1955-1958. II. The clinical disease and its sequelae. New Eng. J. Med. 266:1188-1193.

Swartz, M. N. and P. R. Dodge. 1965. Medical Progress. Bacterial meningitis—a review of selected aspects. I. General clinical features, special problems and unusual meningeal reactions mimicking bacterial meningitis. New Eng. J. Med. 272:725-731.

# 11

# Demyelinating Diseases
# of the Nervous System

LEONARD BERG, ROBERT L. CHESANOW,
AND ARTHUR L. PRENSKY

## INTRODUCTION

The term "demyelinating disease" has been applied to a diverse assortment of acquired illnesses in which there is a loss of myelin from the nervous system, while such other elements of nervous tissue as axons, astrocytes, and blood vessels are relatively well preserved in the diseased areas. The tendency to discuss these disorders as a group should not lead to the inference that they share a common etiology. That their causes are poorly understood will become apparent in the following discussion of a representative member of the group.

### Multiple sclerosis

Multiple sclerosis is the most common demyelinating disease. Its prevalence in the United States and Canada ranges from 40 to 60 per 100,000 population. Because multiple sclerosis tends to attack individuals between 20 and 40 years of age, when people are economically most productive, and because, in most instances, it cripples rather than kills, the disease has a socioeconomic impact disproportionate to its prevalence.

This acquired disease of the central nervous system is characterized by discrete, irregularly shaped demyelinated lesions called plaques. The lesions are scattered throughout the central nervous system and do not appear simultaneously. These features have led to the clinical aphorism that the disease should be diagnosed only when the signs and symptoms indicate that lesions are "separated in time and space."

Plaques may occur without clinical symptoms, but the appearance of well-defined neurological dysfunction can usually be correlated with a lesion in the appropriate area of the central nervous system, as dictated by classic neurological localization. Typical examples of this sometimes exquisite correlation are as follows.

1. Loss of central vision in one eye and edema of the optic disc (papillitis), followed by pallor; demyelination of the optic nerve. If the acute lesion occurs in the optic nerve behind the globe (retrobulbar neuritis), the disc appears normal in the early stages, but the same pallor and demyelination result.

2. Diplopia and nystagmus, mainly of the abducting eye, and weakness of the medial rectus muscle on one side (syndrome of internuclear ophthalmoplegia); plaque in the medial longitudinal fasciculus of the brain stem ipsilateral to the medial rectus.

3. Tingling and/or numbness in one arm and clumsiness and loss of proprioception in the hand; demyelination in the ipsilateral posterior column (fasciculus cuneatus) of the cervical cord.

4. Numbness and/or tingling below the waist, loss of proprioception in the feet, spastic paraparesis, and bilateral Babinski's signs; plaques in the posterior and lateral columns of the thoracic cord.

5. Loss of pain and temperature sensibility below the waist on the right, spastic weakness and hyperreflexia of the left leg, and a left Babinski's sign (partial Brown-Sequard syndrome); plaque in the anterior and lateral regions of the mid-thoracic cord on the left involving the spinothalmic and corticospinal tracts.

6. Attacks of lancinating pain in one side of the face (trigeminal neuralgia); plaque at the root entry zone of the trigeminal nerve in the pons.

Typically a young adult develops periodic attacks of central nervous system dysfunction resulting from lesions in various locations. Common symptoms are blurred vision, diplopia, vertigo, imbalance, numbness or tingling in the limbs, trunk, or face, focal weakness or incoordination, difficulty with urination and/or partial impotence. (It ought to be emphasized, for your peace of mind, that these symptoms in medical and paramedical students indicate anxiety, migraine, or nerve compression much more often than multiple sclerosis!). The onset of the disability is rapid, reaching its peak in hours or days; rarely, the onset is very abrupt, a matter of minutes. Characteristically, the initial symptoms are present only for a few days or weeks, followed some months or years later by different transient symptoms. Multiple symptoms and signs occur later with less complete remission. Common signs include loss of central vision, pallor of the optic disc, nystagmus, impaired extraocular movements, dysarthria, ataxia, weakness of limbs, spasticity, hyperreflexia, clonus, Babinski's sign, and sensory loss.

Remember that one must search for diagnoses other than multiple sclerosis, despite a remittent course, when signs and symptoms, no matter how complex, can be ascribed to a single lesion.

Multiple sclerosis can be a very benign disorder. Typical lesions may be found at autopsy of persons who never had neurological signs or symptoms. Other individuals may have one or more attacks of the disease with remission and never have further symptoms during their lifetime. Demyelinated plaques may be quite profuse at autopsy despite the paucity of residual clinical defects.

Another interesting feature of the disorder is the occurrence of symptoms lasting only a few minutes. This pattern is frequently seen in patients who have had attacks involving the optic nerve. There may be a brief reappearance of a central scotoma when the body temperature is raised, as by a hot bath. Other focal symptoms (extremity weakness or numbness) may also be present during this temperature-related exacerbation. Another type of "mini-attack" involves spontaneous repetitive brain-stem dysfunction (vertigo, nystagmus, and dysarthria). These symptoms resemble transient ischemic attacks in the vertebrobasilar distribution, yet they occur in patients with normal circulation. Such variations from the typical clinical pattern complicate the task of explaining the mechanisms of the disease and refute the oversimplified notion that symptoms appear when a region loses myelin and disappear with regeneration of myelin.

EPIDEMIOLOGY

Population studies have shown that multiple sclerosis is rare in the tropics and that, with some exceptions, its incidence increases with increasing distance from the equator, being highest in the industrialized countries of northern Europe. Among the many factors that can be correlated with this geographic distribution, apart from average temperature and sunshine, are soil composition, degree of industrialization, sanitation, and infant mortality.

Surveys in South Africa and, most recently, in Israel have compared the frequency of multiple sclerosis in natives of and in immigrants to these nations. The most detailed epidemiological studies have been performed in Israel. Multiple sclerosis is common in European immigrants to Israel, but rare among immigrants from Afro-Asian countries. Migrants after puberty coming from a region of high incidence entail the same risk of acquiring the disease that they would have had in their country of origin. Those migrating before they reach puberty have the same incidence as the native-born Israeli population. The suggestion has therefore been made that multiple sclerosis results from exposure to some environmental agent during childhood or adolescence. The fact that Israeli-born offspring of both Afro-Asian and European immigrants have identical age-specific prevalence rates favors the suggestion that environmental factors are important. The Israeli studies also suggest that geoclimatic factors are less important than socioeconomic factors in determining the incidence of the disorder. This conclusion arises from the observation that (1) prevalence rates are as high among native Israelis as among the European immigrants; (2) geoclimatic conditions in Israel are similar to those of neighboring countries with low rates; and (3) socioeconomic conditions in Israel resemble those in European countries with high multiple sclerosis rates.

## PATHOLOGY

The pathology of multiple sclerosis helps explain some of its clinical features, but it also raises further questions regarding its pathogenesis. Small fresh plaques appear to develop around venules and probably enlarge in a centrifugal direction. In the acute stage, perivenular cuffs of inflammatory cells, both lymphocytes and plasma cells, have been seen. (An analogy has been drawn with the perivenular inflammation, called sheathing, that is sometimes seen in the retina of multiple sclerosis patients.) There is evidence that the active changes include three nearly concurrent processes: lysis of oligodendrocytes, breakdown of myelin lamellar structure, and activation of astroglial processes. Acute lesions may also be marked by edema and the presence of immunoglobulins. The detailed sequence of these findings, which might illuminate the mechanism of the demyelination, is still unknown.

Chronic, inactive lesions do not exhibit inflammation or edema. Many lesions are almost certainly associated with some degree of remyelination, but it is not known to what degree such regeneration is possible. The most characteristic feature of the chronic lesion is a proliferation of astrocytic processes that transforms the acute lesion into a hard sclerotic plaque, giving the disorder its name, which results in a glial scar. As lesions increase in age, the lipid products of myelin breakdown are phagocytosed, and, in the oldest lesions, only traces of lipid are noted in scattered macrophages around the blood vessels. The presence or absence of inflammation, the location and number of macrophages filled with breakdown products of lipids, and the degree of gliosis help date the lesion.

Most multiple sclerosis patients who come to postmortem examination exhibit lesions at many levels of the central nervous system, some being acute and others subacute or chronic. Note the correlation with the usual clinical features of the disease, i.e., their dissemination in time and space. The plaques have a predilection for certain regions of the central nervous system—optic nerves, cerebral white matter close to the ventricular surface, tracts of the brain stem and spinal cord—but they also may be widespread in the cerebral cortex and cerebellum.

It is not known whether the onset of clinical dysfunction results from any of the recognized changes in the acute lesion (inflammation, edema, change in glia, immunoglobulin accumulation, and myelin breakdown). The tendency toward remission can probably be explained, in part, by subsidence of the inflammatory response and edema seen in the acute phase of the disorder and possibly by some degree of remyelination of denuded axons. In many instances, however, the return of function is greater and more rapid than one might expect from the limited remyelination. This discrepancy suggests that axons denuded of myelin over short distances may still be able to transmit impulses. Experimental evidence indicates that axons retaining only a thin layer of their myelin sheath can still conduct normally.

The brief reappearance of clinical symptoms under stress of body temperature rise suggests that axons in a demyelinated region have a reduced "safety factor" maintaining their ability to conduct impulses normally. Damaged axons can be shown in the laboratory to be blocked more easily by temperature rise than healthy axons. The lability of function of damaged tracts in multiple sclerosis patients can be demonstrated also by the transient improvement in neurological deficits that results from lowering body temperature or decreasing the serum calcium concentration or blood pH. We, therefore, are considering a pathological process in which symptoms and signs can fluctuate rapidly and reversibly, as a variety of physical, chemical, and possibly immunochemical factors influence axonal function. Note the possibility of future development of symptomatic therapy that could improve transmission in tracts that remain demyelinated.

### PATHOGENESIS

Although the gross and microscopic pathology helps explain some of the clinical features of multiple sclerosis, the pathogenesis of the disease remains obscure. One must account for its geographic distribution, the incidence in migrant populations, the rarity of onset before age 15 and after age 55, the extreme variability in clinical course, the distribution of lesions—perivenular sites with many lesions in cerebral white matter near the ventricles, the predominant destruction of myelin and oligodendroglia.

Theories concerning the possible pathogenesis of multiple sclerosis have been based upon clinical, epidemiological, and pathological data but have also relied upon biochemical examination of patients' tissues and body fluids, animal models of demyelinating disease, and the study of demyelination in tissue culture. The following theories have been put forth: (1) multiple sclerosis may result from an abnormality in the composition of myelin, which predisposes it to destruction; (2) it may be an autoimmune disease of the delayed hypersensitivity type, with the antigen a normal constituent of myelin or its supporting glia or an exogenous factor incorporated into central nervous system tissues; (3) it may result from viral infection with delayed sequelae, mediated either by immunological mechanisms or by persistent viral infection ("slow virus"); or (4) myelin and its supporting glial cells may be susceptible to unknown toxic factors capable of penetrating or breaking down the blood-brain barrier.

Each of these proposals has some experimental support but has met with evidence to the contrary.

1. The suggestion that abnormal myelin is synthesized by persons who develop multiple sclerosis is derived from biochemical observations made upon white matter and myelin obtained at autopsy. Samples were taken from regions that, on careful sectioning, contained no macroscopic evidence of plaques. There have been claims that lecithin and cerebroside isolated from these samples had abnormalities of fatty acid composition. These claims are difficult to accept on a theoretical basis, since other diseases in which demyelination results from the synthesis of abnormal myelin are genetic. Furthermore, mechanisms would have to be invoked to explain why myelin of abnormal chemical composition was attacked in discrete episodes over periods of many years. Since, in addition, the results described above have recently been contradicted (Suzuki et al.), it seems highly unlikely that multiple sclerosis results from the synthesis of abnormal myelin. More likely explanations for the finding of abnormal lipid or protein composition in "normal" white matter and myelin in multiple sclerosis patients are that the investigators have overlooked microscopic plaques or that remyelination is more extensive than hitherto appreciated and results in myelin of different chemical composition.

2. Several lines of investigation suggest that multiple sclerosis may be an immunological disease. First, many disorders thought to have an immunological basis result in multiple discrete clinical exacerbations. Second, the perivenular site of the early lesions suggests that the insult may be mediated via the bloodstream. Third, increased amounts of gammaglobulin are found in the spinal fluid of many patients with multiple sclerosis, and immunoglobulins have been found deposited in and around plaques. Fourth, serum drawn from these patients (especially those with active disease) is capable of causing reversible demyelination of organotypic long-term cultures of rat or mouse cerebellum, spinal cord, or cerebrum. This complement-dependent myelinotoxic activity is rarely found in sera of control patients except for a high incidence in patients with amyotrophic lateral sclerosis, a finding that negates its specificity

for multiple sclerosis. Fifth, it is possible to produce a demyelinating disease, experimental allergic encephalomyelitis, by an immunological insult.

Experimental allergic encephalomyelitis, mediated by sensitized lymphocytes, results from subcutaneous inoculation of laboratory animals with whole brain tissue, white matter, or purified myelin. The inoculum is more potent when coupled with Freund's adjuvant. One component of myelin, basic protein (so named because of its solubility in acid solution), is the only substance thus far isolated from the nervous system capable of inducing this encephalomyelitis in a reproducible, dose-related fashion when injected systemically. Basic protein is therefore called the encephalitogenic protein of brain. It appears that only a small part of the protein molecule is sufficient to produce the disorder. In the guinea pig, a peptide fraction of basic protein containing only nine amino acids can produce the disease. The same peptide, however, is not encephalitogenic when injected into the monkey, a species in which an entirely different sequence of amino acids derived from basic protein is active. Thus, it is theoretically possible that demyelination could result from sensitization to a specific small peptide.

The relevance of basic protein to the problem of multiple sclerosis is suggested by microchemical studies of the margin of acute plaques. These margins show a considerably increased activity of acid proteinase, an enzyme capable of breaking down basic protein. This activity is accompanied by the loss of basic protein at the plaque margin and a decrease of basic protein concentration in a zone surrounding the visible plaque, a zone that appears to be normally myelinated otherwise. A further similarity between experimental allergic encephalomyelitis and multiple sclerosis is the finding in both disorders of the serum complement-dependent myelinotoxic antibodies described above. There is also the striking finding of a reversible complement-dependent serum factor, which blocks polysynaptic transmission of action potentials in central nervous system tissue culture without causing any visible alteration of structure. This "antineuronal antibody" is present in the serum of animals with experimental allergic encephalomyelitis and patients with multiple sclerosis.

Arguments against a purely immunological basis for multiple slerosis include the relatively discrete plaques, the possibility that

an immune response is the result of prior damage to myelin, the
failure to prove hypersensitivity to neural antigens in multiple sclerosis patients as compared with controls, and the failure to produce
a clinically similar disease by injection of brain or any of its constituents. Experimental allergic encephalomyelitis resembles more
the acute encephalomyelitis of man seen after an immunization or
viral infection. The latter, like the former, is typically a monophasic acute illness, as opposed to the chronic relapsing-remitting
syndrome of multiple sclerosis. The relevance of experimental allergic encephalomyelitis to multiple sclerosis is still hotly debated.

3. Recently there has been considerable interest in the possibility that multiple sclerosis results from a viral infection. Evidence in
favor of this idea may be summarized briefly. First, the geographic
variation in the incidence of multiple sclerosis resembles that of the
viral disease paralytic poliomyelitis before a vaccine became available. Second, epidemiological data suggest that the agent responsible for the disease is acquired in childhood, although symptoms
appear later in life. This sequence would be compatible with a persistent viral infection that acted either directly on oligodendroglial
cells or indirectly by periodic release of an encephalitogenic factor
that evoked an autoimmune response. Third, viral demyelinating
diseases have been recognized in animals (visna in sheep, distemper
in dogs, JHM virus in rodents) and man (progressive multifocal
leukoencephalopathy, to be discussed later). Fourth, spinal fluid
immunoglobulins are found in elevated amounts in multiple sclerosis and in subacute sclerosing panencephalitis, a disease in which
chronic viral (measles) infection is strongly incriminated as causal.

Numerous objections have been raised to the viral hypothesis.
Despite repeated attempts, no viral agent has been definitely identified on microscopic study of brain tissue from multiple sclerosis
patients. Inoculation of multiple sclerotic brain tissue into tissue
culture has failed to reveal signs of viral infection in these cultures.
Primates inoculated with brain tissue from patients with active
multiple sclerosis have been followed for more than 5 years and
have yet to develop any sign of disease. Furthermore, animal and
human models of virus-induced demyelination show an inexorable
progression. This pattern is seen in only a small minority of patients who have multiple sclerosis. The restricted age-incidence
curve (sharp peak from age 20 to age 40) is also unlike the known

slow virus models in which the host has no immunity at any age.

These objections are partially met by two recent observations. Using a cell-fusion technique, investigators isolated an infectious agent related to the group-1 parainfluenza virus from cell cultures of brain tissue obtained from two patients with multiple sclerosis. Electron microscopic observations of formalin-fixed brain material obtained from another patient revealed nuclear and cytoplasmic particles resembling paramyxovirus nucleocapsids. Both observations are yet to be confirmed, and, unless the results can be repeated consistently, the chance of coincident infection remains high. It is pertinent to note, in contrast, that clear evidence of persistent viral infection of the brain is being found regularly now in progressive multifocal leukoencephalopathy and subacute sclerosing panencephalitis by the same techniques that regularly give negative results in multiple sclerosis.

The possibility that a low-grade, relatively localized viral infection periodically initiates a more widespread autoimmune response remains interesting, but purely speculative.

4. The hypothesis that multiple sclerosis is a disease that results from the toxic destruction of myelin and/or oligodendroglial cells is one of long standing. Toxic agents might either be periodically ingested or normally present in the bloodstream, entering the brain because of a breakdown in the blood-brain barrier. Facts consistent with this theory are the perivenular sites of the lesions, experimental axon-sparing demyelination induced by various agents (cyanide, cholic acid, and bacterial products), the increased proteolytic activity and early loss of basic protein associated with acute plaques, and an occasional positive brain scan in multiple sclerosis, suggesting penetration of labeled molecules through a faulty blood-brain barrier.

Arguments against the hypothesis are the failure to isolate a toxic agent despite repeated searches, the lack of epidemiological evidence of periodic contacts with toxic agents, and the difficulty of explaining how the action of a toxic agent could account for the highly variable natural history of the disease and the damage to selected areas of the central nervous system.

Strong objections can be raised to each of the theories of multiple sclerosis thus far advanced and to combinations of these theories, but the most attractive theory at present is the suggestion that an

initial viral insult is followed by a secondary (probably immunological) mechanism.

PATHOPHYSIOLOGY

We have already mentioned some aspects of disturbed function
of the nervous system in multiple sclerosis. These points included
an altered conduction in demyelinated tracts, the blocking effect of
multiple sclerosis serum on synaptic transmission *in vitro*, a reduced
"safety factor" for damaged nerve fibers, a lability of function of damaged tracts, and questions of mechanism of onset of symptoms and
their remission. In order to correlate the earlier discussion of pathogenesis with the pathophysiology of multiple sclerosis, we propose a
five-part scheme.

1. Initiating agent. A viral infection of the brain at or before puberty. The virus is capable of directing an immune response against
the oligodendroglial cell/myelin sheath complex after a prolonged
latency. It is desirable, but not essential, that the virus-initiated immune response affect neuronal membrane also.

2. Alteration of blood-brain and/or cerebrospinal fluid-brain
barrier. This change can explain the selective localization of multiple sclerosis lesions, their perivenular distribution, and the periodic exacerbations of the disease. Breakdown of the barrier could
result from the action of virus, toxins, sensitized lymphocytes, or
humoral antibodies.

3. Antibody that disrupts conduction in the central nervous system. An antineuronal antibody blocking conduction and/or synaptic transmission can easily explain the acute onset and rapid fluctu-
ation of symptoms without invoking structural change.

4. Antibody that attacks central nervous system myelin. Such an
antibody can explain the pathological lesions and can also account
for prolonged clinical episodes or progressive deterioration. Limited remyelination is possible if antibody action ceases. Mini-attacks
are explained by the effect of physical or chemical factors on vulnerable (demyelinated or partially demyelinated) nerve fibers.

5. Chronic plaque formation. Glial sclerosis of a demyelinated
zone represents the morphological end-stage of the disease. The degree to which a densely gliotic plaque can interrupt conduction is
not known, but some conduction is theoretically possible if axons
persist.

These five steps do not necessarily occur in this sequence. Variations in the rapidity, extent, or severity of the process at any step could account for the variability in age of onset, pattern of attack, clinical course, and degree of correlation of signs with observed tissue pathology in the individual patient. The scheme describes a sequence of events by which the epidemiological facts are explained more easily than by either a chronic viral infection or an immunological process alone. Whereas non-immunological viral demyelinative activity has been demonstrated in other diseases, the observed facts in multiple sclerosis are poorly explained by direct viral action alone.

This scheme also allows for the early and/or periodic influence of toxic substances in altering blood-brain barriers and for toxic or immunological activation of acid proteinase to hydrolyze basic myelin protein.

The five-step formulation weaves together many of the facts about multiple sclerosis. Holes in the fabric are also evident. We should especially avoid premature closure of the list of possible candidates for etiological agents and pathogenic mechanisms.

## Possible variants of multiple sclerosis

Two acquired diseases that affect myelin, Schilder's disease and Devic's disease, may be variants of multiple sclerosis. Each differs from the usual pattern either in age of onset, clinical course or location, and extent of morphological pathology. These differences are important to the clinician and pathologist, but do not necessarily exclude consideration of the disease as part of the multiple sclerosis spectrum.

Schilder's disease (myelinoclastic diffuse sclerosis) is a disorder mainly of children and young adults. It is characterized by subacute or chronic signs of widespread dysfunction of cerebral white matter. Ataxia, hemiparesis or quadriparesis, aphasia, agnosia, and impairment of sight and hearing (cortical blindness and deafness) may result. The pathology consists of large areas of demyelination that are often symmetrical in both cerebral hemispheres. The brain stem, cerebellum, and spinal cord are often, but not invariably, spared.

One could postulate that the same mechanisms operating in multiple sclerosis are at work here, except that the course is more rapid and severe, and the diffuse pathology overshadows the multifocal type.

Devic's disease (neuromyelitis optica) may be another variant of multiple sclerosis, restricted in time course and localization of lesions. Severe loss of vision occurs because of acute lesions in one or both optic nerves, and this is soon followed by a devastating syndrome of spinal cord dysfunction, often amounting to total interruption of cord function. The tissue destruction tends to be extensive, often proceeding beyond demyelination to necrosis.

Although classical multiple sclerosis commonly affects the spinal cord and optic nerves, the involvement does not coincide so closely in time nor is it so fulminating as in Devic's disease. There is, however, no compelling reason to invoke completely novel mechanisms to explain the illness.

## Other demyelinating diseases

### PROGRESSIVE MULTIFOCAL LEUKOENCEPHALOPATHY

This chronic disorder of the brain mainly occurs in association with systemic diseases of the leukemia and lymphoma type. There is a stepwise development of such clinical signs as confusion, upper motor neuron weakness, ataxia, aphasia, agnosia, and homonymous visual field defects. The dysfunction correlates with large, irregular foci of demyelination in cerebral white matter. These lesions contain bizarre hypertrophied glial nuclei and inclusions that suggest viral particles. Special culture techniques have added weight to the evidence in favor of a viral origin of this disorder in persons who have an altered immunological state.

The pathogenesis of this disease appears to include continuing infection of oligodendroglia by papovavirus, a multifocal demyelinating process in the cerebrum, and an altered immune state, which allows virus infection in the central nervous system to flourish. A secondary immune response to altered glia need not be invoked. Selective central nervous system vulnerability should be postulated, however, to explain the predilection of progressive multifocal leukoencephalopathy for the white matter of the cerebral hemispheres.

## ACUTE DISSEMINATED ENCEPHALOMYELITIS

This disorder occurs in association with various infectious diseases and immunization procedures. It has been recognized most readily with viral exanthems of childhood (measles and chickenpox, particularly) and as a consequence of active immunization against rabies (especially when the antirabies vaccine was derived from central nervous system tissue). One sees an acute illness with headache, confusion, stupor, convulsions, and focal signs indicating widespread lesions in the cerebral hemispehres, brain stem, cerebellum, and spinal cord. Pathological findings include acute inflammation and demyelination in a perivenous distribution throughout the central nervous system.

This disease closely resembles experimental allergic encephalomyelitis in both its clinical and pathological aspects. As described earlier, there is good evidence that this experimental disease is an immunological disorder mediated by sensitized lymphocytes that attack myelin. The association of the human disease with an infectious state may indicate an immunological reaction to the infection, but there is also evidence that the infectious agent may directly attack the nervous system.

## ACUTE IDIOPATHIC POLYNEURITIS

Known also as Guillain-Barré syndrome and postinfectious polyneuritis, this is a special type of acute peripheral nerve syndrome. Symmetrical motor and sensory loss in the extremities, areflexia, and, sometimes, cranial nerve palsies (and especially bilateral facial paralysis) mark the clinical picture. The cerebrospinal fluid protein content is elevated, sometimes to levels of over 1000 mg%, but the cell count of the fluid tends to be normal. Widespread inflammation and demyelination occur throughout the peripheral nervous system.

Just as acute disseminated encephalomyelitis has its animal model, acute idiopathic polyneuritis is well replicated by an experimental allergic neuritis, which can be produced by inoculation of animals with peripheral nerve constituents. In experimental allergic neuritis, there is good evidence that an autoallergic mechanism, mediated by sensitized lymphocytes, leads to the peripheral nerve damage. Active mononuclear cells have been seen "peeling away" the myelin lamellae from axons in the animal's peripheral nerves. There is mounting evidence that similar immunological mechanisms may be operant in the human disease.

A minority of patients with acute idiopathic polyneuritis have had relapses, sometimes when challenged with the inciting antigen. Peripheral nerve myelin is chemically different from central nervous system myelin and does not enjoy the degree of immunological privilege that the latter does. Yet a relapsing and remitting course followed by chronic progression is the exception in idiopathic polyneuritis. There appears to be no satisfactory peripheral nerve analogue to the central nervous system disease called multiple sclerosis.

## General references

Alter, M. 1971. When is multiple sclerosis acquired? Neurology 21:1030-1036.

Behan, P. O. et al. 1972. Cell-mediated hypersensitivity to neural antigens: Occurrence in human patients and nonhuman primates with neurological diseases. Arch. Neurol. 27:145-152.

Behan, P. O. et al. 1973. Immunologic mechanisms in experimental encephalomyelitis in nonhuman primates. Arch. Neurol. 29:4-9.

Brody, J. A. 1972. Epidemiology of multiple sclerosis and a possible virus etiology. Lancet II:173-176.

Davis, F. A. et al. 1970. Effect of intravenous sodium bicarbonate, disodium edetate, and hyperventilation on visual and oculomotor signs in multiple sclerosis. J. Neurol. Neurosurg. Psychiat. 33:723-732.

Einstein, E. R. et al. 1972. Proteolytic activity and basic protein loss in and around multiple sclerosis plaques: Combined biochemical and histochemical observations. J. Neurochem. 19:653-662.

Field, E. J., T. M. Bell, and P. R. Carnegie, eds. 1972. Multiple sclerosis: Progress in research. North-Holland Publishing Co. Amsterdam.

Leibowitz, U. 1971. Multiple sclerosis: Progress in epidemiologic and experimental research. J. Neurol. Sci. 12:307-318.

Leibowitz, U. et al. 1973. The changing frequency of multiple sclerosis in Israel. Arch. Neurol. 29:107-110.

Lumsden, C. E. 1971. The immunogenesis of the MS plaque. Brain Res. 28:365-390.

McAlpine, D., C. E. Lumsden, and E. D. Acheson, eds. 1972. Multiple sclerosis, a reappraisal. Williams & Wilkins, Baltimore.

Prineas, J. W. 1972. Acute idiopathic polyneuritis, an EM study. Lab. Invest. 26:133-147.

Rasminsky, M. 1973. The effects of temperature on conduction in demyelinated single nerve fibers. Arch. Neurol. 28:287-292.

Rowland, L. P., ed. 1971. Immunological disorders of the nervous system. Res. Publ. Ass. Nerv. Ment. Dis., vol. XLIX.

Rucker, C. W. 1972. Sheathing of the retinal veins in multiple sclerosis. Mayo Clin. Proc. 47:335-340.

Shapira, R. et al. 1971. Encephalitogenic fragment of myelin basic protein: Amino acid sequence of bovine, rabbit, guinea pig, monkey and human fragments. J. Biol. Chem. 246:4630-4640.

Suzuki, K. 1973. Myelin in multiple sclerosis. Arch. Neurol. 28:293-297.

Vinken, P. J. and G. W. Bruyn, eds. 1971. Handbook of clinical neurology, vol. 9. Multiple sclerosis and other demyelinating diseases. North-Holland Publishing Co. Amsterdam.

Weiner, L. P. et al. 1973. Viral infections and demyelinating diseases. N. Eng. J. Med. 288:1103-1110.

Wolfgram, F., G. W. Ellison, J. G. Stevens, and J. M. Andrews, eds. 1972. Multiple sclerosis: Immunology, virology and ultrastructure. New York, Academic Press.

Symposium. 1970. Multiple sclerosis. Modern Treatment 7:879 ff.

# 12

# Disorders in the Circulation of Spinal Fluid

## PATHOPHYSIOLOGY OF THE CEREBROSPINAL FLUID

LAWRENCE A. COBEN

The cerebrospinal fluid mechanically preserves the shape of the jelly-like brain and protects the brain from impacts; although it does not nourish the brain, it does function significantly in brain homeostasis. For diagnostic purposes, the measurement of certain cerebrospinal fluid constituents can be useful.

## Circulation

The cerebrospinal fluid circulation is impelled by its active formation. It moves from the cerebral ventricles to the subarachnoid space. Having entered the subarachnoid space via the three exit foramina of the fourth ventricle (the two lateral foramina of Luschka and the midline foramen of Magendie), cerebrospinal fluid flow bifurcates. One path enters the spinal subarachnoid space where mystery enshrouds its sluggish circulation. The other path ascends in the subarachnoid space of the brain stem and cerebral hemispheres to be re-absorbed at the arachnoid villi of the superior sagittal sinus. When arterial or venous pressure changes (e.g., as with cardiac systole, coughing, breathing, etc.), the cerebrospinal fluid surges into the cervical subarachnoid space (the spinal dura is elastic), then back into the subarachnoid space of the head. This helps the cerebrospinal fluid mix and also move.

## HOW SOLUTES CROSS CELL MEMBRANES

The movement of large molecules between blood, brain, and cerebrospinal fluid is controlled at five layers, each one cell thick, where an ultrastructural tight junction seals each contiguous pair of cells together. Thus, large molecules (horseradish peroxidase, mol. wt. 43,000; microperoxidase, mol. wt. 2000) cannot cross the cell layer in either direction.

The brain extracellular fluid and the cerebrospinal fluid are isolated from the extracellular fluid of the dura and of the rest of the body by two of the five tight-junction layers: the outer layer of arachnoid and the endothelium of the arachnoid villus (Fig. 12-1). The other three tight-junction layers severely limit the interchange of large molecules between blood and brain extracellular fluid (endothelium of brain capillary); between blood and cerebrospinal fluid in the ventricle (epithelium of choroid plexus); and between blood and cerebrospinal fluid in the subarachnoid space (endothelium of subarachnoid artery) (Fig. 12-1).

Large and small molecules diffuse easily through the open intercellular junctions of the pia-glia layer (Fig. 12-1) ($C_2$) and the ventricular ependyma (Fig. 12-1) ($C_1$).

Only in a few specialized brain regions (choroid plexuses, area postrema, etc.) do the capillary endothelial cells show greatly thinned segments, the fenestrae (Fig. 12-2, inset G) that allow both sizes of peroxidase to escape. These regions are thus potential sites for a "functional leak" of large molecules into the cerebrospinal fluid from blood via the extracellular fluid of the plexus and brain (Fig. 12-1) (E).

The control of small molecule and ion movement involves several factors. Lipid-soluble solutes quickly diffuse across cell membranes, and water itself diffuses very easily.

Water-soluble solutes cross cell membranes by non-ionic diffusion, which increases if the solute is lipid soluble and binds poorly to plasma proteins. The ionized form of an ionizable solute is almost unable to diffuse across. Ion-trapping causes an excess of weak organic acids in the more basic of two adjacent compartments

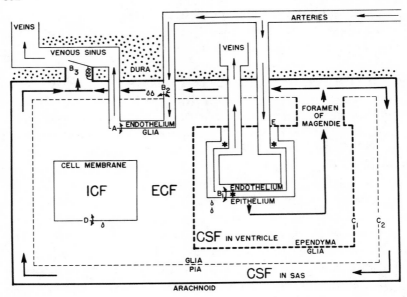

**Fig. 12-1** Diagram of the brain and its fluids. Neurons and glia, whose cell membranes (D) enclose the intracellular fluid (ICF), are bathed in brain extracellular fluid (ECF). The extracellular fluid composition is finely regulated by the extracellular fluid stat, which consists of blood-brain (A), blood-cerebrospinal fluid ($B_1$, $B_2$, $B_3$), and brain-cerebrospinal fluid ($C_1$, $C_2$) barriers; composition is thus kept optimal for neuron and glia function despite perturbations due to nutrient uptake, catabolite discharge, etc. and to relatively wide swings in blood composition. A, brain capillary-glia complex; $B_1$ choroid plexus; $B_2$ subarachnoid (cranial and spinal) artery; $B_3$ arachnoid villus endothelium; $C_1$, ventricular ependyma; $C_2$, pia-glia; D, cell membrane of neurons and glia; E, the potential (functional) leak at the attachment of choroid plexus to the ventricular wall.

Cerebrospinal fluid (CSF) is formed from blood at the choroid plexus ($B_1$); the thick arrows show its circulation and the thin arrows blood circulation. The subarachnoid source of cerebrospinal fluid is indicated by drops at $B_2$ (actual site not known). Minor formation of cerebrospinal fluid in brain from glucose oxidation shown by single drop at D. The sink action of cerebrospinal fluid on brain extracellular fluid (ECF) occurs via intimate diffusion contact across ependyma, allowing extracellular solutes to enter the cerebrospinal fluid flow to be removed by bulk reabsorption of cerebrospinal fluid through the arachnoid villi. Solutes in brain extracellular fluid can easily diffuse into ventricular or subarachnoid space cerebrospinal fluid and vice versa depending upon whether the sink is in the cerebrospinal fluid or in the brain. In hydrocephalus, bulk cerebrospinal fluid moves "backwards" from the ventricle into brain extracellular fluid and then, presumably, to the subarachnoid space (SAS) for absorption via the arachnoid villi. Restricted diffusion, solid line boundaries; relatively free diffusion, dashed line boundaries; one-way open flow (one-way valve effect) through arachnoid villus, spring-loaded door at $B_3$; curved double-headed arrows at A, $B_1$, $B_2$, D, sites of carrier-mediated transport of solutes (cranial and (blood) and of weak organic bases in the more acid one (cerebrospinal fluid). An example is the run-out of phenobarbital, a weak acid, from brain cells into plasma, when the pH difference between plasma and brain is increased by plasma alkalinization.

Carrier-mediation is a means of increasing the rate at which a water-soluble solute traverses a membrane. It results in either uphill (active) transport (solute movement from a compartment having a lower concentration to one having a higher concentration or against an electrochemical gradient) or facilitated diffusion, which ordinarily can only go downhill. Thus, although they are capable of fairly rapid unmediated diffusion through tight junctions, several important classes of small solute (e.g., glucose and amino acids) use the faster carrier-mediation to circumvent the junction (Fig. 12-2, inset G, dashed arrow). Carrier mechanisms are known to reside at the sites labeled A, B1, B2, and D in Fig. 12-1. Carrier-mediated transport can be saturated by increasing the concentration of the solute, and can thus behave as a barrier.

## Formation

Cerebrospinal fluid formation occurs at the choroid plexuses of the ventricles and at as yet unknown sites in the cranial and spinal subarachnoid space. At least 90% comes from blood and less than 10% from oxidation of glucose by the brain.

The normal adult human range of total craniospinal cerebrospinal fluid volume is about $120 \pm 30$ ml. Less than 25% is in the ventricles. The mean rate of net formation of cerebrospinal fluid is 0.35-0.40 ml/minute (about 0.3%/minute) or 530 ml/24 hours.

The functional unit of a choroid plexus consists of an unusually wide capillary separated from its ensheathing single layer of epithelial cells by a collagen-containing extracellular space (Fig. 12-2, inset G).

Water and salts might filter rapidly through the fenestrae of

---

spinal subarachnoid space sites are not known but indicated at B2). Asterisks are in the extracellular space of the choroid plexus.

The ventricular system is shown as a single cavity; the choroid plexuses as a single plexus; and the arachnoid villi as a single villus; etc. Of the three exit foramina of the fourth ventricle, only the foramen of Magendie is shown.

Compare Fig. 12-2, which has a similar view.

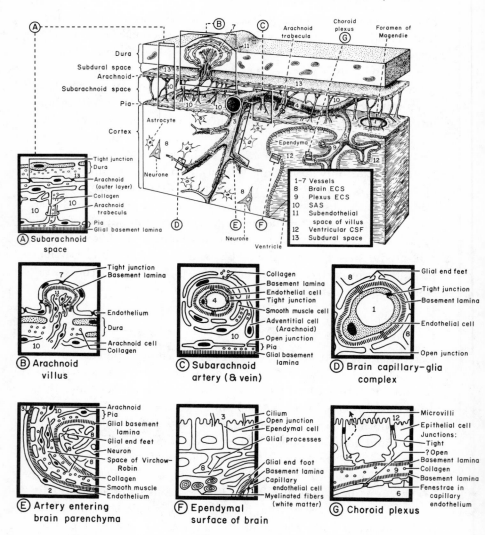

**Fig. 12-2** Schema of the brain and its fluids. Compare with Fig. 12-1. The arachnoid sheath of subarachnoid (4) and intracerebral arteries (3,2) is omitted from the main figure but shown in insets C and E. The entire ventricular system is shown as a single cavity (12) and only the foramen of Magendie is shown. Not labeled in the main figure are the long extracellular channel and basal infoldings of the choroid plexus epithelium (inset G, 14) and the perivascular space of Virchow-Robin (inset E). The plexus epithelium is modified (secretory) ependyma. Cells of pial origin in the extracellular space of the choroid plexus are not shown. The plexus extracellular space (9) does not actually open into the

choroid plexus capillaries into the extracellular space. An isosmolar new cerebrospinal fluid could arise by local osmosis if a cation, $Na^+$ for example, were actively transported from the extracellular space of the chroid plexus across the epithelium by carriers located at the long intercellular channels between adjacent epithelial cells (Fig. 12-3, inset G, dashed arrow). Water (plus $Cl^-$ and $HCO^-_3$?) would be dragged along to establish isosmolality (and electroneutrality?) with the plasma.

## Absorption

Cerebrospinal fluid absorption normally occurs mainly at the arachnoid villi of the superior sagittal sinus as judged from the pattern of flow as seen by cisternography, a procedure in which an external scanner detects the gamma radiation from a tagged substance (e.g., radioiodinated serum albumin) after its injection into the spinal subarachnoid cerebrospinal fluid. Other villi lie on the floor of the cranium and alongside some spinal nerve roots.

Absorption is due to the difference in pressure between the cerebrospinal fluid and the superior sagittal sinus. The mean "opening pressure" (sinus pressure) for absorption in humans is 68 mm (of cerebrospinal fluid); above this, absorption increases linearly with pressure. Villi collapse to prevent reflux of blood into the subarachnoid space whenever the sagittal sinus venous pressure exceeds the subarachnoid pressure, giving a one-way valve effect. Continuous absorption of cerebrospinal fluid occurs in bulk; water and all solutes enter the venous blood together.

Cerebrospinal fluid can be absorbed at least three to four times

---

subarachnoid space (10). Blood supplies to the plexus and brain parenchyma arise in parallel from the subarachnoid space arterial system. Veins are not shown except for dural venous sinus. CSF, cerebrospinal fluid; ECS, extracellular space of brain; SAS, subarachnoid space.

The basement membranes (parallel lines) (insets) are shown pulled away from adjacent cells for clarity, except for the longer lines that indicate the true relationship. The subdural space is potential.

Redrawn and modified from Tschirgi, R. D. Chemical environment of the central nervous system. In: Field, J., Magoun, H. W., and Hall, V. E. (Eds.), Handbook of Physiology, Section 1: Neurophysiology. Vol. 3. Baltimore: Williams & Wilkins, 1960.

as fast as the maximal rate of new formation. Thus, hydrocephalus occurs much more often from blocked absorption than from hypersecretion of cerebrospinal fluid.

## The extracellular fluid of the brain

### THE BRAIN ECF STAT

The brain (and spinal cord) is a collection of neurons and glia, which requires a rigidly controlled environment, the brain extracellular fluid, to prevent irrelevant signals ("noise"). When bathed in a high $K^+$ fluid, for example, a neuron spuriously fires axonal action potentials (noise). The extracellular fluid also provides the brain cells with nutrients and receives from them such potentially toxic solutes as lactate. The regulation of extracellular fluid composition thus becomes a necessity.

Three interfaces, the blood-brain barrier, the blood-cerebrospinal fluid barrier, and the brain-cerebrospinal fluid barrier, cooperate to regulate the extracellular fluid composition. We therefore group these barriers under the term "brain extracellular fluid stat" (Fig. 12-1), designating the homeostatic mechanisms for the fine adjustment of the neuronal environment. (The coarse homeostasis of blood solutes allows wider fluctuations than brain cells can tolerate.)

In the rhesus monkey (Table 12-1), the cerebrospinal fluid leaves the fourth ventricle and enters the subarachnoid space of the cisterna magna, where the $Mg^{++}$ concentration is higher than that of blood. As the cerebrospinal fluid circulates upward around the brain stem and over the cerebral cortex in the subarachnoid space, it should keep losing $Mg^{++}$ to the blood of the brain capillaries (since relatively free diffusion can occur from the subarachnoid space across the pia-glia into the brain extracellular space and thence to the brain capillary). But the cerebrospinal fluid does not lose $Mg^{++}$ as it circulates; it gains $Mg^{++}$, as shown by the fact that fluid taken from the subarachnoid space of the cerebral convexity has a higher $Mg^{++}$ concentration than does cisternal fluid. Thus, there must be a barrier at the brain capillary where an active carrier mechanism continually moves $Mg^{++}$ from blood into brain extracellular fluid. From there, the extra $Mg^{++}$ is free to diffuse into the cerebrospinal fluid in the subarachnoid space of the cerebral convexity.

For $K^+$, the same explanation holds, except that $K^+$ moves by carrier in the opposite direction, leaving the brain extracellular fluid to enter the blood of the brain capillary, thus further lowering the concentration of $K^+$ in the subarachnoid cerebrospinal fluid of the cerebral convexity.

Actually, these data do not precisely fix the site of regulation. The site could be at the capillary-glia complex, at the subarachnoid artery or vein, or even at the first intracerebral portion of the artery or vein.

## THE BLOOD-BRAIN BARRIER

The blood-brain barrier site is the capillary system within the brain plus its sheath of astroglial feet—the brain capillary-glia complex. A coupling of severely restricted diffusion, enzymatic traps (see below), and solute-specific carrier transport comprises the blood-brain barrier. Regional variations (Table 12-1) show that extracellular fluid cations are regulated by carriers. Brain extracellular fluid $K^+$, $Ca^{++}$, and $Mg^{++}$, controlled by the brain extracellular fluid stat, change minimally despite severe plasma shifts to concentrations compatible with life but not with normal neuronal function. Four carrier systems moving solute into brain from blood are those for glucose, essential neutral amino acids, essential basic amino acids, and pyruvate (as well as lactate). They could enhance

TABLE 12-1  *Regional Variation of Cerebrospinal Fluid Cations in the Adult Monkey*[a]

|  | $Mg^{++}$ (Meq/kg $H_2O$) | $K^+$ (Meq/kg $H_2O$) |
|---|---|---|
| Lateral ventricle | 1.99[b] | 2.57 |
| Cistern | 1.86 | 2.55 |
| Cerebral convexity | 2.00[b] | 1.99[b] |
| Lumbar region | 1.78[b] | 2.56 |
| Plasma | 1.18[b] | 4.41[b] |

[a] From L. Z. Bito and R. E. Myers. The ontogenesis of haematoencephalic cation transport processes in the rhesus monkey. J. Physiol. 208:153-170, 1970.
[b] Significantly different from cisternal cerebrospinal fluid concentration.

or limit entry into brain or provide egress, but the details are not yet known. The glucose carrier is not the rate-limiting step in cerebral glucose use.

It is not known whether $HCO_3^-$ is the ion actively transported across the brain capillary-glia complex (and across the blood-cerebrospinal fluid barrier) to regulate brain pH, but clearly $HCO_3^-$ and $H^+$ cross more slowly than does $CO_2$. Thus, in metabolic acidosis, the use of $HCO_3^-$, even when necessary to prevent cardiovascular collapse, may cause transient paradoxical cerebrospinal fluid acidosis and obtundation, despite rising serum $HCO_3^-$ levels, because $CO_2$ enters the cerebrospinal fluid faster than does $HCO_3^-$. Also, in respiratory acidosis with serum pH 7.30, the patient may be comatose due to a lumbar cerebrospinal fluid pH of 7.20.

Putative neuro-transmitters (biogenic amines and amino acids) enter the brain from blood minimally or not at all. It is not known whether a carrier is responsible for the limited transport. The precursors of some of these neuro-transmitters (dopa, 5-hydroxytryptophan), however, enter in significant amounts.

Dopa can cross the endothelium into the brain via the neutral amino acid carrier, but dopa is also trapped by an endothelial decarboxylase and changed into dopamine, which cannot cross. The trap, which can be overcome by high blood levels of L-dopa, varies in strength, being relatively weak in striatum and substantia nigra, for example, and thus allowing the dopaminergic neurons there to be supplied with the appropriate precursor for their preferred transmitter. A similar enzymatic trap at the brain capillary system has been suggested for 5-hydroxytryptophan, the precursor of serotonin, and a third is known for $\gamma$-aminobutyric acid (GABA).

### THE BRAIN-CEREBROSPINAL FLUID BARRIER

With only minor restrictions, the cerebrospinal fluid is in intimate diffusionary contact with the brain extracellular fluid across the ventricular ependyma and pia-glia (brain-cerebrospinal fluid barrier) (Fig. 12-1) ($C_1$, $C_2$), so that the composition of the two fluids is quite similar.

### THE BLOOD-CEREBROSPINAL FLUID BARRIER

The interface separating cerebrospinal fluid from blood occurs in three separate regions, namely, the arachnoid villi, the subarachnoid blood vessels, and the choroid plexuses (Fig. 12-1). These comprise the blood-cerebrospinal fluid barrier. The best studied of these, the choroid plexus, has low passive permeability to water-soluble solutes; the major barrier is the epithelial layer, but this layer also has carriers for seven classes of solute: inorganic and organic cations and anions, hexoses, amino acids, and purines. Often the plexus and capillary-glia carriers have an identical action; for example, iodide is removed from cerebrospinal and brain extracellular fluid, thus keeping the iodide concentration low in both fluids. Since many of these carriers move solutes from cerebrospinal fluid to blood, they contribute to the sink function of the cerebrospinal fluid. Protein exemplifies solutes for which the extracellular fluid stat assures a lower concentration (sink) in the cerebrospinal than in the extracellular fluid, by secreting a solute-poor cerebrospinal fluid and continually reabsorbing it into the blood. The cerebrospinal fluid is thus the brain's lymph, providing bulk drainage for solutes that enter the extracellular fluid but cannot exit by reversing their entry path. Such solutes diffuse downhill into the cerebrospinal fluid sink, whence reabsorption occurs. For a second group of solutes, the brain extracellular fluid stat achieves sink action by adding carrier exodus at the choroid plexus to the passive lymph function. Additional carriers, located downstream, remove such solutes from the cranial and the spinal subarachnoid spaces.

## Solutes of the cerebrospinal fluid

The normal concentration of solutes in a cerebrospinal fluid sample is only partly fixed by the concentrations in the newly formed fluid. As the cerebrospinal fluid circulates, solutes are added or subtracted by diffusional interchange (see Table 12-1) with brain (Fig. 12-1) and by carrier transport across the choroid plexus and in the subarachnoid spaces (Fig. 12-1).

Compared to plasma, normal human lumbar cerebrospinal fluid contains (1) a higher concentration of $Mg^{++}$, $H^+$, $Cl^-$, myoinositol lactate, $CO_2$, tension, ethanolamine, and some proteins; (2) an equal concentration of $Na^+$, osmolality, and glutamine; and (3) a lower concontains (1) a higher concentration of $Mg^{++}$, $H^+$, $Cl^-$, myoinositol, lactate, $CO_2$ (tension) ethanolamine, and some proteins; (2) an equal and lipids) also, the pH is lower, about 7.31.

Only a few of these solutes ordinarily are important in patient care; these are total protein, gammaglobulin, and glucose; in special circumstances, pH is important.

### CEREBROSPINAL FLUID PROTEIN IN HEALTH AND DISEASE

The total protein concentration in normal adult lumbar cerebrospinal fluid is 15-45 mg%, giving a cerebrospinal fluid/blood ratio of 1/200. Values over 55 mg% are definitely abnormal in adults. Values up to 150 mg% are seen in neonates but soon drop to 10-30 mg%, then slowly rise to adult values. Almost all the cerebrospinal fluid proteins are serum proteins, which normally leak into the cerebrospinal fluid, the largest molecular weight normally being about 200,000.

An increased total protein content is accompanied by an increased white blood cell count in infections and other inflammatory diseases either adjacent to (aseptic meningeal reaction) or within the subarachnoid space or ventricle.

When the protein content is increased, but the cell count is normal or nearly normal, there are five categories of pathogenesis: (1) direct alteration of the blood-brain barrier (e.g., intracranial neoplasm) or of the blood-cerebrospinal fluid barrier (fungal meningitis); (2) toxic or metabolic states in which the mechanism is not defined (uremia); (3) diffusion from serum when serum gammaglobulin is increased (sarcoid); (4) blocked cerebrospinal fluid absorption (intraspinal tumor obstructing the subarachnoid space); (5) increased gammaglobulin synthesis in the central nervous system (a few cases of multiple sclerosis, but here the total cerebrospinal fluid protein is borderline or only slightly elevated).

A decrease in cerebrospinal fluid total protein concentration below about 15 mg% is less common than an increase. In benign intracranial hypertension, such a decrease possibly results from an increased bulk flow removal of protein by the normal absorption pathway due to the increased intracranial pressure.

A normal cerebrospinal fluid total protein, but an increased gammaglobulin with normal serum proteins, occurs commonly only in a few diseases, including multiple sclerosis. The nervous system may manufacture an abnormal gammaglobulin in these few diseases.

## CEREBROSPINAL FLUID GLUCOSE IN HEALTH AND DISEASE

The normal cerebrospinal fluid-blood glucose ratio is about 0.6 to 0.7, and cerebrospinal fluid concentrations below 40 mg% are definitely abnormal.

When blood sugar rises (or falls) acutely, the rise (or fall) in cerebrospinal fluid glucose lags unpredictably. Thus, simultaneous cerebrospinal fluid and blood sugar samples should be taken in the fasting state.

High cerebrospinal fluid glucose values are non-diagnostic, showing only that blood sugar had been elevated within the prior few hours.

Low cerebrospinal fluid glucose values are important in diagnosis and occur commonly in (1) acute purulent bacterial meningitis; (2) meningitis due to tuberculosis or to such fungi as *Cryptococcus* and *Coccidioides;* (3) meningitis due to sarcoid, metastatic carcinoma, or related diseases that infiltrate the meninges in cellular sheets; and (4) hypoglycemia.

Low cerebrospinal fluid glucose occurs occasionally in a number of other disorders, e.g., acute mumps meningoencephalitis.

In the pathogenesis of low cerebrospinal fluid glucose, the major factors are (1) an increased use of glucose in anaerobic glycolysis by nearby nervous tissue and polymorphonuclear leukocytes, especially during phagocytosis (cerebrospinal fluid lactate is usually increased in purulent meningitis) and (2) the inhibition of carrier-mediated entry of glucose into the cerebrospinal fluid from blood.

These factors probably interact in different degrees in different illnesses that cause low cerebrospinal fluid sugar. Carrier inhibition may be important when the polymorphonuclear cell count and lactate concentration are only mildly raised, as in carcinomatous meningitis.

## General references

Davson, H. 1972. Dynamic aspects of cerebrospinal fluid. Develop. Med. Child. Neurol. (Suppl.) 27:1-16.

Fishman, R. A. 1971. Cerebrospinal fluid. Chapter 5 *in* A. B. Baker, ed. Clinical neurology. Vol. 1. Hoeber Harper & Row, New York.

Katzman, R. and H. M. Pappius. 1973. Brain electrolytes and fluid metabolism. Williams & Wilkins, Baltimore. Especially Chapters 2, 3, 4.

Oldendorf, W. H. 1972. Cerebrospinal fluid formation and circulation. Progr. Nucl. Med. Vol. 1, pp. 336-358. Karger, Basel and University Park Press, Baltimore.

Prockop, L. D. 1973. Disorders of cerebrospinal fluid and brain extracellular fluid. Pages 229-263 *in* G. E. Gaull, ed. Biology of brain dysfunction. Vol. 1. Plenum Press, New York.

## PATHOPHYSIOLOGY OF HYDROCEPHALUS

MARVIN A. FISHMAN

### Pathology and pathophysiology

In hydrocephalus there is an excessive amount of cerebrospinal fluid within the ventricular system of the brain. The excess is caused by an imbalance between the amount of fluid formed within the system and the amount absorbed. As described in the preceding section, the absorptive capacity normally exceeds the productive capacity by at least threefold. Thus, most cases of hydrocephalus are the result of a decrease in absorption, usually because of an obstruction in the circulation of cerebrospinal fluid from one of its major sites of formation, the choroid plexii of the ventricular system, to its major site of absorption, the arachnoidal villi of the superior sagittal sinus, or because of a functional disturbance in absorption at the villi.

If there is obstruction within the ventricular system, the ventricles proximal to the block become dilated. With stenosis of the aqueduct of Sylvius, for instance, the lateral and third ventricles become dilated, whereas obstruction of the exit foramina of the fourth ventricle results in an enlargement of the fourth ventricle and the aqueduct. When there is an obstruction within the ventricular system, the ventricular fluid does not communicate with the subarachnoid fluid, and the condition is thus termed noncommunicating or obstructive hydrocephalus. When the obstruction lies outside the ventricular system, all the ventricles are enlarged, but free communication exists between the ventricular and subarachnoid fluid. This is termed communicating hydrocephalus.

The pathology of hydrocephalus consists of changes produced by the primary disease process and secondary changes in the ventricular system and brain parenchyma. The ventricle may reach enormous size if the dilation progresses slowly and the cranial sutures have not fused, as in neonates and young infants. In older patients, enlargement of the ventricles is usually less dramatic because the cranium has a fixed capacity. With dilation of the ventricular system, there is stretching of the ventricular surface and disruption of the lining ependyma. This may allow for the transventricular absorption of greater than normal amounts of cerebrospinal fluid. The underlying white matter undergoes atrophy and, in severe cases, may be reduced to a thin ribbon. There is selective preservation of the gray matter, and, when the ventricles have obtained enormous size, the width of the cortical gray matter appears relatively normal.

There are several reasons for the dilation of the ventricular system in hydrocephalus; the most important is the accumulation of fluid under increased pressure within the ventricles. The ventricular pulse wave, which presumably is due to a transmission of the arterial pulse by the choroid plexus, has also been thought to be responsible, in part, for dilation of the ventricular system by transiently increasing the intraventricular pressure. Recent investigations, however, have disclosed only modest reduction in the pulse wave following plexectomy (which may arrest ventricular enlargement), and there is no consistent relationship between pulse pressure and chronic elevations in intraventricular pressure. It has been thought that the circulation of cerebrospinal fluid from the ventricular system to the basal cisterns results, in part, from the transmission of the arterial pulse wave through the ventricular system, because the pulse is highest in the ventricles and dampened distally, which would tend to create a gradient forcing fluid out of the ventricles. In communicating hydrocephalus, however, despite the ventricular pulse wave, the flow of fluid is reversed and proceeds into the ventricular system, as evidenced by studies with isotopic tracers injected into the lumbar cerebrospinal fluid (isotope cisternography). Therefore, the pulse pressure and transmission of the arterial pulse by the choroid plexus do not appear to be major factors in the development of ventricular dilation.

It is obvious that none of the defects of cerebrospinal fluid absorption and circulation in hydrocephalus are complete. Formation of fluid exceeds the entire capacity of the ventricular system every 6 to 8 hours, and a total lack of absorption would be incompatible with survival. Absorption by other than usual means must exist, and the transependymal route is the most likely outlet. Ventricular dilation results in the disruption of the normal ependymal lining of the walls of the cavities, and this permits increased absorption. This route of cerebrospinal fluid movement has been demonstrated by the migration of dyes from the ventricular system into the sub-ependymal white matter and by the detection of radioisotopes in the brain parenchyma adjacent to the ventricles after their intra-ventricular instillation; it has been corroborated by the observation of histological changes. If this collateral route plus some residual absorptive capacity through normal channels is adequate to prevent progressive ventricular dilation, a state of compensation may exist; this occurs most often in communicating hydrocephalus. In arrested hydrocephalus, the cessation of progressive ventricular dilation and abnormal cranial enlargement is followed by the resumption of nor-mal growth when the head size returns to within the normal range. The mechanism by which the process stabilizes is unknown, and its relation to the role of increased transventricular cerebrospinal fluid absorption is speculative.

Normal pressure hydrocephalus is a chronic condition in which neurological function is impaired. The pathophysiology of this con-dition remains to be elucidated, but several theories have been pro-posed. With slowly progressive ventricular dilation, the pressure within the cavities may be reduced as the system enlarges. This is thought to result from the increase in the surface area of·the ven-tricles, thereby dissipating the increased pressure according to the following physical principle: $P = F/A$, where $P =$ pressure, $F =$ force, and $A =$ area. Other explanations have been based on the structural properties of the ventricular walls themselves, and recent studies of patients with this syndrome have demonstrated intermit-tently increased cerebrospinal fluid pressure during sleep, which might be sufficient to account for the ventricular dilation.

## Etiology

The patient's age at onset of hydrocephalus is variable, ranging from the intrauterine period to adulthood. The etiology is also rather variable and includes congenital maldevelopment of the ven-tricular system, outlet foramina of the fourth ventricle, meninges, or skull. Masses, intra- or extracerebral, congenital or acquired, may obstruct the ventricular system and result in hydrocephalus. Inflammatory lesions, infectious or noninfectious, obstruct the aqueduct and basal cisterns or lead to fibrosis of the meninges, thereby interfering with the flow and absorption of cerebrospinal fluid. Infrequently, hydrocephalus may be caused by such genetic factors as a sex-linked disorder or chromosomal malformation.

## Signs and symptoms

The signs and symptoms of hydrocephalus depend upon the age of the patient and the rapidity with which the ventricular dilation occurs. In infants, accelerated growth of the cranium and abnormally large heads are found. Examination of the skull may reveal craniofacial disproportion and abnormal configuration of the cranium with frontal bossing. The veins over the scalp may be distended due to increased intracranial venous pressure, and percussion of the head may reveal a cracked-pot sound because of the increased volume of fluid under increased pressure within the cranium. Transillumination is often abnormal, especially in cases of congenital aqueductal stenosis when the occipital and frontal horns may be massively dilated and the cortical mantle severely reduced in thickness. In addition, since the skull bones are relatively thin, the beam of light is diffused through a fluid-filled cavity. Palpation of the head may reveal separation of the cranial sutures and tenseness of the anterior fontanel. Papilledema is unusual in infants because of the ability of the cranium to expand, but optic atrophy occurs in chronic hydrocephalus, often because of direct pressure of the dilated third ventricle on the optic chiasm or as a nonspecific response to high intracranial pressure. Examination of the eyes may disclose palsies of the abducent (cranial nerve VI) and less frequently the oculomotor (cranial nerve III) nerves due to compression of the nerves in their course through the skull by the expanding brain. The abducent nerve is most susceptible to stretch, since it is fixed in position as it passes through the tentorial notch. The eyes may be deviated downward (the setting sun sign) because of thinning and inferior displacement of the roof of the orbits and/or pressure on the quadrigeminal plate from the enlarged ventricular system resulting in a paralysis of upward gaze. Spasticity is usually present and is greater in the lower than the upper extremities, due to stretching of the paracentral motor fibers around the dilated ventricles. Corticospinal fibers to the legs lie closest to the surface of the lateral ventricle and thus are affected earlier and more severely than fibers to the upper extremities. Ataxia can occur with enlargement of the fourth ventricle and stretching of the cerebellar peduncles. Vomiting, lethargy, and irritability are symptoms of increased intracranial pressure. Adults often have many of the features described above and, in addition, may complain of headaches. Endocrine changes, including alterations in sexual development and obesity, have been reported and may be due to pressure on the hypothalmic centers by the dilated third ventricle. Intellectual impairment is often present, but the pathophysiological mechanisms responsible are uncertain. Reduced cerebral blood flow occurs in hydrocephalus, but its contribution to the neurological dysfunction remains to be defined. Normal pressure hydrocephalus presents with dementia, gait disturbances, and incontinence (signs and symptoms usually not associated with increased intracranial pressure), ventricular enlargement, and normal cerebrospinal fluid pressure as measured by routine lumbar puncture.

### Diagnosis and treatment

The diagnosis and treatment of hydrocephalus are based on pathophysiological principles. The history and physical findings may suggest increasing head size or an elevated intracranial pressure. Radiographs of the skull may reveal useful information. In addition to skull size, signs of increased intracranial pressure can be demonstrated. These include widening of the cranial sutures, erosion of the clinoid processes or dorsum sellae, and increased convolutional markings. A definitive diagnosis, however, can only be made by demonstration of the size of the ventricular system and the potency of the cerebrospinal fluid pathways, which requires contrast encephalography by instilling air either into the lumbar subarachnoid space (if intracranial pressures are not extremely high) or the lateral ventricle. The air displaces the cerebrospinal fluid and, as air has a different density than brain or cerebrospinal fluid, the cerebrospinal fluid pathways can be outlined radiographically. Frequently, both procedures are necessary to determine the level of an obstruction to fluid flow with certainty. Recently, isotope cisternography and ventriculography have been employed to gain further information regarding cerebrospinal fluid dynamics and flow pattern. A radionuclide is introduced into the lumbar subarachnoid space or the ventricles, and its natural flow is monitored over the subsequent 24 to 48 hours. No maneuvering of the position of the patient is required. This procedure may be especially helpful in the evaluation of normal pressure hydrocephalus. If the isotope injected into the lumbar subarachnoid space enters into the lateral ventricles in any quantity and remains, communicating hydrocephalus probably exists.

The treatment of hydrocephalus is primarily surgical. Procedures have been designed to relieve abnormally increased intraventricular pressure by diverting the excessive cerebrospinal fluid from the ventricular system to other body cavities from which it can be absorbed. The two most widely used methods are ventriculo-peritoneal and ventriculo-atrial shunts. In both methods, a catheter is inserted into the ventricular system. The catheter is connected to a valve that directs the flow of cerebrospinal fluid and regulates the pressure within the ventricles by opening within a pre-set range and allowing the cerebrospinal fluid to be diverted from the ventricles. A distal catheter connected to the valve assembly directs the diverted fluid into the peritoneal cavity or the right atrium. No satisfactory long-term medical management of the problem is yet available. Drugs have been administered in attempts to decrease production (e.g., acetazolamide and digoxin) or increase absorption (e.g., such osmotic agents as isosorbide) but without sustained success.

## General references

Matson, Donald D. 1969. Neurosurgery of infancy and childhood. Charles C. Thomas, Springfield, Ill.

Blattner, Russell T. 1965. Hydrocephalus. J. Ped. 67:1216.

Milhorat, Thomas H. 1972. Hydrocephalus and cerebrospinal fluid. Williams & Wilkins, Baltimore.

Russell, Dorothy S. 1949. Observation on the pathology of hydrocephalus. Medical Research Council Special Report Series No. 265. Her Majesty's Stationery Office, London.

# 13
# Metabolic Encephalopathies

WILLIAM E. DODSON

Encephalopathy may be defined as a state of dysfunction of the central nervous system, resulting in diffuse and/or multifocal alterations of neurological function caused by derangement in the metabolic functions of nerve cells in response to such systemic insults as renal, hepatic, or endocrine diseases or in response to toxins or toxic agents. Although severe disturbances in function may be entirely reversible early in the course of an encephalopathy, there is little doubt that with repeated or sustained insults, permanent changes in the structure of the central nervous system occur.

A complete discussion of all etiologies is beyond the scope of this chapter. Rather, I shall focus on the more common encephalopathies seen in hepatic failure, cardiopulmonary disorders, and uremia and attempt to relate them to fundamental neurochemical and neurophysiological mechanisms where these are known.

## Hepatic encephalopathy

Encephalopathy due to hepatocellular failure may occur on an acute or a chronic basis. The acute reversible syndrome is associated with disturbances of mentation and consciousness, ranging from confusion to frank coma, and disturbances of movement and tone. The latter include a flapping, asynchronous, irregular tremor of the extended limbs—asterixis. This is characterized electromyographically by transient loss of tone in muscle groups attempting to maintain posture. Other movement disorders consist of paratonia, perseveration of assumed postures, and slowness of movement with facial grimacing. The electroencephalogram in these states shows symmetrical, bifrontal, and generalized high-amplitude slow activity.

Pathologically acute hepatic encephalopathy is characterized by an increase in the number and size of protoplasmic astrocytes (Alzheimer type II cells), with a characteristic, enlarged vesicular nucleus and a prominent, large nucleolus. These cells appear to be specific for states associated with elevated blood ammonia, and they are the most consistent pathological finding in hepatic coma. They occur in a characteristic distribution involving the gray matter of the cerebral cortex, basal ganglia, red nucleus, substantia nigra, thalamic and subthalamic nuclei, tectum of midbrain, roof nuclei of cerebellum, and dentate and inferior olivary nuclei. There is sparing of white matter and motor nuclei. The severity of involvement of the astrocytes correlates with the severity of the clinical picture. In the most severe cases, neuronal loss is seen in the cortex, thalami, basal ganglia, and red nucleus. More severe involvement of the frontal cortex and extrapyramidal nuclei correlates with the movement disorder noted above. The diffuse cortical changes probably underlie the mental disturbances.

A progressive neurological syndrome occurs in patients with chronic functional or surgical shunting of blood around the liver. Clinically, these patients with portal-systemic shunts demonstrate global defects in cognitive function, cerebellar signs with appendicular dysmetria, as well as ataxic gait and dysarthria. A movement disorder may also be seen, characterized by fine and coarse tremors, asterixis, and a spectrum of involuntary movements from fidgetiness to frank choreoathetosis. About one-half of these patients show mild corticospinal signs such as hyper-reflexia or extensor plantar reflexes. The pathological findings consist of pseudolaminar necrosis of the cortex, which is maximal in the parietal, occipital, and frontal regions, and convolutional atrophy. Microscopically, there is an increased number of Alzheimer type II astrocytes, and intranuclear glycogen inclusions are seen. There is a generalized patchy parenchymal degeneration in deep layers of the cortex and underlying subcortical white matter. Similar degeneration is also seen in the basal ganglia and cerebellum with mild involvement of the thalamus and red nuclei. The astrocytic proliferation is most common in the deep cortical layers, in the nuclei of the extrapyramidal system, and in the molecular layer of the cerebellum. Bizarre astrocytes (Alzheimer type I) are seen in areas of parenchymal degeneration. Poor correlation has been found between lesions in the basal ganglia and the clinical occurrence of choreoathetosis. It is felt, in these cases, that the movement disorder possibly has its basis in the frontoparietal lesions or in metabolic alterations not reflected in overt pathological change.

Some aspects of the pathophysiology of these changes can be explained by examining the neuropathology in rats with Eck-type portocaval shunts. When tissue is fixed by rapid perfusion methods at the time of death, Alzheimer type II astrocytes have irregular, lobulated nuclei. The ballooned appearance of these cells is due to the postmortem accumulation of fluid, suggesting the presence of increased tonicity resulting from increased metabolic hyeractivity. In astrocytes with giant multilobulated nuclei (Alzheimer type I cells)— cells found in areas of parenchymal degeneration in chronic hepatic encephalopathy—there is an increased DNA content, with abnormal mitotic figures characterized by an absence of the spindle apparatus, contractions of the chromatids, and a separation of the arms of the chromosomes. Similar changes have been observed in cells treated with colchicine or grown in high ammonia media, procedures that interfere with microtubule formation. The spindle apparatus is composed of microtubules. Microtubules are also involved in rapid axoplasmic flow, a process that transports metabolites from the perikaryon through the axon to the synaptic region. It is, therefore, suggested that elevated serum ammonia may interfere with polymerization of microtubular components to prevent the formation of normal microtubules. This could produce alterations of axoplasmic flow and disturb neuronal metabolism and function. Abnormal neuronal microtubular structures, however, have been seen in oligodendroglia, but not in neurons. Thus, the pathology of hepatic encephalopathy is characterized by reversible changes in astrocytes suggesting metabolic hyperactivity, as well as by cellular alterations suggesting abnormal function of microtubular systems in glial cells, but structural correlations of neuronal dysfunction are yet to be defined prior to those changes resulting in cell death.

Among the many clinical derangements that may be found in hepatic coma and chronic hepatic encephalopathy, elevation of serum ammonia correlates best with the clinical degree of neurological dysfunction, although a clear correlation between the severity of symptoms and ammonia levels is not defined. Ammonia administration can clearly precipitate coma in susceptible patients. Experiments in primates infused chronically with ammonia have demonstrated electroencephalographic abnormalities and charcteristic astrocytic changes. How hyperammonemia might disrupt cerebral metabolism has been the subject of much discussion and study. In the brain, most ammonia fixation is by incorporation into glutamine. Brain and cerebrospinal fluid glutamine increase in the presence of elevated serum ammonia. It has been suggested that detoxification in the brain of 1 mole of ammonia, by removal of 1 mole of alpha-ketoglutarate from the tricarboxylic acid (TCA) cycle would result in the consumption of up to 28 moles of ATP/mole of glucose metabolized. Thus, one might expect to find decreased levels of alpha-ketoglutarate, high energy phosphate, and other metabolites of the TCA cycle. In rats made symptomatic by chronic exposure to ammonia by inhalation, there is decreased oxygen consumption. Phosphocreatine levels are decreased 13% in the frontal lobe, and 16% in the cerebellum, but levels are normal in the brain stem; ATP was decreased in all three areas with an associated net decrease in total adenylate groups. Alpha-ketoglutarate is not significantly depleted but shows a downward trend in the frontal cortex and cerebellum. Malate was increased in all regions. These results also suggest increased glycolysis, as indicated by elevated lactate pyruvate levels. Alternatively, there may be a block in the transfer of pyruvate into acetyl coenzyme A or oxaloacetate. The equivocal changes in alpha-ketoglutarate demonstrate the difficulty in drawing conclusions about metabolic hyperactivity, using whole brain. The brain is divided into metabolic compartments into which metabolites have differing rates of entry and exit and different rates of turnover. Turnover studies with delineation of compartmental kinetics should further elucidate the mechanism of ammonia detoxication and its effects on intermediary metabolism. It is hypothesized

that that metabolic compartment most concerned with the formation of neuro-transmitters may be most susceptible to the metabolic
changes produced by hyperammonemia.

Other possible toxic agents and pathophysiological mechanisms
are suggested by the finding that brain tissue from cirrhotic animals
does not detoxify ammonia to glutamine to the extent that brain
slices from normal animals do. Additionally, it has been shown that
there is less incorporation of $^{14}$C-glucose into glutamine in cirrhotic
than normal rat brain slices. Other suggested central nervous system
toxic agents have included methionine, tryptophan, tryptophan metabolites, and false neuro-transmitters. Methionine may act as
substrate for increased ammonia release. Derangements in tryptophan metabolism might decrease serotonin levels, but therapy
with serotonin precursors in patients in hepatic coma has not produced measurable clinical changes. It has been suggested that, by
accumulation of tyrosine and catechol metabolites, false neuro-
transmitters may be produced, which interfere with central dopanergic pathways. Such false transmitters would have sufficient
structural resemblance to normal transmitters to obstruct the function of the latter. It is hypothesized that aromatic amines normally
metabolized in the liver by monamine oxidase might escape degradation in hepatic failure and achieve beta-hydroxylation by nonspecific enzymes. Baldessarini and his associates have found that
isolated nerve endings will take up and store beta-phenylethylamine,
tyramine, and octopamine, although in lesser amounts than norepinephrine. In addition, urinary excretion of octopamine is greater
in patients in hepatic coma than in patients with asterixis and confusion only. The suggestion that these compounds might be interfering with dopanergic activities of the extra-pyramidal system is
enticing but remains unsubstantiated. Several groups have reported
brief, transient clinical improvement after L-dopa administration to
patients in hepatic coma. The role of false transmitters will remain
unclear, until it can be determined whether or not they accumulate
at the same site as active transmitter, if they are held in storage sites
and released by appropriate stimulation, and if they are subject to
depletion by agents that deplete normal transmitters.

In hepatic coma, as well as in coma of other etiologies, reduced
cerebral blood flow and reduced brain oxygen consumption are well
documented. In hepatic coma, this is often associated with a mixed

alkalosis with or without hypoxia. Serum alkalosis has been shown to increase the uptake of ammonia into the brain. Hypokalemia occurring from renal potassium loss can further contribute to the clinical picture. The suggestion of intracellular acidosis occurring in association with extracellular alkalosis has not yet been confirmed in experimental animals, although cerebrospinal fluid acidosis occurs. Attempts to increase cerebral blood flow in hepatic coma by inhalation of 5% $CO_2$ have only produced further reduction of cerebral blood flow and oxygen consumption, yet therapy with bicarbonate infusion has improved cerebral blood flow and oxygen consumption by an unexplained mechanism. The clinical improvement and increase in cerebral blood flow and consumption after bicarbonate administration is contradictory to the notion that alkalosis increases brain uptake of ammonia. These problems await further resolution.

There occurs, in children, a parainfectious illness of extremely acute onset, with fatty infiltration of the viscera, disturbed hepatocellular function, variable hypoglycemia, and usually dramatic central nervous system dysfunction associated with cerebral edema—Reye's syndrome. There is no clear correlation between the degree of the hepatic abnormalities and the degree of the central nervous system dysfunction, and alterations of serum ammonia are transient. The mechanisms of this syndrome are not clear, although there is some evidence suggesting that it is due to a mitochondrial insult that interferes with the metabolism of fatty acids and gluconeogenesis, to produce hypoglycemia. High levels of free fatty acid may result in cerebral edema. Why the adult is protected from this insult is uncertain.

## Cardiopulmonary disorders

### CARDIOPULMONARY INSUFFICIENCY

This insufficiency, with alveolar hypoventilation, presents with variable degrees of hypoxia, hypercapnea, polycythemia, and congestive heart failure with cor pulmonale. It may be associated with encephalopathy manifest by headache, papilledema, alterations of cognitive function and consciousness, tremor, twitching, and, occasionally, asterixis. The brain is edematous with increased weight, flattened gyri, and obliterated sulci.

Elevation of $PCO_2$ produces elevated intracranial pressure, possibly by increased cerebrospinal fluid production secondary to increased cerebral blood flow and by increased size of the intracranial vascular compartment secondary to vasodilation. The retinal changes of papilledema and dilated tortuous vessels may relate to increased intracranial pressure, but these changes can be produced directly by increased $PCO_2$ alone. Cerebral blood flow is linearly related to the $PCO_2$ over the physiological range. Thus, increased $PCO_2$ produces vasodilation and a lowering of cerebrovascular resistance. Increased cerebral blood flow is often seen in pulmonary insufficiency. Experimental animals made hypoxic and hypercapnic have heightened vulnerability to drops in systemic blood pressure from a loss of the autoregulatory mechanism maximally dilated by increased $PCO_2$.

The acid-base balance of the brain is rapidly affected by changes in $PCO_2$ because $CO_2$ has a greater diffusability than $H^+$ or $HCO_3^-$. The buffering capacity of the brain is probably intermediate between that of blood and cerebrospinal fluid, with the latter showing a relatively poor buffering capacity and greater pH swings for given changes in $PCO_2$. Because of the difficulty in measuring brain tissue pH, clinical data have, for the most part, been obtained on the spinal fluid in studies of central nervous system acid-base balance. In respiratory acidosis with elevated $PCO_2$, a cerebrospinal fluid pH of less than 7.25 is generally associated with the clinical picture of an encephalopathy. Decreases in cerebrospinal fluid pH or jugular venous pH are better correlates of central nervous system dysfunction in chronic pulmonary encephalopathy than is arterial $PCO_2$. Although a range of arterial $PCO_2$ can be seen in relation to the onset of central nervous system symptomatology, in general, acute symptoms will appear with a rapid rise of the $PCO_2$ to above 7.0, and, in chronic respiratory acidosis, an arterial pH of less than 7.14, with a $PCO_2$ greater than 130 mm Hg, is associated with coma.

In experimental animals, the jugular $PO_2$ does not correlate with altered cerebral metabolism, although, clinically, values of less than 19 mm Hg are usually associated with the appearance of cerebral symptoms. In the presence of graded hypotension, metabolic aberrations may be seen above this level. Conversely, a jugular $PO_2$ at or below this level is not necessarily associated with depletion of high energy phosphate compounds. With mild degrees of hypoxia, experimental animals show an activation of central nervous system glycolytic pathways with an increased production of pyruvate and lactate and an increase in the lactate to pyruvate ratio reflecting the altered redox state.

Hypercapnic acidotic cats show an inhibition of glycolytic activity with no change in brain glucose, glucose-6-phosphate, high energy phosphate, or lactate to pyruvate ratios, but with a decrease in alpha-ketoglutarate, malate, lactate, and pyruvate. Animals made both hypercapnic and hypoxic show a cellular metabolic protective effect of hypercapnia. There is less hypoxic activation of glycolysis and no high energy phosphate depletion. In addition, there is less tissue acidosis in brain than in the non-acidotic animal with a similar degree of hypoxia, although serum and spinal fluid acidosis may be more marked. The intracellular acidosis evoked by an elevated $PCO_2$ is compensated for by an increased buffering capacity, and intracellular acidosis is less marked than with hypoxia alone, due to a reduction of lactate. It seems that the protective effect of hypercapnia associated with hypoxia is due to improved cerebral perfusion, although cerebral blood flow has not been measured directly under these experimental conditions. Hypercapnia combined with hypoxia in experimental animals heightens the vulnerability to drops in perfusion pressure in excess of the vulnerability to hypotension in either hypoxia or hypercapnia alone.

Patients with major cerebrovascular disease and cardiopulmonary insufficiency show a greater propensity to electroencephalogram abnormalities, with greater jugular venous acidosis for a given rise in arterial $PCO_2$. Cerebrovascular disease may limit vasodilation from hypercapnia. In addition, cerebral blood flow may be reduced by shunting of blood to other organs in hypercapnia with systemic vasodilation. Failing cardiac output as a result of congestive heart failure may further limit cerebral perfusion. Thus, a system being maximally driven by hypercapnia has a limited capacity to respond to changes in perfusion pressure with further autoregulation. It is probably a combination of these factors that predispose a patient to cerebral metabolic alterations and manifest encephalopathy. Further studies of cerebral blood flow and central nervous system glycolytic products will elucidate these problems.

An encephalopathy may be precipitated by bicarbonate therapy in milder states of respiratory acidosis. In this situation, the bicarbonate may partially correct the systemic acidosis, diminish alveolar ventilation, and raise serum $PCO_2$; the $CO_2$ then diffuses into the central nervous system more rapidly than $HCO_3^-$ and exceeds the buffering capacity of brain tissue and cerebrospinal fluid. Thus, despite partial correction of the serum pH, cerebral acidosis worsens.

## Hypertensive encephalopathy

This relatively rare condition is manifested by headache and disturbances of mentation and consciousness with seizures, coma, papilledema, and multifocal neurological signs. This occurs in the clinical setting of an acute increase in blood pressure and is generally associated with proteinuria. It is often symptomatic of such diseases as acute glomerulonephritis or toxemia but may occur out of a background of essential hypertension. It is generally associated with diastolic blood pressures greater than 200 mm Hg. Pathologically, the encephalopathy is characterized by cerebral edema and scattered hemorrhages and infarctions.

Cerebral blood flow remains constant over a wide range of blood pressures through autoregulation. With a rapid increase in blood pressure, there is an initial brief distention of arterioles to produce a microvascular hyperemia. This is shortly followed by vasoconstriction with both generalized and segmental narrowing of arterioles. If appropriate injections of dyes, fluorescent-labeled proteins, or enzymes are made, leakage of labeled substances can be demonstrated at regions of arteriolar dilation. The overdistention of the microvasculature (that takes place in the brief time interval prior to establishing protective vasoconstriction) produces smooth muscle and endothelial injury. Vascular leakage is not observed with gradual changes in blood pressure of a comparable degree. In addition to leakage of proteins and fluids, small areas of hemorrhage can be observed in experimental animals or pathological specimens. Tissue acidosis from hypercapnia or long-standing untreated hypertension may limit the upper range of autoregulation, increasing the vulnerability of the microvasculature to overdistention. Overstretched, damaged vascular endothelial cells then leak fluid and protein to produce cerebral edema. With a rapid rise of blood pressure, cerebral blood flow may be reduced or normal. If ischemia and tissue hypoxia occur and produce acidosis, a further breakdown of protective mechanisms occurs, with a vicious cycle of progressive cerebral edema. Severe prolonged ischemia can result in micro infarcts.

## Uremia

Uremic encephalopathy is characterized clinically by fluctuations in mental status, increased muscular tone, and movement disorders consisting of twitches, tetany, tremulousness, and, occasionally, asterixis. Coma may be accompanied by decorticate, and, less often, decerebrate posturing. Seizures are not uncommon, and terminal seizures often result from disturbed cardiac rhythms. The electroencephalographic is often abnormal at times when the blood urea nitrogen (BUN) is greater than 60 mg%, although the BUN level is by no means directly related to electroencephalographic abnormalities. Abnormal electroencephalographic features consist of diffuse slowing with paroxysmal slow bursts and, in more severe states, multifocal spiking. Seizures occur in 15% of uremic patients, and some workers have been able to correlate their occurrence with an elevated potassium to calcium ratio.

Gross neuropathological findings are few in uremic encephalopathy. Occasionally, petechial hemorrhages are seen. Cerebral edema is not a feature. Microscopically, neuronal changes are noted with chromatolysis, vacuolations, swelling of dendrites, pyknosis, and cell loss. In addition, 60% of patients dying with uremia show necrosis of the granular layer of the cerebellum, but this is believed to be a terminal, possibly hypoxic, event. The neuronal cellular changes are generalized but maximal in the sensory nuclei of the brain stem, reticular formation, and cerebral cortex. Glial proliferations, perivascular cellular accumulations, and occasional endothelial changes also occur.

The severity of uremic encephalopathy does not correlate clearly with any single biochemical or pathological abnormality. Such diverse etiologies of uremia as polyarteritis, polycystic disease, and hypertension often are associated with cerebrovascular pathology, which complicates the picture. Associated metabolic acidosis, hyperosmolality, hypocalcemia, and anemia further contribute to the problem.

Metabolic studies in uremic animals have shown elevated ATP, phosphocreatine, and organic phosphate in brain tissue. A partial block in glycolysis at the phosphofructokinase step has been observed in experimental animals. It is felt that this inhibition may result from the elevated levels of high energy phosphate. Fishman and his associates have shown that there is an increased rate of potassium influx and a decreased rate of sodium influx into the central nervous system. At the same time, the central nervous system sodium and potassium content are increased. There is increased permeability to inulin and sucrose, although brain water is not increased. These findings suggest an increase in brain permeability without cerebral edema. Studies measuring the activity of sodium/potassium-dependent ATPase have yielded variable results.

The search for the toxic agent in uremia has produced many candidates, although no single compound has been found that, alone, can account for the clinical and metabolic findings. Compounds proposed have included free amino acids, urea, ornithine derivatives, aromatic amines, indoles, phenols, and organic acids, all of which show increased levels in renal disease. The phenolic acids have been shown to inhibit a variety of enzymes, and they also reduce anaerobic glycolysis, although the amounts required have been well above those observed in patients. When these compounds are given to uremic rats, lowering of seizure threshold and twitching, similar to that seen on uremia, are produced. Similarly, methylguanidine may produce uremic symptoms in dogs similar to those seen in uremic man, but doses above the physiological range are required. Twitching in man does seem to correlate with high cerebrospinal fluid phosphate levels. It is likely that the cerebral symptoms of uremia relate to the altered permeability of the capillary membrane, which permits toxic agents to enter the central nervous system. How these agents disrupt neuronal function is not clear. It is clear, however, that the symptoms of uremic encephalopathy are not related to the blood urea level.

The treatment of uremic encephalopathy carries with it some of the same dangers noted in the treatment of cardiopulmonary encephalopathies. Rapid correction of the acidosis may increase the acidosis noted in brain tissue fluids and in cerebrospinal fluid. Furthermore, rapidly lowering the blood osmolality may result in a rapid influx of water into brain, with cerebral edema and an exacerbation of symptoms.

## General references

Austin, F. K., M. W. Carmichael, and R. D. Adams, 1957. Neurologic manifestations of chronic pulmonary insufficiency. New Eng. J. Med. 257:579.

Cavanaugh, J. B. 1972. Cellular abnormalities in the brain in chronic liver disease. Pages 238-247 *in* I. Gilliland and J. Francis, eds. Scientific basis of medicine: annual reviews. Humanities Press, Inc., New York.

Lassen, N. A. and A. Agnoli. 1972. The upper limits of autoregulation of cerebral blood flow—on the pathogenesis of hypertensive encephalopathy. Scand. J. Clin. Lab. Invest. 30:113.

# Contributors

**Leonard Berg,** M.D., Professor (Clinical) of Neurology, Department of Neurology, Washington University School of Medicine, St. Louis, Missouri

**Saul Boyarsky,** M.D., Professor of Genitourinary Surgery, Department of Surgery, Washington University School of Medicine, St. Louis, Missouri

**John E. Brooks,** M.B., Ch.B., Assistant Professor of Neurology, Department of Neurology, Washington University School of Medicine, St. Louis, Missouri

**Ronald M. Burde,** M.D., Professor of Ophthalmology, Department of Ophthalmology, Washington University School of Medicine, St. Louis, Missouri

**Robert L. Chesanow,** M.D., Assistant Professor of Neurology, Department of Neurology, Washington University School of Medicine, St. Louis, Missouri

**Lawrence A. Coben,** M.D., Associate Professor of Neurology, Department of Neurology, Washington University School of Medicine, St. Louis, Missouri

**William S. Coxe,** M.D., Professor of Neurological Surgery, Department of Surgery, Washington University School of Medicine, St. Louis, Missouri

**Hallowell Davis,** M.D., Research Professor Emeritus and Lecturer in Otolaryngology, Professor Emeritus of Physiology, Research Associate and Director of Research Emeritus, Central Institute for the Deaf, St. Louis, Missouri

**Darryl C. DeVivo,** M.D., Associate Professor of Pediatrics and Neurology, Departments of Pediatrics and Neurology, Washington University School of Medicine, St. Louis, Missouri

**Philip R. Dodge,** M.D., Professor and Head, Department of Pediatrics and Professor of Neurology, Department of Neurology, Washington University School of Medicine, St. Louis, Missouri

**W. Edwin Dodson,** M.D., Instructor in Pediatrics, Department of Pediatrics, Washington University School of Medicine, St. Louis, Missouri

**Sven G. Eliasson,** M.D., Ph.D., Professor of Neurology, Department of Neurology, Washington University School of Medicine, St. Louis, Missouri

381

**Carl Ellenberger,** M.D., Fellow in Neuro-Ophthalmology, Department of Ophthalmology, Washington University School of Medicine, St. Louis, Missouri

**Ralph D. Feigin,** M.D., Professor of Pediatrics, Department of Pediatrics, Washington University School of Medicine, St. Louis, Missouri

**James A. Ferrendelli,** M.D., Associate Professor of Neurology and Pharmacology, Departments of Neurology and Pharmacology, Washington University School of Medicine, St. Louis, Missouri

**Marvin A. Fishman,** M.D., Associate Professor of Pediatrics and Neurology, Departments of Pediatrics, Neurology and Preventive Medicine, Washington University School of Medicine, St. Louis, Missouri

**Sidney Goldring,** M.D., Professor of Neurological Surgery, Department of Surgery, Washington University School of Medicine, St. Louis, Missouri

**Phillip Green,** M.D., Assistant and Fellow (NINDS) in Neurology, Department of Neurology, Washington University School of Medicine, St. Louis, Missouri

**Robert L. Grubb,** M.D., Assistant Professor of Neurological Surgery, Department of Surgery, Washington University School of Medicine, St. Louis, Missouri

**William B. Hardin, Jr.,** M.D., Assistant Professor of Neurology, Department of Neurology, Washington University School of Medicine, St. Louis, Missouri

**George H. Klinkerfuss,** M.D., Associate Professor of Neurology, Department of Neurology, Washington University School of Medicine, St. Louis, Missouri

**William M. Landau,** M.D., Professor and Head, Depratment of Neurology, Washington University School of Medicine, St. Louis, Missouri

**Richard M. Merson,** Ph.D., Speech Pathologist, Central Institute for the Deaf, St. Louis, Missouri

**Arthur L. Prensky,** M.D., Professor of Pediatrics and Neurology, Departments of Pediatrics and Neurology, Washington University School of Medicine, St. Louis, Missouri

**Marcus E. Raichle,** M.D., Assistant Professor of Neurology and Radiology, Departments of Neurology and Radiology, Washington University School of Medicine, St. Louis, Missouri

**Malcolm H. Stroud,** F.R.C.S., Professor of Otolaryngology, Department of Otolaryngology, Washington University School of Medicine, St. Louis, Missouri

**Joseph J. Volpe,** M.D., Assistant Professor of Pediatrics and Neurology, Departments of Pediatrics and Neurology, Washington University School of Medicine, St. Louis, Missouri

# Index

Acetylcholine, 63-67, 141, 142, 158; hypersensitivity to, 52; injection of, 65

Acetyl coenzyme A, in metabolic encephalopathy, 371

Achromatopsia, 177

Acidosis, and central nervous system infection, 316; metabolic, 251; in metabolic encephalopathy, 375-78

Acid proteinase, in multiple sclerosis, 341, 345

Acromegaly, and eosinophilic adenoma, 281; and release of growth hormone, 281-82

ACTH, and basophilic adenoma, 281; in myasthenia, 69

Acute glomerulonephritis, with hypertensive encephalopathy, 376

Acute rheumatic fever, and focal nodular myopathy, 85

Addison's disease, with myopathy, 86

Adenosine diphosphate (ADP), 10, 279, 307

Adenosine monophosphate (AMP), 279; cyclic, 197

Adenosine triphosphate (ATP), 159, 167-69, 279, 307, 371, 377-78

Adipsia, hypothalamic mechanisms of, 106

Adynamia episodica hereditaria, 88

Agnosia, 127, 154, 170, 172, 174, 175, 345-46; apperceptive, 175-76; associative, 175-76; tactual, 176; visual, 176-77

Albuminocytological dissociation, 360

Alexander's leukodystrophy, 41

Alkalosis, in coma, 373

Alpha-adrenergic receptor, 97

Alpha-ketoglutarate, in metabolic encephalopathy, 371, 375

Alveolar hypoventilation, with encephalopathy, 373

Amaurosis fugax, 203

Amblyopia, 200-201

Amenorrhea, with intracranial lesions, 282

Amines, as agent in uremia, 378; in hepatic failure, 372

Amino acid concentration, in developing brain, 9

Amino acids, as agent in uremia, 378; branch chained content depression in experimental hyperphenylalaninemia, 44; disturbances in metabolism of, 43

Ammonia, in cerebrospinal fluid, 359; elevated, in coma, 369-73

Amnesia, 179, 298, 300

Amniotic fluid, aspiration and neonatal central nervous system infection, 311-13

Amyloidosis, in autonomic disturbances, 99; and hypertrophic muscle, 86

Amyotrophic lateral sclerosis, 53

Anencephaly, 11-12, 16, 18; after occlusion, 22; after radiation, 18

Aneurysm, 192-93, 203, 253, 261-62; of Charcot-Bouchard, 262; mycotic, 262, 324, 329

Angiography, 332

Angulated fibers, in myopathy, 81

383